Endocrine Therapy
in Breast Cancer

Endocrine Therapy in Breast Cancer

edited by

William R. Miller
Western General Hospital
Edinburgh, Scotland

James N. Ingle
Mayo Clinic
Rochester, Minnesota

MARCEL DEKKER, INC.   NEW YORK · BASEL

ISBN: 0–8247–0787-7

This book is printed on acid-free paper.

Headquarters
Marcel Dekker, Inc.
270 Madison Avenue, New York, NY 10016
tel: 212-696-9000, fax: 212-685-4540

Eastern Hemisphere Distribution
Marcel Dekker AG
Hutgasse 4, Postfach 812, CH-4001 Basel, Switzerland
tel: 41-61-261-8482; fax: 41-61-261-8896

World Wide Web
http://www.dekker.com
The publisher offers discounts on this book when ordered in bulk quantities. For more information, write to Special Sales/Professional Marketing at the headquarters address above.

Preface

The knowledge that hormones influence both the risk of developing and the natural history of breast cancer is not new (indeed, Beatson, working in Scotland over a century ago, made the pioneering observation that ovarian ablation in premenopausal women produced regression of breast cancer). However, the recent development of new specific and highly potent endocrine agents makes it timely to examine the "new horizons" they create. To this end, 50 clinicians and basic scientists—experts at the forefront of endocrine research in breast cancer—convened a workshop in Gleneagles, Scotland, to evaluate progress and to assess future potential and needs. This volume summarizes the developments discussed in that workshop.

Part I sets the scene with Chapter 1 addressing the question "Why endocrine therapy?" The book is then divided into four interrelated subject areas: advanced breast cancer, early breast cancer, neoadjuvant therapy, and chemoprevention.

The status of endocrine agents in the treatment of advanced breast cancer is discussed in Part II by individual experts with firsthand experience in their use: tamoxifen (Chap. 2); aromatase inhibitors (Chap. 3); other selective estrogen receptor modulators (SERMs) (Chap. 4), as well as other endocrine agents and therapies directed at molecular targets (Chap. 5). Part III uses the same approach to cover early breast cancer: tamoxifen (Chap. 6); aromatase inhibitors (Chap. 7); and other SERMs (Chap. 8). In addition, because treatment of early breast cancer often involves adjuvant therapy over relatively long periods of time, surrogate markers of response to, and side effects of, treatment are reviewed in Chapter 9.

While the conventional sequence of treatment in most patients with early breast cancer is surgery followed by systemic therapy, Part IV reviews primary or neoadjuvant therapy, in which drug treatment is given prior to surgery with the tumor still within the breast. This strategy offers both potential clinical benefits to patients and unique opportunities for research. Until recently, the use of endocrine therapy in this setting had been relatively ignored, but this gap is filled in Chapter 10 (which presents the subject from a medical perspective); Chapter 11 (from a surgical perspective); and Chapter 12 (from a pathological perspective). Chapter 13 focuses on research opportunities.

Neoadjuvant therapy may also be exploited to study mechanisms of resistance (which is a major obstacle to increasing survival by endocrine measures), but other model systems are providing interesting results. These data are covered in Chapter 14.

Part V is concerned with chemoprevention. The etiology of breast cancer has a strong hormonal component. Chapter 15 reviews the epidemiological basis for believing endocrine manipulation may prevent most breast cancers. Evidence that estrogen may have a direct carcinogenic effect and initiate breast cancer is presented in Chapter 16. The relative advantages and disadvantages of using either antiestrogens or aromatase inhibitors are summarized in Chapters 17 and 18. Throughout this volume, discussion sessions are presented in an unabridged form so that the areas of controversy can be identified and points of detail clarified.

A consensus was reached at the workshop in Gleneagles. First, it was agreed that these are momentous times in terms of the development of new endocrine agents. On the one hand, the new generation of aromatase inhibitors can inhibit estrogen biosynthesis more potently and specifically than ever before. On the other hand, the SERMs can block the mechanism of estrogen action differentially in different tissue, thus offering the promise of selectively turning off the estrogen stimulus to malignant growth while maintaining the same signal in normal tissues. Results from clinical trials in advanced disease have established that aromatase inhibitors such as letrozole, anastrozole, and exemestane are at least as efficacious as other endocrine agents when used as second-line therapy after tamoxifen and, indeed, may be superior to tamoxifen when used as first-line therapy. Similar promising clinical benefits have been observed when, for example, letrozole was compared with tamoxifen in the neoadjuvant setting. Indeed, when used neoadjuvantly against estrogen-receptor-rich tumors, clinical and pathological response can be remarkable high, rivaling that previously seen only after chemotherapy. The benefits of neoadjuvant therapy stretch beyond clinical outcomes because of the opportunity to have easy and sequential access to the tumor. Combining this approach with molecular technology will allow us to define accurately the phenotype of responsive tumors and the mechanism of endocrine resistance; thus treatment will be optimized.

The transfer of these observations to earlier stages of the disease and cancer prevention is underway and, in the next few years, we will know whether the newer SERMs and aromatase inhibitors can continue the trend of improved survival attributed to tamoxifen.

The epidemiology and etiology of breast cancers suggest that hormonal measures, if implemented earlier and used correctly, can prevent the appearance of breast cancer. The challenge is to identify high-risk groups and develop acceptable regimes (perhaps by offering other health benefits such as contraception at the same time). In this context, if estrogens are genotoxic carcinogens, aromatase inhibitors (by reducing levels of estrogen rather than blocking interaction at receptor sites) may be more effective chemopreventatives than tamoxifen and other SERMs.

Since the era of Beatson, there has been no more exciting time to be associated with endocrine therapy. It is thus highly appropriate that this volume emanated from a workshop in Beatson's homeland. It is patently clear that there are unprecedented opportunities for advancing the science and understanding of breast cancer and improving the care of our patients with this disease. We hope this volume will stimulate and extend your horizons in the field of endocrine therapy in breast cancer.

William R. Miller
James N. Ingle

Contents

Preface   *iii*
Contributors   *xi*

Part I.   Introduction

1. Why Endocrine Therapy?   3
    Daniel F. Hayes

Part II.   Advanced Breast Cancer

2. Tamoxifen and Advanced Breast Cancer: An Overview   17
    John F. Forbes

3. Overview of Aromatase Inhibitors and Inactivators in the Treatment
    of Advanced Breast Cancer   33
    Per Eystein Lønning

4. Endocrine Treatment of Advanced Breast Cancer: Selective
    Estrogen-Receptor Modulators (SERMs)   47
    Stephen R. D. Johnston and Anthony Howell

5. Other Endocrine and Biological Agents in the Treatment of
    Advanced Breast Cancer   79
    Jan G. M. Klijn, Els M. J. J. Berns, and John A. Foekens

    Panel Discussion 1:   Advanced Breast Cancer   91
    Manfred Kaufmann and Henning T. Mouridsen, Chairmen

Part III.   Early Breast Cancer

6. Early Breast Cancer: Tamoxifen Overview   125
    Carsten Rose

7. Aromatase Inhibitors and Early Breast Cancer   135
    Paul E. Goss

8. SERMs: Overview in Early Breast Cancer   145
    Ian E. Smith

9. Surrogate and Intermediate Markers in Early Breast Cancer   157
    Mitch Dowsett

    Panel Discussion 2: Early Breast Cancer   171
    Hans-Jorg Senn and William R. Miller, Chairmen

Part IV.   Neoadjuvant Therapy

10. Neoadjuvant Endocrine Therapy for Breast Cancer: A Medical
    Oncologist's Perspective   181
    Matthew J. Ellis

11. Neoadjuvant Therapy: Surgical Perspectives   197
    J. Michael Dixon

12. Pathology of Breast Cancer Following Neoadjuvant
    Endocrine Therapy   213
    Hironobu Sasano, Takashi Suzuki, and Takuya Moriya

13. Neoadjuvant Therapy: Prediction of Response   223
    William R. Miller, T. J. Anderson, S. Iqbal, and J. Michael Dixon

14. Mechanisms of Resistance to Endocrine Therapy   231
    Nancy E. Hynes

Panel Discussion 3: Neoadjuvant Therapy 243
James N. Ingle and Ian E. Smith, Chairmen

Part V. Chemoprevention

15. Epidemiological Basis of Hormonal Chemoprevention of
Breast Cancer 267
Malcolm C. Pike, John R. Daniels, and Darcy V. Spicer

16. Breast Carcinogenesis and Its Prevention by Inhibition of
Estrogen Genotoxicity 287
Joachim G. Liehr

17. Use of Selective Antiestrogens for the Chemoprevention
of Breast Cancer 303
Trevor J. Powles

18. Aromatase Inhibitors and Chemoprevention of Breast Cancer 309
Paul E. Goss

Panel Discussion 4: Chemoprevention 319
Christopher C. Benz and Anthony Howell, Chairmen

Part VI. Conclusion

Panel Discussion 5: Final Discussion and Wrap-Up 337
James N. Ingle and Ajay Bhatnagar, Chairmen

Index *365*

Contributors

T. J. Anderson, M.B., Ch.B., Ph.D., F.R.C.Path. Edinburgh Breast Unit, Western General Hospital, Edinburgh, Scotland

Christopher C. Benz, M.D. Professor and Director, Program of Cancer and Developmental Therapeutics, Buck Institute for Age Research, Novato, California

Els M. J. J. Berns, Ph.D. Laboratory for Tumor Endocrinology, Daniel den Hoed Cancer Center and Erasmus University Medical Center, Rotterdam, The Netherlands

Ajay Bhatnagar, Ph.D. Novartis Pharma AG, Basel, Switzerland

H. Leon Bradlow, Ph.D. Professor, Department of Surgery, Cornell University Medical College, New York, New York

Angela Brodie, M.D. Department of Pharmacy and Therapeutics, University of Maryland School of Medicine, Baltimore, Maryland

John R. Daniels, M.D. Professor, Department of Medicine, Norris Cancer Center, University of Southern California Keck School of Medicine, Los Angeles, California

J. Michael Dixon, M.D., F.R.C.S., F.R.C.S. Ed. Consultant Surgeon, Edinburgh Breast Unit, Western General Hospital, Edinburgh, Scotland

Mitch Dowsett, Ph.D. Professor, Department of Biochemistry, Royal Marsden Hospital NHS Trust, London, England

Wolfgang Eiermann, Prof. Dr. Med. Medical Director, Frauenklinik vom Roten Kreuz, Munich, Germany

Matthew J. Ellis, M.B., Ph.D., F.R.C.P. Associate Professor of Medicine, and Director, Duke University Breast Cancer Program, Department of Medical Oncology, Duke University Medical Center, Durham, North Carolina

John A. Foekens, Ph.D. Head, Laboratory for Tumor Endocrinology, Daniel den Hoed Cancer Center and Erasmus University Medical Center, Rotterdam, The Netherlands

John F. Forbes, F.R.A.C.S., F.R.C.S., M.S., B.Med.Sci. Professor, Department of Surgical Oncology, University of Newcastle, Newcastle, Australia

Michael Gnant AKH-Wien, Vienna, Austria

Paul E. Goss, M.D., Ph.D., F.R.C.P.C., F.R.C.P.(U.K.) Professor, Department of Medicine, University of Toronto, and Director, Breast Cancer Prevention Program, Princess Margaret Hospital, University Health Network, Toronto, Ontario, Canada

Bernd Groner Chemotherapeutisches Forschungsinstitut, Frankfurt, Germany

Daniel F. Hayes, M.D. Clinical Director, Breast Cancer Program, and Professor, Department of Medicine, University of Michigan Comprehensive Cancer Center, Ann Arbor, Michigan

Anthony Howell, M.D., F.R.C.P. Professor, Department of Medical Oncology, Christie Hospital NHS Trust, Manchester, England

Nancy E. Hynes, Ph.D. Senior Staff Member, Friedrich Miescher Institute for Biomedical Research, Basel, Switzerland

James N. Ingle, M.D. Professor, Department of Oncology, Mayo Clinic, Rochester, Minnesota

S. Iqbal, M.B., Ch. B. F.R.C.S., M. Sc. Edinburgh Breast Unit, Western General Hospital, Edinburgh, Scotland

Stephen R. D. Johnston, M.D., F.R.C.P. Senior Lecturer and Honorary Consultant in Medical Oncology, Department of Medicine—Breast Unit, Royal Marsden Hospital NHS Trust, London, England

Manfred Kaufmann, M.D., Ph.D. Professor and Head, Department of Gynecology and Obstetrics, J. W. Goethe University, Frankfurt am Main, Germany

Gary J. Kelloff, M.D. Senior Scientist, National Cancer Institute, National Institutes of Health, Bethesda, Maryland

Jan G. M. Klijn, M.D., Ph.D. Professor, Department of Medical Oncology, Daniel den Hoed Cancer Center and Erasmus University Medical Center, Rotterdam, The Netherlands

Joachim G. Liehr, Ph.D. Chief Pharmacologist, Stehlin Foundation for Cancer Research, Houston, Texas

Per Eystein Lønning, M.D. Professor, Department of Oncology, Haukeland Hospital, University of Bergen, Bergen, Norway

William R. Miller, Ph.D., D.Sc. Professor of Experimental Oncology, Edinburgh Breast Unit, Western General Hospital, Edinburgh, Scotland

Takuya Moriya, M.D., Ph.D. Associate Professor, Department of Pathology, Tohoku University School of Medicine, Sendai, Japan

Henning T. Mouridsen, M.D., M.Sci. Department of Oncology, Rigshospital, Copenhagen, Denmark

Robert I. Nicholson, Ph.D. Director of Research, Tenovus Cancer Research Centre, Cardiff, Wales

Malcolm C. Pike, Ph.D. Professor, Department of Preventive Medicine, Norris Cancer Center, University of Southern California Keck School of Medicine, Los Angeles, California

Trevor J. Powles, Ph.D., F.R.C.P. Professor, Breast Unit, Royal Marsden Hospital, Sutton, Surrey, England

Carsten Rose, M.D. Director, Department of Oncology, Lund University Hospital, Lund, Sweden

Hironobu Sasano, M.D., Ph.D. Professor and Chairman, Department of Pathology, Tohoku University School of Medicine, Sendai, Japan

Hans-Jorg Senn, M.D. Medical and Scientific Director, Center for Tumor Detection and Prevention, St. Gallen, Switzerland

Ian E. Smith, M.D., F.R.C.P.E., F.R.C.P. Professor, Royal Marsden Hospital NHS Trust, London, England

Darcy V. Spicer, M.D. Professor, Department of Medicine, Norris Cancer Center, University of Southern California Keck School of Medicine, Los Angeles, California

Takashi Suzuki, M.D., Ph.D. Assistant Professor, Department of Pathology, Tohoku University School of Medicine, Sendai, Japan

Katia Tonkin Medical Oncologist, Cross Cancer Institute, Edmonton, Alberta, Canada

Rajeshwar Rao Tekmal, Ph.D. Professor, Department of Gynecology and Obstetrics, Emory University School of Medicine, Atlanta, Georgia

Part I

INTRODUCTION

1

Why Endocrine Therapy?

Daniel F. Hayes
University of Michigan Comprehensive Cancer Center
Ann Arbor, Michigan

I. ABSTRACT

As the uncontrolled activation of cellular endocrine systems is characteristic of many breast cancers, endocrine therapy should be an effective and relatively nontoxic treatment. This chapter reviews the role of ablative and additive endocrine approaches to block estrogen synthesis and function. The occurrence of endocrine therapy–resistant cancers as well as the mechanisms involved in such resistance and possible approaches to overcome resistance are also discussed.

II. INTRODUCTION

The question "Why endocrine therapy?" begs a second question, "What is endocrine therapy?" In its purest sense, endocrine therapy is the modulation of signal transduction pathways initiated by interaction of a soluble growth factor with its specific cellular receptor. In its classical sense, endocrine therapy for breast cancer has been understood to imply disruption of the estrogen-estrogen receptor (ER) axis, either by inhibition of function of the estrogen-producing organ (ablative therapies) or by blockade or perturbation of the estrogen-ER interaction (additive therapies). However, the results of basic and clinical research over the last century have expanded this limited definition of endocrine therapy to include additional hormonal axes. These might include steroidal hormone–intracellular receptor signal transduction pathways other than ER, such as those mediated by the progesterone–progesterone receptor (PgR), androgen–androgen receptor (AR), retinoic acid–retinoic acid and related receptors (RAR, RXR), and even glucocorticoid–glucocorticoid receptor (GR). An even broader definition of endocrine therapy would include the peptide growth factors and their cell surface receptors, including insulin-like growth factor–insulin-like growth factor receptors (IGFR) 1 and 2, the four members of the epidermal growth factor receptor family (EGFR, also known as human epithelial receptor, HER, and erbB), various angiogenic factors and their receptors (fibroblast growth factors, vascular endothelial growth factor, etc.), and other less well-characterized peptide growth factors.

Each of these "endocrine axes" has been clearly demonstrated to play an important if not key role in breast cancer oncogenesis and/or progression. Indeed, one might consider breast (and other) cancers to be "endocrinology gone wild." In other words, a variety of genetic insults appear to induce either overproduction or activation of otherwise well-controlled cellular endocrine systems, resulting in uncontrolled growth, invasion, metastases, and survival—the phenotypic hallmarks of malignancy.

Therefore, the concept of therapeutic gain through disruption of one or more of these signal transduction pathways is appealing. Indeed, this statement provides the answer to the interrogative title of this chapter, "Why Endocrine Therapy?" Simply put, if the malignant phenotype is being driven by an aberrant endocrine axis that is relatively tissue- or organ-specific, then disruption of that process should provide effective and relatively nontoxic therapy. This concept has generated considerable enthusiasm in the field of "molecular medicine," in which the observations made by molecular and cellular biologists are used to design effective and efficient therapeutic agents.

III. HISTORICAL PERSPECTIVE OF ENDOCRINE THERAPY

One could argue that the field of molecular medicine was initiated in the late 1890s, when Sir George Thomas Beatson, a surgeon at the Glasgow Infirmary, hypothesized the existence of a link between the breast and the ovary, since castration of dairy cattle enhances lactation [1]. He offered oophorectomy to three young women with what would now be called locally advanced breast cancer. Remarkably, two of these three women experienced regression of their disease. Although Beatson concluded that this effect was secondary to a neurological link between the organs, we now know that he was removing a molecular growth factor (estrogen) from a dependent cancer.

By midcentury, endocrine therapy, consisting of oophorectomy for young women and pharmacological doses of estrogenic compounds for postmenopausal women, was the treatment of choice in advanced disease. Some of the earliest prospective randomized clinical trials in all of medicine addressed adjuvant oophorectomy. These trials demonstrated reductions in distant recurrence and mortality and remain positive to this day [2]. Since then, several surgical and medical approaches have been introduced that have improved the efficacy and safety of endocrine therapy directed toward the ER pathway. Coupled with the high incidence of breast cancer in the western world affecting a relatively young population, the substantial life prolonging benefits of ER-based endocrine therapy may result in more life-years saved than any other active anticancer therapy. Therefore, a thorough understanding of endocrine therapy is essential for any student or practitioner involved with breast cancer and should serve as a primer for the emerging peptide-hormone based therapies during the next decade.

IV. ABLATIVE AND ADDITIVE ENDOCRINE THERAPY

Fundamentally, endocrine therapy has been divided into two categories: ablative and additive (Table 1). Ablative therapies are directed toward removing the sources of estrogen, which are primarily the ovaries in premenopausal women

Table 1 Categories of Steroid Hormone Endocrine Therapies for Breast Cancer

	Additive	Ablative surgical	Medical
Estrogenic compounds	Ethinylestradiol	Oophorectomy	LHRH Agonists/antagonists
	Diethylstilbestrol	Adrenalectomy	Goserelin
Androgens	Fluoxymestrone	Hypophysectomy	Leuprolide
	Methyltestosterone		Aromatase inhibitors
SERMs	Tamoxifen		Aminoglutethamide
	Toremifene		Formestane
	Droloxifene		Fadrozole
	Idoxifene		Anastrazole
	Raloxifene		Letrozole
	EM 800		Exemestane
Pure antiestrogens	Fulvestrant		Vorozole
Progestins	Megestrol acetate		
	Medroxyprogesterone Acetate		
Antiprogestins	Mifepristone		
	Onapristone		

and the adrenal glands in postmenopausal women. Initial ablative therapies were accomplished by surgical or radiation-induced ablation of hormone-producing organs, but more recently the goal of estrogen deprivation can be accomplished by chemical means. Surgical ablative therapies can be direct, such as oophorectomy or adrenalectomy, or indirect, such as hypophysectomy. In premenopausal women, "chemical castration" can be obtained by the administration of agonists and/or antagonists of luteinizing hormone–releasing hormone (LHRH), which prevent production of luteinizing hormone (LH) and therefore block ovarian estrogen production. In postmenopausal women, most if not all estrogen production stems from conversion of adrenal steroid precursors to estradiol by aromatase activity, either in peripheral adipose tissue or even within the tumor itself. First-generation aromatase inhibitors lacked specificity and were associated with substantial toxicity. However, powerful agents that specifically and almost completely inhibit aromatase activity are now in widespread use, and the results of recently published studies suggest that they may be even more effective than tamoxifen [3–9].

Additive endocrine therapies, in principle, function by direct action on the hormonally dependent cancer cell. In that regard, estrogen production persists, but its action is blocked at the cellular level by interfering with estrogen and its receptor. Enigmatically, the first such agents to be used successfully were estrogenic compounds (diethylstilbestrol, ethyinylestradiol) administered at pharmacological doses, although androgenic agents were also found to be marginally effective. Subsequently, estrogenic agents were replaced by the equally active but less toxic triphenylethylamine tamoxifen, which was originally considered to be an "antiestrogen." Subsequent studies have demonstrated that tamoxifen has dualistic agonist and antagonist activity, depending on the tissue of interest. Consequently, tamoxifen and other agents like it have been designated selective estrogen-receptor modifiers (SERMs).

Other hormonal therapies—such as progestational agents (megestrol, medroxyprogesterone acetate) and androgens—have been harder to classify. Both of these types of treatments have been proven to be active against breast cancer, although they have been largely replaced or relegated to third- or fourth-line therapy by newer, more active and tolerable agents. In theory, they might exert their effects at the cellular level and would thus be classified with the SERMs as additive agents. On the other hand, neither progesterone nor androgen receptors appear to be fundamentally important for breast cancer behavior, and neither antiprogestin nor antiandrogen therapy has been particularly successful against breast cancer. Therefore, it has been speculated that the mechanism of action of progestins and androgens may be a consequence of suppression of the hypothalamic-pituitary axis via a feedback mechanism. In this case, one might consider these strategies as ablative.

V. BREAST CANCER RESISTANCE TO ENDOCRINE THERAPY

In spite of the considerable progress made, several important questions regarding ER-directed endocrine therapies remained unanswered. First and foremost, one must wonder why all breast cancers are not equally responsive to ER disruption. The malignant phenotype of a substantial portion (up to 50%) of breast cancers appears to be hormone (estrogen)-independent; therefore, classic ER-directed endocrine therapy provides little or no benefit to such patients. Moreover, many patients whose tumors are initially hormone-dependent ultimately develop disease that is resistant to one or another of the endocrine strategies. Surprisingly, these breast cancers may remain sensitive to alternative hormone treatments for some period of time, but unfortunately most of these women ultimately develop completely hormone-independent disease and are destined to succumb to their malignancy.

A. ER-Dependent Mechanisms of Resistance

1. The Role of ERs in Endocrine Therapy Resistance

Considerable insight into the mechanisms of resistance has been provided by the remarkable advances in knowledge concerning the molecular biology of endocrine-responsive cancers. It is now well established that steroid hormones, such as estradiol, exert their effect by freely diffusing through the plasma membrane and binding to cytoplasmic peptide receptors. Binding of the steroid ligand with the receptor (in this case, estrogen and ER) induces ER homodimerization and phosphorylation, followed by interaction with estrogen response elements (ERE) in the promoter regions of estrogen-dependent genes. Recent work has demonstrated that at least two such ERs exist, ERα and ERβ [10–12]. Specific genetic function is dictated by carefully orchestrated interaction between the ER/ERE and intranuclear coactivating and corepressing proteins. The precise cellular/tissue responses to estrogen or to other ligands such as the SERMs depends on the specific ligand, the balance of ERα and ERβ, and the relative concentrations of multiple coactivators and repressors. Perhaps the best example of this exquisite balance is the apparent difference in tissue specificity between tamoxifen and raloxifene, a more recently introduced SERM. Both have antiestrogenic qualities in breast tissue and in the central nervous system, and both appear to be estrogenic in bone and liver. However, while the estrogenic effects of tamoxifen in the uterus accounts for part if not all of its associated increase in endometrial cancer, raloxifene appears to be an ER antagonist in the endometrium [13–20].

2. The ER as a Marker of Responsiveness to Endocrine Therapy

These advances have led to the adoption of ER and the estrogen-dependent gene PgR as powerful predictive factors for the odds of clinical response to endocrine therapy. It is now well established that hormone receptor–poor and especially negative breast cancers almost never respond to any form of endocrine therapy. That is, these breast cancers are resistant to all forms of endocrine therapy de novo. This resistance almost certainly occurs because the malignant phenotype of such tumors is independent of estrogen and instead dependent on other endocrine pathways. In this rapidly developing field, results suggest that these endocrine pathways are driven by peptide growth factors and/or signal transduction through their cell surface receptors [21–23].

3. Non-ER Markers of Responsiveness to Endocrine Therapy

Presence of the ER is necessary but not sufficient for estrogen dependence. Clinically, endocrine therapy appears to reduce recurrence in the adjuvant setting by only about 40%. Only about 50% of patients with ER-rich metastatic disease will benefit from endocrine therapy, and almost all patients with metastatic disease will ultimately become resistant to all forms of endocrine therapy, even though their tumors may still express ER [24–27]. Therefore, additional predictive factors are needed to help in the selection of patients who are very unlikely to respond to endocrine therapy, so that alternative treatments such as more toxic chemotherapy can be recommended. However, such factors must, like ER, separate these two groups with almost absolute precision, since most patients with breast cancer are willing to accept the relatively low toxicity of endocrine therapy for a very small chance of benefit [28,29]. Thus far, no such factor has been identified. Several relatively weak predictive factors seem to separate ER-positive patients into those who are more or less like to respond, but not with the accuracy that would lead one to withhold endocrine therapy. Of these, the members of the HER family, especially HER-2, appear particularly interesting. Several preclinical and clinical studies (although not universally) have suggested that ER-positive HER-2–positive tumors are less responsive to endocrine agents, suggesting "cross-talk" between the HER peptide growth factor and ER steroid growth factor axes [30].

B. Long-Term Administration of Tamoxifen

Molecular biology of the ER-axis may also explain another puzzling clinical observation. During the first 15 years of tamoxifen use, most clinicians assumed that long-term administration should be more effective than shorter courses. Indeed, prospective randomized trials and a worldwide overview of clinical results have demonstrated that while 1 year of adjuvant tamoxifen improves disease-free and overall survival, 2 years and 5 years provide even more benefit. However, in two prospective trials in which women who reached 5 years on adjuvant tamoxifen were randomly assigned to ongoing maintenance versus discontinuation of the drug, there was no apparent benefit to more than 5 years; there may actually be a higher risk of recurrence and death [31,32]. Recent in vitro studies have demonstrated that, as in bone and liver, tamoxifen can behave in an agonistic manner for the ER in breast cancer tissue, perhaps due to a change in the balance of ERα and ERβ, as well as coactivators and repressors, or to mutations in the ER that render it hypersensitive to tamoxifen [33].

C. Non-ER Mechanisms of Resistance to Endocrine Therapy

Other peptide growth factor pathways are also under investigation as either de novo axes that breast cancer cells might exploit for hormone independence or as upregulated systems that result in emergence of resistance to endocrine therapy. These include the insulin-like growth factors (IGF-1 and IGF-2) and associated receptors [34] and other, less well studied axes, such as that signaled through NOTCH receptors (a highly conserved receptor family involved in the regulation of cell differentiation, proliferation, and apoptosis in many cell types) [35]. Although none of the studies of non-HER pathways has attained clinical utility, it seems likely that future investigations will be fruitful.

VI. OVERCOMING BREAST CANCER RESISTANCE TO ENDOCRINE THERAPY

These considerations raise a second question: "How can resistance to ER-directed therapy be overcome?" A critical subcomponent of this question is whether all breast cancers derive from stem cells that are initially estrogen-dependent or whether two (or more) stem cell components exist: one estrogen dependent and the other not. If the latter is the case, then one might expect that more effective therapies directed toward the ER would substantially reduce or eliminate the burden of breast cancer. Such strategies might include development of new agents that block the estrogen-ER pathway more effectively, either by additive or ablative means. These might include drugs that work via similar mechanisms to existing agents, such as the SERMs, the aromatase inhibitors, or the gonadatropin releasing factor agonists/antagonists. Alternatively, it is conceivable that pharmacological modulation of the ER corepressors and coinhibitors, or of the steroid or peptide growth factor pathways that interact with ER, might be effective strategies. Future preclinical and clinical studies are likely to move in these directions.

Of course, another strategy is to make already existing agents work better by using classical pharmacological maneuvers. In this regard, studies of schedule alterations, dose intensity, and combinations of existing hormone therapies have, until recently, been disappointing [26]. However, an important survival advantage for the combination of goserelin and tamoxifen has been reported in ER-positive premenopausal patients with metastatic disease [36]. This study raises the possibility that combining ablative and additive therapies might be substantially more effective than either approach alone, and it has generated a flurry of clinical trials to test this hypothesis. Indeed, the increasingly sophisticated understanding of the molecular biology underlying resistance to endocrine therapy has led to initiation of several trials comparing ablative strategies (either LH-RH-antagonists or aromatase inhibitors) to tamoxifen, including combination strategies. As the results of these studies become available, the scientific community will further refine our conceptual perspectives of these complex pathways. Perhaps the most successful strategy for improving endocrine (or any systemic anticancer therapy) has been early application. It is now clear that mortality from breast cancer is decreased by 20–30% by the application of adjuvant tamoxifen to ER-rich patients for 5 or more years [24]. Will even earlier application be even more effective? Four prospective randomized clinical trials have compared tamoxifen with placebo for the prevention of new breast cancers. The largest of these, performed by the National Surgical Adjuvant and Breast Project (NSABP) in the United States, has demonstrated a 50% reduction in emergence of new breast cancers after 5 years of therapy [37–39]. However, even this study has not demonstrated a survival benefit, and it is not clear that the benefit/risk ratio favors treatment of an enormous number of women (even if considered "high risk") for suppression of breast cancer in only a few [40]. Moreover, ER-negative cases have emerged at equal rates, supporting the previously discussed theory that two stem cell compartments may give rise to new breast cancers: one estrogen-dependent, the other not. Preliminary results from a recently reported study of molecular fingerprinting using gene expression arrays have suggested that two such compartments do exist; one stemming from "basal" cells, the other from alleged "luminal" cells [41,42]. These results raise two possible avenues of research of chemoprevention of breast cancer: improving ER-directed endocrine therapy and identification and suppression of the other pathways that lead to estrogen-independent phenotypes. A third question regarding the clinical toxicities of ER-directed endocrine therapy needs to be addressed. These are, on the most part, predictable, based on the antiestrogenic (menopausal symptoms, bone loss, sexual dysfunction, possibly heightened cardiovascular risk, and possibly decreased cognitive function) and the estrogenic (thrombosis, uterine cancer, cataract promotion) properties of the respective therapies. A critical observation is that only a fraction of patients suffer each of these, suggesting a considerable pharmacogenomic component to individual response. Studies of germline polymorphisms in the hepatic cytochrome P450 system enzymes, as well as the possibility of germline polymorphisms of the target tissue comodulating factors, are now under way. It is conceivable that, in the future, specific endocrine treatments can be selected for each individual patient.

"Why endocrine therapy?" These days, the question is really "Why not?" The exciting advances in the field of estrogen-ER directed therapies have already led to important quality-of-life and survival advantages. The era of non–ER pathway disruption has now been opened with the introduction of anti-HER2 therapy using trastuzumab [43–46]. It is likely that this is only the first of such "target-directed" therapies that will disrupt other endocrine axes.

REFERENCES

1. Beatson GW. On the treatment of inoperable cases of carcinoma of the mamma: Suggestions for a new method of treatment with illustrative cases. Lancet 1896; 2:104–107, 162–165.
2. Early Breast Cancer Trialists Collaborative Group. Ovarian ablation in early breast cancer: Overview of the randomised trials. Lancet 1996; 348:1189–1196.
3. Buzdar AU, Jonat W, Howell A, et al. Anastrozole versus megestrol acetate in the treatment of postmenopausal women with advanced breast carcinoma: results of a survival update based on a combined analysis of data from two mature phase III trials. Arimidex Study Group. Cancer 1998; 83:1142–1152.
4. Dombernowsky P, Smith I, Falkson G, et al. Letrozole, a new oral aromatase inhibitor for advanced breast cancer: double-blind randomized trial showing a dose effect and improved efficacy and tolerability compared with megestrol acetate (see comments). J Clin Oncol 1998; 16:453–461.
5. Vergote I, Bonneterre J, Thurlimann B, et al. Randomised study of anastrozole versus tamoxifen as first-line therapy for advanced breast cancer in postmenopausal women. Eur J Cancer 2000; 36(suppl 4):S84–S85.
6. Nabholtz JM, Buzdar A, Pollak M, et al. Anastrozole is superior to tamoxifen as first-line therapy for advanced breast cancer in postmenopausal women: Results of a North American multicenter randomized trial. Arimidex Study Group. J Clin Oncol 2000; 18:3758–3767.
7. Bonneterre J, Thurlimann B, Robertson JF, et al. Anastrozole versus tamoxifen as first-line therapy for advanced breast cancer in 668 postmenopausal women: Results of the Tamoxifen or Arimidex Randomized Group Efficacy and Tolerability study. J Clin Oncol 2000; 18:3748–3757.
8. Gershanovich M, Chaudri H, Hornberger U, Lassus M. Comparison of letrozole 2.5 mg (Femara) with megestrol acetate and with aminoglutethimide in patients with visceral disease (abstr). Breast Cancer Res Treat 1997; 46:212.
9. Mouridsen H, Gershanovich M, Sun Y, et al. Superior efficacy of letrozole versus tamoxifen as first-line therapy for postmenopausal women with advanced breast cancer: Results of a phase III study of the International Letrozole Breast Cancer Group. J Clin Oncol 2001; 19:2596–2606.

10. Mosselman S, Polman J, Dijkema R. ER beta: Identification and characterization of a novel human estrogen receptor. FEBS Lett 1996; 392:49–53.
11. Pace P, Taylor J, Suntharalingam S, et al. Human estrogen receptor beta binds DNA in a manner similar to and dimerizes with estrogen receptor alpha. J Biol Chem 1997; 272:25832–25838.
12. Barkhem T, Carlsson B, Nilsson Y, et al. Differential response of estrogen receptor alpha and estrogen receptor beta to partial estrogen agonists/antagonists. Mol Pharmacol 1998; 54:105–112.
13. Love R, Mazess R, Tormey D, et al. Bone mineral density in women with breast cancer treated with adjuvant tamoxifen for at least two years. Breast Cancer Res Treat 1988; 12:297–301.
14. Love R, Newcomb P, Wiebe D, et al. Lipid and lipoprotein effects of tamoxifen therapy in postmenopausal women with node-negative breast cancer. Breast Cancer Res Treatment 1989; 14:183a.
15. Fornander T, Cedermark B, Mattsson A, et al. Adjuvant tamoxifen in early breast cancer: Occurrence of new primary cancers. Lancet 1989; 1:117–120.
16. Fornander T, Rutqvist LE, Wilking N, et al. Oestrogenic effects of adjuvant tamoxifen in postmenopausal breast cancer. Eur J Cancer 1993; 4:497–500.
17. Balfour JA, Goa KL. Raloxifene. Drugs Aging 1998; 12:335–341, 342.
18. Boss SM, Huster WJ, Neild JA, et al. Effects of raloxifene hydrochloride on the endometrium of postmenopausal women. Am J Obstet Gynecol 1997; 177:1458–1464.
19. Cummings SR, Eckert S, Krueger KA, et al. The effect of raloxifene on risk of breast cancer in postmenopausal women: results from the MORE randomized trial. Multiple Outcomes of Raloxifene Evaluation. JAMA 1999; 281:2189–2197.
20. Yang NN, Venugopalan M, Hardikar S, Glasebrook A. Identification of an estrogen response element activated by metabolites of 17-beta-estradiol and raloxifene. Science 1996; 273:1222–1225.
21. Pinkas-Kramarski R, Shelly M, Guarino BC, et al. ErbB tyrosine kinases and the two neuregulin families constitute a ligand-receptor network. Mol Cell Biol 1998; 18:6090–6101.
22. Tzahar E, Yarden Y. The ErbB-2/HER2 oncogenic receptor of adenocarcinomas: From orphanhood to multiple stromal ligands. Biochim Biophys Acta 1998; 1377:M25–M37.
23. Klapper LN, Glathe S, Vaisman N, et al. The ErbB-2/HER2 oncoprotein of human carcinomas may function solely as a shared coreceptor for multiple stroma-derived growth factors. Proc Natl Acad Sci USA 1999; 96:4995–5000.
24. Early Breast Cancer Trialists' Collaborative Group. Tamoxifen for early breast cancer: An overview of the randomised trials. Lancet 1998; 351:1451–1467.
25. Osborne CK. Receptors. In: Harris J, Hellman S, Henderson I, Kinne D, eds. Breast Diseases. Philadelphia: Lippincott, 1991:301–325.
26. Ellis M, Hayes DF, Lippman ME. Treatment of Metastatic Disease. In: Harris J, Lippman M, Morrow M, Osborne CK, eds. Diseases of the Breast. Philadelphia: Lippincott-Raven, 2000:749–798.
27. Hull DP III, Clark GM, Osborne CK, et al. Multiple estrogen receptor assays in human breast cancer. Cancer Res 1983; 43:413–416.

28. Hayes DF, Trock B, Harris A. Assessing the clinical impact of prognostic factors: When is "statistically significant" clinically useful? Breast Cancer Res Treat 1998; 52:305–319.

29. Hayes DF. Do we need prognostic factors in nodal-negative breast cancer? Arbiter. Eur J Cancer 2000; 36:302–306.

30. Yamauchi H, Stearns V, Hayes DF. When is a tumor marker ready for prime time? A case study of c-erbB-2 as a predictive factor in breast cancer. J Clin Oncol 2001; 19:2334–2356.

31. Fisher B, Dignam J, Bryant J, et al. Five versus more than five years of tamoxifen therapy for breast cancer patients with negative lymph nodes and estrogen receptor-positive tumors. J Natl Cancer Inst 1996; 88:1529–1542.

32. Stewart HJ, Prescott RJ, Forrest AP. Scottish adjuvant tamoxifen trial: A randomized study updated to 15 years. J Natl Cancer Inst 2001; 93:456–462.

33. Osborne CK. Tamoxifen in the treatment of breast cancer. N Engl J Med 1998; 339:1609–1618.

34. Ellis MJ. The insulin-like growth factor network and breast cancer. In: Bowcock AM, ed. Breast Cancer: Molecular Genetics, Pathogenesis and Therapeutics. Totowa, NJ: Humana Press, 1999.

35. Jang MS, Zlobin A, Kast WM, Miele L. Notch signaling as a target in multimodality cancer therapy. Curr Opin Mol Ther 2000; 2(1): 55–65.

36. Klijn JG, Blamey RW, Boccardo F, et al. Combined tamoxifen and luteinizing hormone-releasing hormone (LHRH) agonist versus LHRH agonist alone in premenopausal advanced breast cancer: A meta-analysis of four randomized trials. J Clin Oncol 2001; 19:343–353.

37. Fisher B, Costantino JP, Wickerham DL, et al. Tamoxifen for prevention of breast cancer: Report of the National Surgical Adjuvant Breast and Bowel Project P-1 Study. J Natl Cancer Inst 1998; 90:1371–1388.

38. Powles T, Eeles R, Ashley S, et al. Interim anlaysis of the incidence of breast cancer in the Royal Marsden Hospital tamoxifen randomised chemoprevention trial. Lancet 1998; 352:98–101.

39. Veronesi U, Maisonneuve P, Costa A, et al. Prevention of breast cancer with tamoxifen: preliminary findings from the Italian randomised trial among hysterectomised women. Lancet 1998; 352:93–97.

40. Pritchard KI. Is tamoxifen effective in prevention of breast cancer? Lancet 1998; 352:80–81.

41. Perou CM, Jeffrey SS, van de Rijn M, et al. Distinctive gene expression patterns in human mammary epithelial cells and breast cancers. Proc Natl Acad Sci USA 1999; 96:9212–9217.

42. Perou CM, Sorlie T, Eisen MB, et al. Molecular portraits of human breast tumours. Nature 2000; 406:747–752.

43. Baselga J, Tripathy D, Mendelsohn J, et al. Phase II study of weekly intravenous recombinant humanized anti-p185HER2 monoclonal antibody in patients with HER2/neu-overexpressing metastatic breast cancer. J Clin Oncol 1996; 14: 737–744.

44. Vogel C, Cobleigh MA, Tripathy D, et al. First-line, single-agent Herceptin

(trastuzumab) in metastatic breast cancer: a preliminary report. Eur J Cancer 2001; 37(suppl 1):S25–29.

45. Cobleigh MA, Vogel CL, Tripathy D, et al. Multinational study of the efficacy and safety of humanized anti-HER2 monoclonal antibody in women who have HER2-overexpressing metastatic breast cancer that has progressed after chemotherapy for metastatic disease. J Clin Oncol 1999; 17:2639.

46. Slamon DJ, Leyland-Jones B, Shak S, et al. Use of chemotherapy plus a monoclonal antibody against HER2 for metastatic breast cancer that overexpresses HER2. N Engl J Med 2001; 344:783–792

Part II

ADVANCED BREAST CANCER

2

Tamoxifen and Advanced Breast Cancer: An Overview

John F. Forbes
University of Newcastle
Newcastle, Australia

I. ABSTRACT

Tamoxifen has been used to treat advanced breast cancer for 30 years and has been the first-line endocrine therapy of choice for much of this period. It is well tolerated and inexpensive, and serious side effects are uncommon. Survival rates are equivalent to those from chemotherapy, and although initial response rates are lower, it offers a superior quality of life in initial responders. Tamoxifen should not be displaced as a key therapy for advanced breast cancer without substantial and convincing data from large randomized trials. Response rates depend on patient selection and are higher for patients with estrogen-responsive tumors. Tamoxifen alone has efficacy similar to that of estrogens or progestins when used singly or in combination, but it is better tolerated than most alternative endocrine therapies. In premenopausal patients there is good evidence that the combination of tamoxifen and a luteinizing hormone–releasing hormone (LH-RH) analogue is superior to either single agent alone. This benefit of combination endocrine therapy with tamoxifen will not necessarily be translated to postmenopausal patients. Recently, third-generation aromatase inhibitors have been compared with tamoxifen in postmenopausal patients with advanced breast cancer and have been shown to have possibly superior efficacy, with reduced side effects. This opens up new, potentially beneficial strategies using combined endocrine therapies—concurrently and in sequence in both pre- and post-menopausal patients. Given the sequential benefits demonstrated for tamoxifen from advanced to in situ disease and prevention for over 30 years, it seems very likely that aromatase inhibitors will be shown to be effective in all types of endocrine-responsive breast cancer. Future clinical trials testing endocrine therapies in advanced breast cancer should be large, have similar defined populations and biological endpoints, and involve intergroup collaborations similar to those established for adjuvant trials. This is essential to avoid taking another 30 years to evaluate newer endocrine therapies.

II. BACKGROUND

A. Current Clinical Use of Tamoxifen

Tamoxifen has been approved for use in treatment of advanced breast cancer since 1973 in the United Kingdom and 1977 in the United States. This followed the report by Cole in 1971 of a 22% response rate with Nolvadex, the citrate salt of tamoxifen [1]. Since 1971, tamoxifen has been used for more than 10 million patient-years worldwide. It is one of the safest, cheapest, best-tolerated, and most effective of all cancer treatments. Until recently, it has been the first-line treatment for endocrine-responsive advanced breast cancer, and it remains the treatment of choice for early invasive breast cancer and preinvasive breast cancer or duct carcinoma in situ (DCIS). It has also been shown to reduce the incidence of contralateral breast cancer after a diagnosis of invasive breast cancer as well as reducing the occurrence of first clinical breast cancer in women considered to be at increased risk. Tamoxifen, therefore, is widely used clinically for treatment of early and advanced disease, DCIS, and prevention. The U.S. Food and Drug Administration (FDA) approved usages include adjuvant therapy in postmenopausal women with node-positive breast cancer with chemotherapy (1985) and alone (1986); in premenopausal women with estrogen receptor-positive advanced breast cancer (1989); as adjuvant treatment for pre- and postmenopausal women with node-negative estrogen receptor–positive breast cancer (1990); for reduction of risk of breast cancer in high-risk pre- and postmenopausal women (1998); and for adjuvant treatment of ductal carcinoma in situ after surgery and radiotherapy to reduce the incidence of invasive breast cancer (2001). Tamoxifen is clearly a pillar of breast cancer control and has made a substantial contribution to the reduced mortality rate that has been reported in several developed countries since 1990. It will require substantial and strong evidence of efficacy, tolerability, and safety before tamoxifen is replaced by alternative treatments for women with endocrine-responsive breast cancer.

B. Tolerability of Tamoxifen

Tamoxifen is well tolerated, and fewer than 3% of advanced disease patients discontinue therapy [2]. However, tamoxifen does have undesirable effects. Potentially serious effects include an increased risk of venous thrombosis and pulmonary embolism [3] and an increased risk of endometrial cancer [2]. Both are relatively uncommon effects, and risk is largely confined to postmenopausal women. Women with advanced disease are exposed to these risks for a shorter period of time than patients receiving tamoxifen as adjuvant therapy. More common effects consist of menopausal-like symptoms, including hot flashes (27%), night sweats, vaginal dryness, and menstrual irregularity in premenopausal women (13%). If bone metastases are present, some women have a tumor flare soon after beginning tamoxifen [3].

Tamoxifen may reduce the risk of osteoporosis by preserving or increasing bone mineral density [4,5], but this may be confined to postmenopausal women [6]. In addition, it can lower cholesterol and other blood lipids [7]. However, this has not been shown to lead to a reduction of cardiovascular events in women with advanced breast cancer. Individual patients require careful consideration of competing risks and benefits before starting tamoxifen. In general, women with advanced breast cancer have a more favorable balance of potential gain versus serious risks than women with early breast cancer, who require a longer duration of therapy.

III. USE OF TAMOXIFEN ALONE AS TREATMENT OF ADVANCED BREAST CANCER

A. Patient Populations and Early Trials

A large number of clinical trials have evaluated tamoxifen treatment of advanced breast cancer, providing information on response rates, duration of response, and parameters affecting response. Early trials studied patients who had not previously received adjuvant tamoxifen or adjuvant chemotherapy. Most of these trials were not confined to patients with estrogen responsive tumors. A distinction is made between (a) patients with advanced breast cancer who received prior adjuvant tamoxifen and progressed while on treatment and discontinued treatment and (b) those who received tamoxifen as adjuvant therapy and had progression of their tumor at least 12 months after stopping tamoxifen. Patients who have had prior adjuvant chemotherapy may also demonstrate a response to tamoxifen. This is most likely due to the prior determination that their tumors were negative for estrogen receptors.

B. Trial Endpoints

Response rates vary depending on category and the definition of acceptable response; they may have no bearing on true differences in treatment efficacy. Categories of response usually include complete response (CR), partial response (PR), no change (NC), and progressive disease (PD). For comparison of treatments, CR plus PR rates are usually used together to define total or overall response (OR); but increasingly the concept of "clinical benefit," usually defined as CR plus PR plus NC for a minimum period of time—e.g., 24 weeks—may be used. This is a useful concept as it may reflect response duration and time to disease progression, indicating the clinical value of a therapy in advanced disease. It is very important that definitions be clear so that data can be evaluated reliably. Other issues affecting the value of data from clinical trials in advanced breast cancer include sample size, stratification, and methods of patient evaluation [8].

C. Tamoxifen as a First-Line Single Endocrine Agent

The most definitive data on response rates and survival from a randomized trial of tamoxifen alone given to patients with advanced breast cancer and no prior tamoxifen exposure was conducted by the Australian New Zealand Breast Cancer Trials Group (ANZ BCTG) trial ANZ 7802 [9]. Trial ANZ 7801 built on the first trial that incorporated quality-of-life assessment, comparing chemotherapy versus tamoxifen for the treatment of advanced breast cancer in postmenopausal women [10]. ANZ BCTG 7802 commenced in 1978 and randomized 339 postmenopausal patients with advanced breast cancer to initial therapy with tamoxifen (20 mg per day), chemotherapy with AC [doxorubicin (Adriamycin) 50 mg/m^2 IV with cyclophosphamide 750 mg/m^2 IV, 21 day cycles] or tamoxifen plus AC given concurrently. Each treatment was continued until progression or until a maximum defined dose of anthracycline had been given. Documented patient and tumor characteristics included a disease free interval (DFI) >2 years, 51%; <2 years, 36.9%; no prior tamoxifen, 100%; known estrogen receptor (ER)–positive primary tumor, 16.8%; known ER-negative primary tumor, 8.3%; unknown ER status of primary tumor, 74.9%; no prior chemotherapy, 90%; prior phenylalanine mustard, 5.6%; dominant sites of disease soft tissue only, 6.5%; bone, 33.6%; visceral (not liver), 32.2 %; liver, 27.7%.

Response rates (CR plus PR) were tamoxifen, 22.1%; AC, 45.1%; tamoxifen plus AC, 51.3%. Clinical benefit rates (CR+ PR+ stable disease) were 80, 88, and 91%. Despite the differences in response rates, median survival rates [tamoxifen, 22.75 months (95% CI 19.0 to 26.5); AC plus tamoxifen, 22.5 months (17.9 to 27.3); and AC, 19.04 months (16.2 to 22.0), respectively] were not different ($p = 0.49$). Response rates were higher for patients with a longer disease-free interval and lower for patients who had liver disease or received prior adjuvant chemotherapy—probably reflecting a poorer prognosis at the time of diagnosis of the primary tumor. Trials in the future may include patients with exposure to prior adjuvant tamoxifen and known ER status of the primary tumor. Many patients in trial ANZ 7802 had their breast cancer diagnosed prior to the availability of ER assays.

IV. COMPARISON OF TAMOXIFEN WITH OTHER ENDOCRINE THERAPIES

In trials of single-agent comparisons, response rates to tamoxifen average 30 to 35% (CR plus PR) compared with progestins and estrogens. Estrogens, however, are not as well tolerated. Survival durations in advanced breast cancer average around a median of 20 to 25 months.

Early trials compared tamoxifen alone with other endocrine treatments alone or in combination with tamoxifen. Single-agent comparisons have been undertaken with estrogen (ethinyl estradiol and diethylstilbestrol) [11–13], androgen (fluoxymesterone) [14–16], progestins (medroxyprogesterone acetate, megestrol acetate) [17–24], ovarian ablation by surgical oophorectomy [25–27], and more recently the combination of tamoxifen and ovarian suppression by LH-RH analogues and LH-RH analogue alone [28–30]. Recent trials include more patients who had received prior adjuvant systemic therapy and known ER status of tumor, making comparisons of data from these trials with data from earlier trials invalid.

In summary, despite a large number of trials, there is little evidence that response rates of advanced breast cancers to various single endocrine agents differ when compared directly with each other.

Comparison of tamoxifen with oophorectomy in premenopausal patients failed to find any difference for overall response rates, duration of response, time to progression, or survival [25–28]. As no survival differences have been seen with these various single agents, quality-of-life assessment remains an important part of the evaluation to determine the usefulness of endocrine treatments. For example, surgical ovarian ablation is very different from long-term tamoxifen.

V. TAMOXIFEN AND COMBINED ENDOCRINE THERAPIES

No convincing benefit has been demonstrated in survival or response rates for the addition of most endocrine single agents to tamoxifen therapy. The possible exception is the combination of tamoxifen with an LH-RH analogue. A pivotal EORTC trial compared tamoxifen with the LH-RH analogue buserelin and with the combination of both agents as first-line treatment in 161 pre- and perimenopausal women with advanced breast cancer [30]. Patients with negative or unknown tumor steroid receptor status were excluded, as were patients who had a disease-free interval of less than 2 years. This ensured that the population was likely to have endocrine-responsive tumors. The median follow-up was 7.3 years, by which time 76% of patients had died.

It was found that combined treatment with tamoxifen and buserelin was superior to either buserelin or tamoxifen alone: objective response rates, 48, 34, and 28%, $p = 0.01$ (all p values two-sided); median progression-free survival, 9.7, 6.3, and 5.6 months, $p = 0.03$; overall survival, 3.7, 2.5, and 2.9 years, $p = 0.01$. Actuarial 5-year survival percentages were 34.2% (95% confidence interval (CI) 20.4 to 48%], 14.9% (95% CI = 3.9%–25.9%) and 18.4% (95% CI = 7.0%–29.8%), respectively. No significant differences were reported between the two single agents alone. This trial is unique in demonstrating a survival advantage for combination endocrine therapy versus single-agent therapy in premenopausal patients.

An overview of four trials, including the EORTC trial, involving the combination of an LH-RH analogue and tamoxifen compared with LH-RH analogue alone reconfirmed the advantage of this combination [29]. A total of 306 patients were included in the four trials, three compared the LH-RH analogue goserelin (Zoladex) alone with the combination of goserelin and tamoxifen, and the fourth trial compared buserelin with tamoxifen and buserelin (i.e., two arms of the EORTC trial). There was a consistent advantage for the combined therapy. Objective response, 30 versus 39% [odds ratio (OR) 0.67, 95% CI 0.46 to 0.96, $p = 0.03$]; median progression-free survival (months), 5.4 versus 8.7 (OR 0.70, 95% CI 0.58 to 0.85, $p <0.001$); median response duration (months), 11.3 versus 19.4, and median overall survival (years) 2.5 versus 2.9 (OR 0.78, 95% CI 0.63 to 0.96, $p = 0.02$); all favored the combination and appears to be a real advantage.

If this benefit is real, it does not necessarily mean that other combinations of endocrine treatment will also be beneficial. Nor can it be concluded that similar combinations of plasma estrogen–lowering agents with tamoxifen will be equally beneficial in treating postmenopausal women with advanced breast cancer. The combination of tamoxifen and LH-RH analogue results in suppression of plasma estrogen to postmenopausal levels, and the tamoxifen-induced stimulation of the pituitary-ovarian function is avoided. This is markedly different to the combination of a progestin and tamoxifen, which may have similar actions and does not seem to have any advantage in efficacy over tamoxifen alone. In general, other combinations of endocrine agents have not proven to be superior to single agents. In the EORTC trial, the combined treatment and treatment with buserelin alone both caused similar degrees of suppression of plasma estradiol levels, whereas treatment with tamoxifen was associated with a three- to fourfold increase in these levels. The combination of lowered plasma estradiol and tamoxifen antiestrogen activity at the tumor cell, together with a direct antitumor effect of tamoxifen, may all contribute to the benefit. The results also suggest that other combinations of estrogen lowering, by oophorectomy or an aromatase inhibitor, and antitumor effects with tamoxifen or newer antiestrogen agents acting at the cellular level (e.g., Faslodex) may be potentially valuable therapies. It is plausible that tamoxifen is more efficacious when plasma estradiol levels are very low, or that the biology of breast tumor cell growth in premenopausal women is uniquely sensitive to lowering of the estradiol, which at the same time promotes an acute sensitivity to direct tamoxifen cellular effects. In premenopausal patients, alternative combinations could include an LH-RH analogue with an aromatase inhibitor, with or without tamoxifen, and an LH-RH agonist with alternative antiestrogen agents including Faslodex and raloxifene. Sequencing of such agents may be as valuable as combining them.

The large ATAC (Arimidex Tamoxifen Alone or Combined) adjuvant trial comparing single-agent endocrine therapy with tamoxifen, aromatase inhibitor (anastrazole), or both agents given concurrently for ER-positive or ER-unknown early breast cancer in postmenopausal women will address similar questions to the EORTC trial. The fact that the ATAC population is postmenopausal is important, as the tumors will have developed in a relatively low-estrogen environment and will have different biological characteristics. Whether or not the ATAC combined therapy arm (i.e., tamoxifen plus anastrazole) proves to be beneficial in this setting, other combinations with an estrogen-lowering agent and alternative antiestrogen agents to tamoxifen, such as Faslodex, will be important to evaluate, with these given concurrently or in sequence. This will be important both for tamoxifen naïve patients with advanced disease and for tamoxifen-resistant tumors.

VI. TAMOXIFEN VERSUS OTHER COMBINATIONS OF ENDOCRINE THERAPY

Tamoxifen alone has been compared with combinations of tamoxifen with other endocrine agents. There is limited evidence of any advantage for the combination of tamoxifen and progestin [31] or tamoxifen plus the first-generation aromatase inhibitor aminoglutethimide [32,33]. The combination of danazol, aminoglutethimide, and tamoxifen had an increased response rate over tamoxifen alone, but no survival advantage has been reported [34]. The sequence of tamoxifen and medroxyprogesterone may produce a superior response to tamoxifen alone [35], but no evidence of a survival advantage has been seen. A large trial by the ANZ BCTG compared the addition or substitution of medroxyprogesterone acetate to tamoxifen in postmenopausal women who progressed on tamoxifen. There was no difference for overall response rates or survival [36]. Thus, the only convincing evidence for combinations of endocrine therapy over tamoxifen alone is in premenopausal patients when estrogen lowering is combined with tamoxifen.

VII. TAMOXIFEN VERSUS CHEMOTHERAPY

The definitive trial comparing tamoxifen with chemotherapy and the combination of tamoxifen and chemotherapy has been referred to above in the discussion of tamoxifen efficacy. This trial, ANZ 7801 [9], involved patients with advanced breast cancer (metastatic and/or locally advanced) randomized to two single-modality treatment sequences—(a) doxorubicin (Adriamycin) plus cyclophosphamide (AC) followed on failure by tamoxifen (TAM) and (b) TAM followed by AC. These were compared with combined-modality chemoendocrine therapy (TAM plus AC). First-line response data and data on alternative sequences were obtained. Overall response rates (PR plus CR) to TAM, 22.1%, were inferior to those for AC, 45.1%, and that for TAM plus AC, 51.3%. However, patients randomized to the sequence TAM followed by AC on progression had a 42.5% overall tumor response to sequential protocol therapy, similar to the 46.9% for those randomize to AC followed by TAM. Despite the significantly inferior initial response rate, the tamoxifen patients had a comparable survival, with median overall survival (months) of TAM 22.75 (95% CI 19.0 to 26.5%), TAM plus AC 22.5 (95% CI 17.9 to 27.3), and AC 19.04 (95% CI 16.22 to 22.0) [9].

Adverse prognostic factors for survival were liver metastases, short disease-free interval (less than 2 years), poor performance status, and prior adjuvant chemotherapy (5.6% of patients had prior adjuvant phenylalanine mustard). Endocrine therapy with tamoxifen proved particularly effective in postmenopausal patients where chemotherapy had failed. Such patients also experienced a superior quality of life.

Although the population of patients in the ANZ 7801 may have been different from those in advanced breast cancer trials completed more recently, the overall survivals are comparable. This trial remains the only one with direct comparisons of tamoxifen with both chemotherapy and combined-modality therapy. Patients also had sequential therapy with tamoxifen following chemotherapy on tumor progression and vice versa. The conclusion that beginning with endocrine therapy and changing to chemotherapy for those who progress on tamoxifen does not compromise survival and offers a better quality of life remains valid today and is likely to be relevant for treatment with newer aromatase inhibitors. Finally, in trial ANZ 7801, 83.2% of patients had ER-negative or ER-unknown tumors, and this would bias against the tamoxifen therapy.

Other studies, although mostly less informative, have also found a lower response rate for tamoxifen compared with chemotherapy. However, response rates with ER-positive tumors average 45 to 60% and are comparable to chemotherapy response rates in this population. Other trials comparing tamoxifen with combined-modality therapy have also found higher response rates when chemotherapy is included. A small randomized trial comparing TAM with TAM plus CMF (cyclophosphamide, methotrexate,and 5-fluorouracil) in patients with ER-positive tumors found similar response rates for tamoxifen and combined-modality therapy (15/24 versus 17/26) [37].

Similarly, when the combination of tamoxifen and chemotherapy is compared with chemotherapy alone, little advantage is seen beyond an increase in response rate (e.g., with TAM plus CMF response rates were 86/115, 75%, versus 51/105, 49%, for CMF alone [38]; but as in ANZ 7801, no significant survival advantage was seen for the addition of tamoxifen to chemotherapy.

Finally, additional trials have compared combined-modality therapy using tamoxifen and chemotherapy with sequential therapy and failed to identify significant advantages for either. In ANZ 7802, tamoxifen had a lower initial response rate, and this was compensated for by response to subsequent chemotherapy on progression. A durable response to tamoxifen alone, however, may allow a second or third endocrine therapy to be used with potential advantages for patients in terms of quality of life. The first comparison undertaken of chemotherapy versus endocrine therapy documented a lower response rate but superior quality of life for endocrine therapy using linear analogue self-assessment (LASA) scales in cancer patients for the first time [39].

VIII. TAMOXIFEN COMPARED TO AROMATASE INHIBITORS

A. Early Trials

Aromatase, a cytochrome P450-dependent enzyme, converts androgen substrates to estrogens [40]. Blockade of the aromatase enzyme is associated with reduction of estrogen levels and an antitumor effect.

The first report of tamoxifen versus an aromatase inhibitor used aminoglutethimide and involved 117 patients with advanced breast cancer. Response rates and median response durations were similar, but tamoxifen patients had fewer side effects [41]. Subsequently, tamoxifen has been compared with fadrozole, a nonsteroidal imidazole aromatase inhibitor. Tamoxifen had higher response rates and a significantly longer median response duration ($p=0.009$) in one trial [42], and a nonsignificant higher response rate and response duration with a significantly longer time to disease progression in the other trial [43]. Tamoxifen has also been compared with formestane, a "second-generation" steroidal aromatase inhibitor, as first-line endocrine therapy in 409 postmenopausal patients. There was no significant difference in response rates, response duration, or overall survival, but tamoxifen had a significantly longer time to disease progression (294 versus 213 days, $p=0.010$) [44].

B. Tamoxifen Compared to Third-Generation Aromatase Inhibitors as First-Line Therapy

Tamoxifen has been compared with the third-generation aromatase inhibitors letrozole and anastrozole (nonsteroidal) and exemestane (steroidal). These three third-generation aromatase inhibitors have first been compared to megestrol in prospective randomized clinical trials as second-line endocrine therapy for advanced breast cancer. A meta-analysis of all three trials concluded that compared with megestrol, the aromatase inhibitors were associated with a relative risk of death of 0.79 (95% CI 0.69–0.91, $p= 0.001$)—a mean survival gain of 4.1 months per patient, and had a favorable pharmacoeconomic profile [45]. Hence there is a sound basis to compare these agents with tamoxifen as first-line treatment for advanced breast cancer.

Three clinical trials comparing tamoxifen to letrozole and to anastrozole as first-line endocrine treatment of advanced breast cancer in postmenopausal women have been conducted.

1. Letrozole

Letrozole, a third-generation nonsteroidal aromatase inhibitor has been compared with tamoxifen in a large phase III trial [46]. This trial involved 907 postmenopausal women with advanced breast cancer with either estrogen receptor– and/or progesterone receptor–positive tumors or both receptors unknown. Patients were excluded if recurrent breast cancer was diagnosed during adjuvant antiestrogen therapy or within 12 months of prior endocrine therapy for advanced disease. Patients may have had a single prior chemotherapy regimen for advanced disease. For the primary endpoint of median TTP, letrozole was superior, 41 versus 26 weeks (hazards ratio, 0.70, 95% CI 0.60 to 0.82, $p=0.0001$), regardless of dominant site, receptor status, or prior adjuvant antiestrogen therapy. Letrozole also produced a significantly longer TTF, median 40 versus 25 weeks. Overall RR 30 versus 20%, $p=0.0006$, and rate of clinical benefit, 49 versus 38%, $p=0.001$, were both significantly higher for letrozole. No survival data were reported [46]. This is a large trial and documents an advantage for letrozole over tamoxifen as first-line treatment for advanced breast cancer. It remains to be seen whether this will be translated into a survival advantage as well.

2. Anastrozole

Anastrozole is a nonsteroidal third-generation aromatase inhibitor administered by daily oral tablet. Two concurrent prospective randomized double-blind trials have compared anastrozole, 1 mg daily, to tamoxifen, 20 mg daily, in postmenopausal women with advanced breast cancer who had not received any prior endocrine therapy for metastatic disease and who had ceased tamoxifen at least 12 months earlier. Patients were hormone receptor–positive or unknown [47,48]. The first trial (Trial 0027) was a worldwide trial and entered 668 patients, 328 on tamoxifen and 340 on anastrozole. Follow-up was for a median of 19 months. Results were similar for objective response (OR) (CR plus PR): 32.9% for anastrozole, 32.6% for TAM. Clinical benefit (CR + PR + stabilization rates of $\geq$ 24 weeks) were 56.2 and 56.5%, respectively. Median times to progression (TTP) were similar: 8.2 and 8.3 months, respectively. There were less thromboembolic events with anastrozole (4.8% versus 7.3%) and less vaginal bleeds (1.2% versus 2.4%) [47].

The second large trial (Trial 0030) was conducted in North America and randomized 353 patients with similar entry criteria, using the same drug doses as trial 0027. Anastrozole had similar OR rates as tamoxifen, 21 and 17% respectively. Clinical benefit favored anastrozole, 59 versus 46% (two-sided p = 0.0098, retrospective analysis). Anastrozole had a longer median TTP than tamoxifen, 11.1 and 5.6 months, respectively (two-sided p = 0.005, hazards ratio 1.44, lower one-sided 95% confidence limit, 1.16). Thromboembolic events and vaginal bleeding were less common with anastrazole (4.1 vs. 8.2%, and 1.2 vs. 3.8%, respectively). It was concluded from both trials that anastrozole had "satisfied the predefined criteria for equivalance to tamoxifen" and had a significant increase in TTP—as well as less thromboembolic events and vaginal bleeding—and should be considered as first-line therapy for postmenopausal women with advanced breast cancer [48].

Data on 119 patients of 137 in Trial 0027 known to have received tamoxifen after anastrozole was obtained by questionnaire. This indicated that 46 (38.7%) achieved disease stabilization for 24 weeks or more on tamoxifen and 58 (48.7%) obtained clinical benefit (CR, PR, or stable disease for 24 weeks or more) (presented by B. Thurlimann at the Nottingham International Breast Cancer Meeting, September, 2001). This may indicate that the sequence of anastrozole followed by tamoxifen is valuable; however, no data are available on the reverse sequence—i.e., tamoxifen followed by anastrozole on progression.

3. Exemestane

Exemestane is a steroidal third-generation aromatase inactivator. It binds irreversibly to the aromatase enzyme and is a potent inhibitor of aromatization, reducing estrogen synthesis by 97%. Like anastrozole and letrozole, it is safe and well tolerated. It is administered as oral tablets, 25 mg daily. Exemestane has also been compared with tamoxifen as first-line endocrine treatment of advanced breast cancer. Data are awaited with interest. In a smaller study, exemestane seemed to have a substantially higher response rate than tamoxifen.

IX. CONCLUSIONS

For nearly 30 years, tamoxifen has been the first-line endocrine therapy for advanced breast cancer. It produces response rates of 20 to 30% in unselected patients with advanced breast cancer and up to 60% in selected patients with estrogen receptor–positive tumors. Tamoxifen alone has similar efficacy to various combinations and sequences of endocrine therapies. The exception in premenopausal patients is the combination of tamoxifen and an LH-RH analogue, which appears to be superior to both tamoxifen alone and to LH-RH analogue alone. There are unique features of breast cancer in premenopausal patients; however, such combinations or sequencing of endocrine therapies in postmenopausal patients may not have the same advantages. In postmenopausal women the third-generation aromatase inhibitors appear to be at least as good and, in the case of letrozole, superior to tamoxifen alone as first-line endocrine therapy, although not yet for survival. This opens up potentially beneficial new strategies for treatment using aromatase inhibitors with tamoxifen and LH-RH analogues in premenopausal patients and in combination and sequence in postmenopausal patients with new antiestrogens such as Faslodex.

It is essential that advanced breast cancer trials be large and that they have carefully defined populations and standardized evaluation of biological endpoints. This mandates international collaboration, such as has been established for adjuvant trials. This is essential to avoid taking another 30 years to evaluate newer endocrine therapies such as aromatase inhibitors.

REFERENCES

1. Cole MP, Jones CTA, Todd IDH. A new antioestrogenic agent in late breast cancer: An early clinical appraisal of ICI 46,474. Br J Cancer 1971; 25:270–275.
2. Fossati R, Confalonieri C, Torri V, et al. Cytotoxic and hormonal treatment for metastatic breast cancer: a systematic review of published randomised trials involving 31,510 women. J Clin Oncol 1998; 16:3439–3460.
3. Litherland S, Jackson IM. Antioestrogens in the management of hormone-dependent cancer. Cancer Treat Rev 1988; 15:183–194
4. Love RR, Mazess RB, Barden HS. Effects of tamoxifen on bone mineral density in postmenopausal women with breast cancer. N Engl J Med 1992; 326:852–856.
5. Fisher B, Costantino JP, Wickerham DL, et al. Tamoxifen for prevention of breast cancer: report of the National Surgical Adjuvant Breast and Bowel Project P-1 study. J Natl Cancer Inst 1998; 90:1371–1388.
6. Powles TJ, Hickish T, Kanis JA, et al. Effect of tamoxifen on bone mineral density measured by dual-energy x-ray absorptiometry in healthy premenopausal and postmenopausal women. J Clin Oncol 1996; 14:78–84.
7. Love RR, Wiebe DA, Feyzi JM. et al. Effects of tamoxifen on cardiovascular risk

factors in postmenopausal women after 5 years of treatment. J Natl Cancer Inst 1994; 86:1534–1539.

8. Forbes JF. Breast Cancer: Advanced Disease. In: Furr BJA, ed. Clinics in Oncology. Hormone Therapy 1982:149–175.

9. The Australian and New Zealand Breast Cancer Trials Group, Clinical Oncological Society of Australia. Writing Committee: Coates AS, Simpson J, Forbes JF. A randomised trial in postmenopausal patients with advanced breast cancer comparing endocrine and cytotoxic therapy given sequentially or in combination. J Clin Oncol 1986; 4:186–193.

10. Priestman T, Baum M, Jones B, Forbes JF. Comparative trial of endocrine versus cytotoxic treatment in advanced breast cancer. Br Med J 1977 1·1248–1250.

11. Ingle JN, Ahmann DL, Green SJ, et al. Randomised clinical trial of diethylstilbestrol versus tamoxifen in post menopausal women with advanced breast cancer. N Engl J Med 1981; 304:16–21.

12. Beex L, Pieters G, Smals A, et al. Tamoxifen versus ethinyl estradiol in the treatment of postmenopausal women with advanced breast cancer. Cancer Treat Rep 1981; 65:179–185.

13. Ribeiro GG. A clinical trial to compare the use of tamoxifen vs stilboestrol in the treatment of post-menopausal women with advanced breast cancer. Rev Endocr Rel Cancer 1981 (suppl 9):409–414.

14. Nagai R, Kumaoka S. Clinical evaluation of tamoxifen in advanced breast cancer (primary and recurrent)—Double blind study. Clin Eval 1980; 8:321–352.

15. Westerberg H. Tamoxifen and fluoxymesterone in advanced breast cancer: A controlled clinical trial. Cancer Treat Rep 1980; 64:117–121.

16. Wada T, Yoshida M, Senoo T. Clinical Studies of tamoxifen in advanced breast cancer (Japan)—Multi-centre open trial and double blind trial. Rev Endocr Rel Cancer 1981; (suppl 9):293–300.

17. Mattson W. A phase III trial of treatment with tamoxifen versus treatment with high-dose medroxyprogesterone acetate in advanced premenopausal breast cancer. Prog Cancer Res Ther 1980; 15:65–71.

18. Morgan LR, Donley, PJ. Tamoxifen versus megestrol acetate in breast cancer. Rev Endocr Rel Cancer 1981; (suppl 9):301–310.

19. Ingle JN, Ahman DL, Green SJ, et al. Randomised clinical trial of megestrol acetate versus tamoxifen in paramenopausal or castrated women with advanced breast cancer. Am J Clin Oncol 1982; 5:155–160.

20. Pannuti F, Martoni A, Fruet F, et al. Oral high dose medroxyprogesterone acetate versus tamoxifen in postmenopausal patients with advanced breast cancer. In Iacobelli S, ed. The Role of Tamoxifen in Breast Cancer. New York: Raven Press, 1982:85–92.

21. Beretta G, Tabiadon D, Tedeschi L, Luporini G. Hormone therapy of advanced breast carcinoma: Comparative evaluation of tamoxifen citrate versus medroxyprogesterone acetate. In Iacobelli S, ed. The Role of Tamoxifen in Breast Cancer. New York: Raven Press, 1982:113–120.

22. Muss HB, Wells HB, Paschold EH, et al. Megestrol acetate versus tamoxifen in advanced breast cancer: 5-year analysis—A phase III trial of the Piedmont Oncology Association. J Clin Oncol 1988; 6:1098–1106.

23. Parazzini F, Colli E, Scatigna M. Tozzi L. Treatment with tamoxifen and progestins for metastatic breast cancer in postmenopausal women: A quantitative review of published randomised clinical trials. Oncology 1993; 50:483–489.

24. Gill PG, Gebski V, Snyder R, et al. Randomized comparison of the effects of tamoxifen, megestrol acetate, or tamoxifen plus megestrol acetate on treatment response and survival in patients with metastatic breast cancer. Ann Oncol 1993; 4:741–744.

25. Ingle JN, Krook JE, Green SJ, et al. Randomized trial of bilateral oophorectomy versus tamoxifen in premenopausal women with metastatic breast cancer. J Clin Oncol 1986; 4:178–185.

26. Buchanan RB, Blamey RW, Durrant KR, et al. A randomised comparison of tamoxifen with surgical oophorectomy in premenopausal patients with advanced breast cancer. J Clin Oncol 1986; 4:1326–1330.

27. Crump M, Pritchard KI, Sawka CA, et al. An individual patient-based meta-analysis of tamoxifen versus ovarian ablation as first line endocrine therapy for premenopausal women with metastatic breast cancer. Breast Cancer Res Treat 1997; 44:201–210.

28. Jonat W, Kaufman M, Blamey RW, et al. A randomised study to compare the effect of the luteinizing hormone releasing hormone (LHRH) analogue goserelin with or without tamoxifen in pre- and perimenopausal patients with advanced breast cancer. Eur J Cancer 1995; 31A:137–142.

29. Klijn JGM, Blamey RW, Boccardo F, et al. New standard treatment for advanced premenopausal breast cancer: A meta-analysis of the Combined Hormonal Agent Trialists Group (CHAT). Eur J Cancer 1998; 34(suppl 5):S90.

30. Klijn JGM, Beex LVAM, Mauriac L, et al. For the European Organisation for Research and Treatment of Cancer—Breast Cancer Cooperative Group. Combined treatment with buserelin and tamoxifen in premenopausal metastatic breast cancer: a randomised study. J Natl Cancer Inst 2000; 92:903–911.

31. Mouridsen HT, Elleman K, Mattson W, Palshof T. Therapeutic effect of tamoxifen versus tamoxifen combined with medroxyprogesterone acetate in advanced breast cancer in postmenopausal women. Cancer Treat Rep 1979; 63:171–175.

32. Ingle JN, Green SJ, Ahmann DL, et al. Progress report on two clinical trials in women with advanced breast cancer. Trial 1. Tamoxifen versus tamoxifen plus aminoglutethimide. Trial 2. Aminoglutethimide in patients with prior tamoxifen exposure. Cancer Res 1982; 42(suppl 8):3461S–3467S.

33. Ingle JN, Green SJ, Ahmann DL, et al. Randomised trial of tamoxifen alone or in combination with aminoglutethimide and hydrocortisone in women with metastatic breast cancer. J Clin Oncol 1986; 4:958–964.

34. Powles TJ, Ashley S, Ford HT, et al. Treatment of disseminated breast cancer with tamoxifen, aminoglutethimide, hydrocortisone and danazol, used in combination or sequentially. Lancet 1984; 1:1369–1373.

35. Bruno M, Roldan E, Diaz B. Sequential vs simultaneous administration of tamoxifen and medroxyprogesterone acetate in advanced breast cancer (abstr 26). J Steroid Biochem 1983; 19(suppl):87S.

36. Byrne MJ, Gebski V, Forbes JF, et al. Medroxyprogesterone acetate addition or substitution for tamoxifen in advanced tamoxifen-resistant breast cancer: a phase III randomised trial. J Clin Oncol 1997; 15:3141–3148.

37. Bezwoda WR, Derman D, de Moor NG. Treatment of metastatic breast cancer in estrogen receptor positive patients. A randomised trial comparing tamoxifen alone versus tamoxifen plus CMF. Cancer 1982; 50:2247–2250.

38. Mouridsen HT, Rose C, Englesman F. Combined cytotoxic and endocrine therapy in postmenopausal patients with advanced breast cancer. A randomised trial of CMF vs CMF plus tamoxifen. Eur J Cancer Clin Oncol 1985; 21:291–199.

39. Priestman TJ, Baum M, Jones V, Forbes JF. The role of cytotoxic therapy in advanced breast cancer, In: Wicks CJ, ed. The Vinca Alkaloids Centennial Year Symposium, 1978:95–102.

40. Miller WR. Aromatase inhibitors. Endocr Rel Cancer 1996; 3:65–79.

41. Smith IE, Harris AL, Morgan M, et al. Tamoxifen versus aminoglutethimide in metastatic breast cancer: A randomised cross-over trial. Br Med J 1981; 283:1432–1434.

42. Falkson CI, Falkson HC. A randomised study of CGS 16949A (fadrozole) versus tamoxifen in previously untreated postmenopausal patients with metastatic breast cancer. Ann Oncol 1996; 7:465–469.

43. Thurlimann B, Beretta K, Bacchi M, et al. First-line fadrozole HCl (CGS 16949A) versus tamoxifen in postmenopausal women with advanced breast cancer. Prospective randomised trial of the Swiss group for Clinical Research SAKK 20/88. Ann Oncol 1996; 7:471–479.

44. Perez Carrion R, Alberola CV, et al. Comparison of the selective aromatase inhibitor formestane with tamoxifen as first-line hormonal therapy in postmenopausal women with advanced breast cancer. Ann Oncol 1994; 5(suppl 7):S19-S24.

45. Messori A, Cattel F, Trippoli S, Vaiani M. Survival in patients with metastatic breast cancer: Analysis of randomised studies comparing oral aromatase inhibitors versus megestrol. Anticancer Drugs 2000; 11:701–706.

46. Mouridsen H, Gershanovich M, Sun Y, Perez-Carrion R, Superior efficacy of letrozole versus tamoxifen as first-line therapy for postmenopausal women with advanced breast cancer: Results of a phase III study of the International Letrozole Breast Cancer Group. J Clin Oncol 2001; 19: 2596–2606.

47. Bonneterre J, Thurlimann B, Robertson JF, et al. Anastrazole versus tamoxifen as first-line therapy for advanced breast cancer in 688 postmenopausal women: Results of the Tamoxifen or Arimidex Randomised Group Efficacy and Tolerability study. J Clin Oncol 2000; 18:3748–3757.

48. Nabholtz JM, Buzdar A, Pollak M, et al. Anastrazole is superior to tamoxifen as first-line therapy for advanced breast cancer in postmenopausal women: Results of a North Amnerican multicenter randomised trial. Arimidex Study Group. J Clin Oncol 2000; 18;3758–3767.

3

Overview of Aromatase Inhibitors and Inactivators in the Treatment of Advanced Breast Cancer

Per Eystein Lønning
Haukeland Hospital
University of Bergen
Bergen, Norway

I. ABSTRACT

Since the introduction of aminoglutethimide, the first aromatase inhibitor, for breast cancer treatment 30 years ago, these drugs have achieved increasing importance in the therapy of advanced breast cancer and are currently being evaluated in the adjuvant setting. The third-generation aromatase inhibitors and inactivators—principally anastrozole, letrozole, and exemestane—all exhibit potent biochemical efficacy, with 97–99% aromatase inhibition. In addition, these drugs are well tolerated, and clinical studies have revealed their superiority over conventional drugs (aminoglutethimide and megestrol acetate) in second-line therapy.

The results for these agents as a first-line treatment are more varied. Letrozole has been found to be superior to tamoxifen with respect to overall response rate as well as time to progression (TTP). This aromatase inhibitor has, furthermore, been shown to be superior to tamoxifen for particular subgroups, such as for estrogen (ER)/progesterone receptor (PgR)–positive tumors and in patients not exposed to adjuvant endocrine therapy. Anastrozole, on the other hand, has been found to be of equivalent efficacy to tamoxifen in clinical trials, but it is not clear whether it provides superiority. Preliminary results from an ongoing study evaluating exemestane are encouraging, but so far the number of patients is too small to draw any conclusion. The early results with these novel compounds support the hypothesis that their clinical efficacy is related to the degree of estrogen suppression they produce. The observation from in vitro studies that tumor cells may adapt to low estrogen concentrations indicates that therapeutic advantage may be found in using more potent estrogen-suppressing drugs. The observed lack of cross-resistance between aromatase inhibitors and inactivators (formerly called steroidal aromatase inhibitors) represents a key subject for further investigation.

II. INTRODUCTION

Aromatase inhibitors suppress estrogen synthesis by blocking the final step in the synthetic pathway aromatization of an androgen to an estrogen. Although the aromatase enzyme found in the ovaries and peripheral tissue (the site of E_1 synthesis in postmenopausal women) is the same, the early results using aminoglutethimide found that ovarian estrogen blockade was overruled by gonadotrophin secretion [1]. This was also found for the second-generation aromatase inactivator formestane [2]; therefore, it has become accepted that these drugs are unsuitable for treatment of premenopausal women. This still remains to be proven for the third-generation inhibitors/inactivators; considering their much greater potency, the possibility exists they will also block the ovarian aromatase activity.

The pathways of estrogen synthesis in postmenopausal women have been described [3] and are not given in detail here. Briefly, it should be recalled that circulating androgens (mainly androstenedione), synthesized in the adrenal glands and (to a lesser extent) in the ovaries, are converted into estrogens in different peripheral tissues like muscle, connective tissue, skin, and liver [3,4]. Estrogen synthesis also occurs in normal breast tissue as well as in breast tumors [5]. It is interesting that in contrast to what is seen in premenopausal individuals, tissue estradiol concentrations are much higher than plasma levels in postmenopausal women [6]. Whether this is related to local synthesis, active uptake mechanisms, or both is currently unknown [7–9].

III. DEVELOPMENT OF AROMATASE INHIBITORS AND INACTIVATORS FOR CLINICAL THERAPY

The development of aromatase inhibition as a therapeutic strategy in breast cancer is interesting from a historical perspective. Aminoglutethimide was developed as an antiepileptic compound, but because of its toxic effects, in particular on the adrenal gland [10], the drug was subsequently withdrawn. Since it was known for a long time that surgical adrenalectomy could cause dramatic remissions in postmenopausal breast cancer patients, aminoglutethimide was subsequently reintroduced in an attempt to achieve "a medical adrenalectomy" in patients with advanced breast cancer [11–13]. It took a further 10 years or so before its mechanism of action was fully elucidated, revealing it to be a potent aromatase inhibitor in vivo yet allowing sustained androgen secretion [14,15]. Similarly testololactone, the first-generation aromatase inactivator, was evaluated in breast cancer therapy before it was subsequently shown to be an aromatase inhibitor [16,17].

Both of these drugs have now been withdrawn from clinical treatment, for although aminoglutethimide was in use for more than 20 years and was effective, it was highly toxic, causing neurological side effects and skin rash [18]. Testololactone had a rather low efficacy [16] in addition to its poor toxicity profile and was consequently also withdrawn.

IV. SECOND-GENERATION AROMATASE INHIBITORS AND INACTIVATORS

Based on the encouraging antitumor effect but high toxicity profile of aminoglutethimide, a lot of effort has been spent on developing novel less toxic compounds. These various aromatase inhibitors are now often referred to by their "generation" (Table 1). The second-generation aromatase inhibitors and inactivators, like fadrozole and formestane, were found to be less toxic than aminoglutethimide, but they did not exhibit improved efficacy as compared with conventional drugs as second-line [19,20] or first-line [21,22] therapy.

Table 1   The Development, Generation, and Family Characteristics of the Antiaromatase Agents

	Nonsteroidal inhibitors	Steroidal inhibitors
Characteristics	"AG" or triazole class	Androgen derivatives
	Bind to heme part of enzyme	Bind to substrate-binding site
	Reversible	Irreversible
First generation	Aminoglutethimide	Testololactone
Second generation	Fadrozole	Formestane
Third generation	Anastrozole	Exemestane
	Letrozole	

V. THIRD-GENERATION AROMATASE INHIBITORS AND INACTIVATORS—SECOND-LINE THERAPY

Currently three third-generation compounds are available, all with acceptable toxicity profiles. Anastrozole and letrozole both belong to the triazole class of drugs (Fig. 1) and are so-called type 2 inhibitors causing reversible inhibition of the aromatase enzyme. In contrast, the aromatase inactivator exemestane binds irreversibly to the substrate-binding site of the enzyme (type 1 inhibitor) (Table 1). These compounds have all shown some kind of clinical superiority compared with conventional therapy [23–26]. Each of them has been compared with megestrol acetate, while one study compared letrozole to aminoglutethimide (Table 2). In all cases the new compounds were superior or at least equal to the comparator in terms of overall survival and time to failure.

However, as no head-to-head comparisons of these compounds have been conducted, it is not clear whether any one of these third-generation aromatase inhibitors/inactivators exhibits superiority over the others [27].

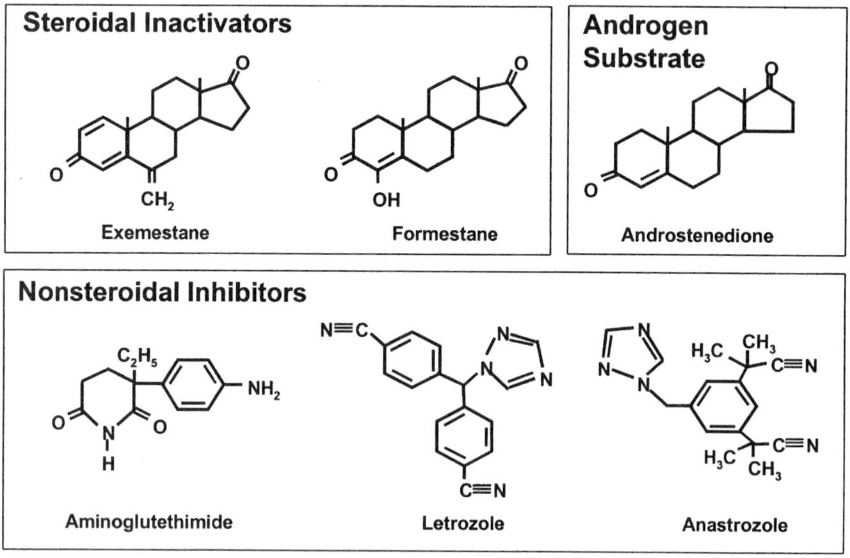

Figure 1 Chemical structures of nonsteroidal aromatase inhibitors and aromatase inactivators together with the key substrate for the aromatase enzyme androstenedione.

Table 2 Results of Phase III Studies Comparing Letrozole (Let), Anastrozole (Ana), and Exemestane (Ex) to Conventional Therapy of Megestrol Acetate (MA) or Aminoglutethimide (AG)[a]

	Let–MA [24]	Let–AG [25]	Ana–MA [23]	Ex–MA [26]
RR	Yes*	No	No	No
Benefit	No	No	No	No
TTP	No	Yes*	No	Yes*
TTF	Yes*	Yes***	No	Yes*
Survival	No	Yes***	Yes**	Yes*

[a]The figures in brackets are the publication references and the superiority of the aromatase inhibitor to control is indicated with p values (*$p<0.05$, **$p<0.025$, ***$p<0.01$). RR, response rate; TTP, time to progression; TTF, time to drug failure.

VI. THIRD-GENERATION COMPOUND—FIRST-LINE RESULTS COMPARED WITH TAMOXIFEN

In first-line therapy for advanced breast cancer, we have the results of three phase III studies. Two studies enrolling a total of 1021 patients compared anastrozole with tamoxifen and one compared letrozole with tamoxifen in 907 patients [28–30]. Although the letrozole trial revealed superiority of the aromatase inhibitor over tamoxifen, with respect to the different parameters, the two anastrozole trials reached conflicting conclusions. The detailed results of these trials are summarized in Table 3.

Among the problems encountered in comparing these trials were the differences in the requirements for patient enrollment. In particular, the proportion of patients who had received endocrine therapy in the adjuvant setting was about 10% for the European anastrozole study [28] and about 20% for the other two. In addition, the percentage of patients with receptor-unknown tumors (ER as well as PgR unknown) varied substantially between 11 and 55%. These differences tend to make comparisons between the trials more difficult.

In terms of the major endpoint, time to progression (TTP), the trial evaluating letrozole and the American (but not the European) trial evaluating anastrozole revealed superiority compared with tamoxifen. For the secondary endpoint, response rate, the letrozole study was the only study to show any significant difference. If one looks at just the ER+ subgroup in the European trial, there was a small nonsignificant improvement in median TTP for anastrozole. This modest change when compared with what was seen for the total population suggests the bulk of ER/PgR-unknown tumors were actually receptor-positive. Thus the lower proportion of receptor-known tumors in the European study is not likely to

Table 3 Results from the Phase III First-Line Therapy Trials of Anastrozole (Ana) Versus Tamoxifen (Tam) and Letrozole (Let) Versus Tam[a]

	Anastrozole Europe [28]		Anastrozole USA [29]		Letrozole [30]	
Number of patients	668		353		907	
Treatment	Ana	Tam	Ana	Tam	Let	Tam
Adj Endo (%)	12.0	1.7	21.1	18.1	19.0	18
ER/PgR?	54.4	55.8	11.1	11.0	34.0	33
RR %	32.9	32.6	21.1	17.0	30.0	20.0****
RR ER+	?	?	?	?	31.0	21.0***
RR no adj tam			?	?	31.0	23.0*
Benefit	56.2	55.5	69.1	45.6**	49.0	38.0****
TTP (months)	8.2	8.3	11.1	5.6***	9.4	6.0#
TTP ER+	8.9	7.8	?	?	9.6	6.0****
TTP no adj tam			?	?	9.6	6.0#

[a]Adj Endo (%), percent of population who received adjuvant Tam; ER/PgR?, percent of population with unknown hormone receptor status; RR%, response rate; RR ER+, response rate in ER-positive group; TTP, time to progression. Significant differences from Tam treated (*$p<0.05$, **$p<0.01$, ***$p<0.005$, ****$p<0.001$, #$p<0.0001$).

explain the difference between this and the American trial. Other factors may also contribute. Potentially, the higher frequency of patients exposed to adjuvant tamoxifen in the American trial may have reduced the response to tamoxifen in the metastatic disease setting, whereas the response to anastrozole would be unaffected by this.

The conclusion at this stage is that letrozole appears superior to tamoxifen as first-line therapy, but the result for anastrozole is equivocal. While it is obvious anastrozole is not inferior to tamoxifen, it is not possible to conclude that it is superior, nor can we say for certain whether there is any real difference between anastrozole and letrozole. The high number of ER/PgR-unknown tumors in the largest anastrozole study is a confounding factor. Yet it should be remembered that in the letrozole study, one-third of the patients enrolled belonged to the same category. A key difference with the letrozole study, however, is the very careful way in which it has been analyzed with respect to subgroups, separating out not only the effect on ER/PgR-positive tumors but also the potential impact of adjuvant endocrine therapy. A full review with respect to all these parameters for the combined anastrozole studies would be highly welcome.

VII. THE IMPORTANCE OF BIOCHEMICAL EFFICACY OF AROMATASE INHIBITORS/INACTIVATORS TO THE CLINICAL OUTCOME

An interesting observation with regard to estrogen-suppression therapy of advanced breast cancer is that response seems independent of pretreatment serum hormone levels. Thus, while ovarian ablation works in premenopausal women, aromatase inhibitors/inactivators are effective in postmenopausal women and may even work in patients who have undergone adrenalectomy or hypophysectomy who have very low pretreatment estrogen levels [31].

Although the mechanism of action of progestins is not fully understood [32], megestrol acetate administered at its therapeutic dose of 160 mg daily suppresses adrenal as well as ovarian androgen production, causing about 80% suppression of plasma estrogen levels in postmenopausal breast cancer patients [33]. It is essential to assess the biochemical efficacy of different aromatase inhibitors and aromatase inactivators in vivo. Although efficacy may be assessed by in vitro assays, the efficacy in vivo clearly depends on other parameters, such as drug disposition [34]. Methodological difficulties in measuring estrogen levels in the plasma and tissue of postmenopausal women are known and have been discussed elsewhere [35]. Due to its high concentration, suppression of plasma estrone sulfate may be detected with a median of 99% [36]. In general, however, plasma estrone and estradiol will reach the detection limit of the assay when suppressed by 85–90%. On the other hand, direct assessment of in vivo aromatization following injections of 3H-labeled androstenedione and 14C-labeled estrone allows detection of ≥99.1% inhibition in most patients [37].

The inhibition of aromatase in vivo using some of the various inhibitors and inactivators was assessed in a joint program (Table 4) [38–46]. It is notable that the three third-generation compounds—anastrozole, letrozole, and exemestane—are in a class of their own, causing >97% aromatase inhibition. On the other hand, a substantial interindividual variation excludes direct comparisons between different studies. In one study, however, a crossover design was used to compare the biochemical efficacy of anastrozole and letrozole head to head [46]. This revealed that letrozole produces a significantly better aromatase inhibition and also better suppression of plasma estrone sulfate than anastrozole.

However, the problems associated with assay sensitivity may restrict our assessment of aromatase inhibitor/inactivator efficacy in target tissues of patients undergoing endocrine therapy [36,47,48].

Table 4 The Efficacy of Aromatase Inhibitors and
Inactivators in Suppressing In Vivo Enzymatic Activity[a]

Drug	Percentage Aromatase Inhibition
Rogletimide	51% / 64% / 74%
Formestane oral	62% / 70% / 57%
Fadrozole	82% / 93%
Formestane i.m.	85% / 92%
Aminoglutethimide	91.0%
Formestane + AG	94.0%
Letrozole	98.4% / 98.9% / **99.1%**
Anastrozole	96.7% / 98.1% / **97.9%**
Exemestane	97.9%

[a]The sensitivity limit is theoretically 99.1% [37]. The only direct comparison was between letrozole and anastrozole [46] (figs. in bold).
Sources: Refs. 37–46.

VIII. LACK OF CROSS-RESISTANCE TO DIFFERENT AROMATASE INHIBITORS/INACTIVATORS IN SECOND- AND THIRD-LINE THERAPY

The apparent lack of complete cross-resistance between aromatase inhibitors (which are nonsteroidal) and the inactivators (which are steroidal) is an interesting phenomenon, which for the moment remains unexplained [49–52]. Three trials (Fig. 2) revealed a response to a steroidal compound after a nonsteroidal one [49,51,52], while in another small retrospective study anastrozole was found to stabilize disease in patients failing on formestane [50]. Although one can hypothesize that patients may respond to exemestane after treatment with aminoglutethimide, owing to a better estrogen deprivation afforded by the third-generation drug [51,52], the positive response to formestane in aminoglutethimide failures [49] or to exemestane in patients failing a third-generation nonsteroidal compound [52] may not be explained in this way. Only a limited number of studies have attempted to address the intratumoral effects of aromatase inhibitors/inactivators on estrogen synthesis [47, 53–55]. Although they have found suppression of tissue estrogens, none has compared the effects of different compounds in a head-to-head or crossover design. The problem of measuring low levels of estrogens in tissue even with the use of sensitive assays [48] places a severe limitation on our research [55].

One should also consider possibilities other than a difference in plasma estrogen concentration to explain the lack of cross-resistance found for some of these compounds. Neither the lack of complete cross-resistance between aminoglutethimide and megestrol acetate given in either order [56] nor the re-

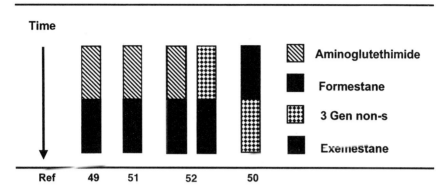

Figure 2 Lack of cross-resistance between steroidal aromatase inactivators and nonsteroidal aromatase inhibitors. In the four trial designs shown schematically, four of the treatment arms (trials 49, 51, and 52) used a switch from a nonsteroidal inhibitor [either aminoglutethimide or a third-generation inhibitor (3 Gen non-s)] to a steroidal compound (either formestane or exemestane) and found clinical effects. The fifth treatment arm used a switch from a steroidal compound (formestane) to a nonsteroidal compound (3 Gen non-s) and also found stable disease.

sponse to hypophysectomy in patients failing aminoglutethimide [57] is likely to be due to this. The fact that steroidal aromatase inactivators express modest androgenic effects on the liver, especially when administered by the oral route, may well be significant. This has been found for formestane [58] as well as for exemestane (its 17 hydro-metabolite) [59] by observation of a slight drop in plasma levels of sex-hormone binding globulin. Further investigations in vitro have revealed a complex cross talk between the estrogenic and androgenic pathways (see references and discussion in Ref. 60). Finally, it has been shown that MCF-7 cells adapt to estrogen withdrawal by developing hypersensitivity [61]. Thus it is possible that estrogen-deprived cells could also be sensitized to androgen stimulation, and it is anticipated that further investigation, using different aromatase inhibitors/inactivators in sequence along with core biopsies and gene expression analysis, will provide a way forward in resolving this issue.

IX. CONCLUSIONS AND FUTURE DIRECTIONS

Third-generation aromatase inhibitors/inactivators have earned their place in first- as well as second-line therapy for advanced breast cancer. Ongoing trials assessing their role in adjuvant therapy and their potential for breast cancer prevention are discussed in other chapters herein. Key targets for future development in advanced disease may include strategies to enhance the degree of hormone suppression, assessment of the potential role of aromatase inhibition in premenopausal breast cancer, and investigation of the optimal sequential use of the different compounds. A greater understanding of mechanisms and consequences of hormone suppression in normal breast tissue and tumor cells will help us achieve these goals.

NOTE ADDED IN PROOF

During the preparation of this chapter, two important articles appeared in the literature. Thus the article by Buzdar et al. [62] found no superiority for letrozole compared to megestrol with respect to either response rates or TTP or survival in a phase III study enrolling 602 patients (see Table 2). Bonneterre et al. [63] have analyzed the combined data from the two studies comparing anastrozole to tamoxifen [28,29]. Although there was a trend for superiority for anastrozole compared to tamoxifen in most subgroups, only in the subgroup of ER-positive tumors did the difference reach a level of statistical significance.

REFERENCES

1. Santen RJ, Samojlik E, Wells SA. Resistance of the ovary to blockade of aromatisation with aminoglutethimide. J Clin Endocrinol Metab 1980; 51:473–477.
2. Dowsett M, Stein RC, Coombes RC, Aromatization inhibition alone or in combination with GmRH agonists for the treatment of premenopausal breast cancer patients. J Steroid Biochem Mol Biol 1992; 43:155–159.
3. Lønning PE, Dowsett M, Powles TJ. Postmenopausal estrogen synthesis and metabolism: Alterations caused by aromatase inhibitors used for the treatment of breast cancer. J Steroid Biochem 1990; 35:355–366.
4. Sluijmer AV, Heineman MJ, De Jong FH, Evers JL. Endocrine activity of the postmenopausal ovary: The effects of pituitary down-regulation and oophorectomy. J Clin Endocrinol Metab 1995; 80:2163–2167.
5. Lønning PE, Lien E. Mechanisms of action of endocrine treatment in breast cancer. Crit Rev Oncol/Haematol 1995; 21:158–193.
6. Van Landeghem AAJ, Poortman J, Nabuurs M, Thijssen JHH. Endogenous concentration and subcellular distribution of estrogens in normal and malignant breast tissue. Cancer Res 1985; 45:2900–2904.
7. Masamura S, Santner SJ, Gimotty P, et al. Mechanism for maintenance of high breast tumor estradiol concentrations in the absence of ovarian function: Role of very high affinity tissue uptake. Breast Cancer Res Treat 1997; 42:215–226.
8. James VHT, Reed MJ, Adams EF, et al. Oestrogen uptake and metabolism in vivo. In: Beck JS, ed. Oestrogens and the Human Breast. Proc R Soc Edinburgh 1989:95B, 185–193.
9. Miller WR. Importance of intratumour aromatase, and its susceptibility to in-

hibitors. In: Dowsett M, ed. Aromatase inhibition—Then, Now and Tomorrow. London: Parthenon Publishing Group, 1994:43–53.

10. Hughes SWM, Burley DM. Aminoglutethimide: A "side-effect" turned to therapeutic advantage. Postgrad Med J 1970; 46:409–416.

11. Dao TL, Huggins C. Bilateral adrenalectomy in the treatment of cancer of the breast. Arch Surg 1955; 71:645–657.

12. Cash R, Brough AJ, Cohen MNP, Satoh PS. Aminoglutethimide (Elipten-Ciba) is an inhibitor of adrenal steroidogenesis: Mechanism of action and therapeutic trial. J Clin Endocrinol Metab 1967; 27:1239–1248.

13. Santen RJ, Lipton A, Kendall J. Successful medical adrenalectomy with aminoglutethimide. JAMA 1974; 230:1661 1665.

14. Samojlik E, Veldhuis JD, Wells SA, Santen RJ. Preservation of androgen secretion during estrogen suppression with aminoglutethimide in the treatment of metastatic breast carcinoma. J Clin Invest 1980; 65:602–612.

15. Santen RJ, Santner S, Davis B, et al. Aminoglutethimide inhibits extraglandular estrogen production in postmenopausal women with breast carcinoma. J Clin Endocrinol Metab 1978; 47:1257–1265.

16. Volk H, Deupree RH, Goldenberg IS, et al. A dose response evaluation of delta-1-testololactone in advanced breast cancer. Cancer 1974; 33:9–13.

17. Barone RM, Shamonki IM, Siiteri PK, Judd HL. Inhibition of peripheral aromatization of androstenedione to estrone in postmenopausal women with breast cancer using 1-testoloclactone. J Clin Endocrinol Metab 1979; 49:672–676.

18. Lønning PE, Kvinnsland S. Mechanisms of action of aminoglutethimide as endocrine therapy of breast cancer. Drugs 1988; 35:685–710.

19. Buzdar AU, Smith R, Vogel C, et al. Fadrozole HCL (CGS-16949A) versus megestrol acetate treatment of postmenopausal patients with metastatic breast carcinoma. Results of two randomized double blind controlled multiinstitutional trials. Cancer 1996; 77:2503–2513.

20. Thürlimann B, Castiglione M, HsuSchmitz SF, et al. Formestane versus megestrol acetate in postmenopausal breast cancer patients after failure of tamoxifen: A phase III prospective randomised cross over trial of second-line hormonal treatment (SAKK 20/90). Eur J Cancer 1997; 33:1017–1024.

21. Perèz-Carrión R, Candel VA, Calabresi F, et al. Comparison of the selective aromatase inhibitor formestane with tamoxifen as first-line hormonal therapy in postmenopausal women with advanced breast cancer. Ann Oncol 1994; 5:S19–S24.

22. Thürlimann B, Beretta K, Bacchi M, et al. First-line fadrozole HCl (CGS 16949A) versus tamoxifen in postmenopausal women with advanced breast cancer—Prospective randomised trial of the Swiss Group for Clinical Cancer Research SAKK 20/88. Ann Oncol 1996; 7:471–479.

23. Buzdar AU, Jonat W, Howell A, et al. Anastrozole versus megestrol acetate in the treatment of postmenopausal women with advanced breast carcinoma: Results of a survival update based on a combined analysis of data from two mature phase III trials. Cancer 1998; 83:1142–1152.

24. Dombernowsky P, Smith I, Falkson G, et al. Letrozole, a new oral aromatase inhibitor for advanced breast cancer: Double-blind randomized trial showing a dose

effect and improved efficacy and tolerability compared with megestrol acetate. J Clin Oncol 1998; 16:453–461.

25. Gershanovich M, Chaudri HA, Campos D, et al. Letrozole, a new oral aromatase inhibitor: Randomised trial comparing 2.5 mg daily, 0.5 mg daily and aminoglutethimide in postmenopausal women with advanced breast cancer. Ann Oncol 1998; 9:639–645.

26. Kaufmann M, Bajetta E, Dirix LY, et al. Exemestane is superior to megestrol acetate after tamoxifen failure in postmenopausal women with advanced breast cancer: results of a phase III randomized double-blind trial. J Clin Oncol 2000; 18:1399–1411.

27. Hamilton A, Piccart M. The third-generation non-steroidal aromatase inhibitors: A review of their clinical benefits in the second-line hormonal treatment of advanced breast cancer. Ann Oncol 1999; 10:377–384.

28. Bonneterre J, Thurlimann B, Robertson JFR, et al. Anastrozole versus tamoxifen as first-line therapy for advanced breast cancer in 668 postmenopausal women: Results of the tamoxifen or arimidex randomized group efficacy and tolerability study. J Clin Oncol 2000; 18:3748–3757.

29. Nabholtz JM, Buzdar A, Pollak M, et al. Anastrozole is superior to tamoxifen as first-line therapy for advanced breast cancer in postmenopausal women: Results of a North American multicenter randomized trial. J Clin Oncol 2000; 18:3758–3767.

30. Mouridsen H, Gershanovich M, Sun Y, et al. Superior efficacy of letrozole versus tamoxifen as first-line therapy for postmenopausal women with advanced breast cancer: Results of a phase III study of the International Letrozole Breast Cancer Group. J Clin Oncol 2001; 19:2596–2606.

31. Samojlik E, Santen RJ, Worgul TJ. Suppression of residual oestrogen production with aminoglutethimide in women following surgical hypophysectomy or adrenalectomy. Clin Endocrinol 1984; 20:43–51.

32. Lundgren S. Progestins in breast cancer treatment. Acta Oncol 1992; 31:709–722.

33. Lundgren S, Helle SI, Lønning PE. Profound suppression of plasma estrogens by megestrol acetate in postmenopausal breast cancer patients. Clin Cancer Res 1996; 2:1515–1521.33.

34. Bhatnagar AS, Hausler A, Schieweck K. Inhibition of aromatase in vitro and in vivo by aromatase inhibitors. J Enzyme Inhib 1990; 4:179–186.

35. Lønning PE. Stepwise estrogen suppression manipulating the estrostat. J Steroid Biochem Mol Biol 2001. In press.

36. Lønning PE, Ekse D. A sensitive assay for measurement of plasma estrone sulphate in patients on treatment with aromatase inhibitors. J Steroid Biochem Mol Biol 1995; 55:409–412.

37. Jacobs S, Lønning PE, Haynes B, et al. Measurement of aromatisation by a urine technique suitable for the evaluation of aromatase inhibitors in vivo. J Enzyme Inhib 1991; 4:315–325.

38. Dowsett M, Jones A, Johnston SRD, et al. In vivo measurement of aromatase inhibition by letrozole (CGS 20267) in post menopausal patients with breast cancer. Clin Cancer Res 1995; 1:1511–1515.

39. Lønning PE, Jacobs S, Jones A, et al. The influence of CGS 16949A on peripheral aromatisation in breast cancer patients. Br J Cancer 1991; 63:789–793.

40. Jones AL, MacNeill F, Jacobs S, et al. The influence of intramuscular 4-hydroxyan-

drostenedione on peripheral aromatisation in breast cancer patients. Eur J Cancer 1992; 28A:1712–1716.

41. MacNeill FA, Jones AL, Jacobs S, et al. The influence of aminoglutethimide and its analogue rogletimide on peripheral aromatisation in breast cancer. Br J Cancer 1992; 66:692–697.

42. MacNeill FA, Jacobs S, Lønning PE, et al. Combined treatment with 4-hydroxyandrostenedione and aminoglutethimide: Effects on aromatase inhibition and oestrogen suppression. Br J Cancer 1994; 69:1171—1175.

43. MacNeill FA, Jacobs S, Dowsett M, et al. The effects of oral 4-hydroxyandrostenedione on peripheral aromatisation in post-menopausal breast cancer patients. Cancer Chemother Pharmacol 1995; 36:249–254.

44. Geisler J, King N, Dowsett M, et al. Influence of anastrozole (Arimidex), a selective, non-steroidal aromatase inhibitor, on in vivo aromatisation and plasma oestrogen levels in postmenopausal women with breast cancer. Br J Cancer 1996; 74:1286–1291.

45. Geisler J, King N, Anker G, et al. In vivo inhibition of aromatization by exemestane, a novel irreversible aromatase inhibitor, in postmenopausal breast cancer patients. Clin Cancer Res 1998; 4:2089–2093.

46. Geisler J, Haynes B, Anker G, et al. Influence of letrozole and anastrozole on total body aromatization and plasma estrogen levels in postmenopausal breast cancer patients evaluated in a randomized cross-over–designed study. J Clin Oncol 2001. In press.

47. Miller WR, Telford J, Love C, et al. Effects of letrozole as primary medical therapy on in situ oestrogen synthesis and endogenous oestrogen levels within the breast. Breast 1998; 7:273–276.

48. Geisler J, Berntsen H, Lonning PE. A novel HPLC-RIA method for the simultaneous detection of estrone, estradiol and estrone sulphate levels in breast cancer tissue. J Steroid Biochem Mol Biol 2000; 72:259–264.

49. Murray R, Pitt P. Aromatase inhibition with 4-OH androstenedione after prior aromatase inhibition with aminoglutethimide in women with advanced breast cancer. Breast Cancer Res Treat 1995; 35:249–253.

50. HarperWynne C, Coombes RC. Anastrozole shows evidence of activity in postmenopausal patients who have responded or stabilised on formestane therapy. Eur J Cancer 1999; 35:744–746.

51. Thürlimann B, Paridaens R, Serin D, et al. Third-line hormonal treatment with exemestane in postmenopausal patients with advanced breast cancer progressing on aminoglutethimide: A phase II multicentre multinational study. Eur J Cancer 1997; 33:1767–1773.

52. Lønning PE, Bajetta E, Murray R, et al. Activity of exemestane (Aromasin) in metastatic breast cancer after failure of nonsteroidal aromatase inhibitors: A phase II trial. J Clin Oncol 2000; 18:2234–2244.

53. Reed MJ, Aherne GW, Ghilchik MW, et al. Concentrations of oestrone and 4-hydroxyandrostenedione in malignant and normal breast tissue. Int J Cancer 1991; 49:562–565.

54. de Jong PC, van de Ven J, Nortier HWR, Thijssen JHH, et al. Inhibition of breast cancer tissue aromatase activity and estrogen concentrations by the third-generation aromatase inhibitor vorozole. Cancer Res 1997; 57:2109–2111.

55. Geisler J, Berntsen H, Ottestad L, et al. Neoadjuvant treatment with anastrozole (Arimidex) causes profound suppression of intra-estrogen levels. Clin Cancer Res 2001; 7:1230–1236.

56. Garcia-Giralt E, Ayme Y, Carton M, et al. Second and third line hormone therapy in advanced post-menopausal breast cancer: A multicenter randomized trial comparing medroxyprogesterone acetate with aminoglutethimide in patients who have become resistant to tamoxifen. Breast Cancer Res Treat 1992; 24:139–145.

57. Bundred NJ, Eremin O, Stewart HJ, et al. Beneficial response to pituitary ablation following aminoglutethimide. Br J Surg 1986; 73:388–389.

58. Dowsett M, Mehta A, King N, et al. An endocrine and pharmacokinetic study of four oral doses of formestane in postmenopausal breast cancer patients. Eur J Cancer 1992; 28:415–420.

59. Johannessen DC, Engan T, Salle ED. et al. Endocrine and clinical effects of exemestane (PNU 155971), a novel steroidal aromatase inhibitor, in postmenopausal breast cancer patients: A phase I study. Clin Cancer Res 1997; 3:1101–1108.

60. Geisler J, Lønning P. Resistance to endocrine therapy of breast cancer: Recent advances and tomorrows challenges. Clin Breast Cancer 2001; 1:297–308.

61. Masamura S, Santner SJ, Heitjan DF, Santen RJ. Estrogen deprivation causes estradiol hypersensitivity in human breast cancer cells. J Clin Endocrinol Metab 1995; 80:2918–2925.

62. Buzdar A, Douma J, Davidson N, Elledge R, Morgan M, Smith R, et al. Phase III, multicenter, double-blind, randomized study of letrozole, an aromatase inhibitor, for advanced breast cancer versus megestrol acetate. J Clin Oncol 2001;19:3357–3366.

63. Bonneterre J, Buzdar A, Nabholtz J-M, Robertson J, Thürlimann B, von Euler M, et al. Anastrozole is superior to Tamoxifen as first-line therapy in hormone receptor positive advanced breast carcinoma. Cancer 2001;2247–2258.

4

Endocrine Treatment of Advanced Breast Cancer: Selective Estrogen-Receptor Modulators (SERMs)

Stephen R. D. Johnston
Royal Marsden Hospital NHS Trust
London, England

Anthony Howell
Christie Hospital NHS Trust
Manchester, England

I. ABSTRACT

The ability of tamoxifen to antagonize estrogen-dependent growth factor by binding estrogen receptors (ERs) and inhibiting breast epithelial cell proliferation make it one of the most effective treatments for breast cancer. However, tamoxifen has estrogenic agonist effects in other tissues, such as bone and endometrium, where liganded ERs can activate target genes. Several novel antiestrogen compounds and older high-dose estrogens have been developed that are also selective ER modulators (SERMs). These SERMs have altered agonist profiles on breast and gynecological tissues and offer the potential for enhanced efficacy and reduced toxicity compared with tamoxifen. In advanced breast cancer, clinical data exist for four groups of SERMs. These are high-dose estrogens [e.g., diethylstilbestrol (DES), ethinylestradiol], the triphenylethylene estrogen analogues in addition to tamoxifen (e.g., toremifene, droloxifene, idoxifene, GW5638), the "fixed ring" compounds (e.g., raloxifene, arzoxifene, EM-800, and ERA-923), and the "pure antiestrogen" [e.g., fulvestrant (ICI 182780), SR 16234, ZK 191703]. High-dose estrogens show similar response rates to tamoxifen and are active after tamoxifen failure. In phase II trials of the other triphenylethylene SERMs, 263 patients resistant to tamoxifen have been treated. The median objective response rate to these SERMs was 5% (range 0 to 15%), with stable disease for $\geq$ 6 months in an additional 18% (range 9 to 23%). As first-line therapy for advanced breast cancer, the median response rate was 31% (range 20 to 51%), with a median time to progression of 7 months. Randomized phase III trials in over 1500 patients for toremifene and idoxifene showed no significant difference compared with tamoxifen. Fewer clinical data exist for the fixed-ring SERMs (raloxifene, arzoxifene, EM-800, and ERA-923), although a similarly low median response rate of 6% (range 0 to 14%) was seen in phase II trials in tamoxifen-resistant patients. It remains unclear whether any clinical advantage exists for the fixed-ring SERMs over tamoxifen as first-line therapy.

At present, data are available only for fulvestrant, a member of the pure antiestrogen class of SERMs. Fulvestrant is active in tamoxifen failure and in phase III trials has been shown to be at least equivalent to anastrozole as second-line treatment for advanced disease after failure with tamoxifen. With the emergence of potent aromatase inhibitors (AIs), which are superior to tamoxifen, the clinical questions in advanced disease have shifted to which antiestrogens may be effective following failure of AIs, and whether any merit exists for combined AI/SERM therapy. The main advantage for SERMs such as tamoxifen and raloxifene probably remains in early-stage disease (adjuvant therapy or prevention), whereas more clinical trial data are required to determine the place of pure antiestrogens and high-dose estrogens.

II. INTRODUCTION

Ever since evidence emerged that human breast carcinomas may be associated with estrogen, attempts have been made to block or inhibit estrogen's biological effects as a therapeutic strategy for women with breast cancer. Estrogen has important physiological effects on the growth and function of hormone-dependent reproductive tissues, including normal breast epithelium, uterus, vagina, and ovaries, as well as preserving bone mineral density and reducing the risk of osteoporosis, protecting the cardiovascular system by reducing cholesterol levels, and modulating cognitive function and behavior. Thus, a strategy to block or reduce estrogen function in an attempt to treat/prevent breast cancer could have a severe impact on a woman's health by interfering with normal estrogen-regulated tissues.

For over 50 years, synthetic estrogens and antiestrogens have been developed as treatment for estrogen receptor (ER) positive breast cancer. The synthetic estrogen diethylstilbestrol and the triphenylethylene trichlorophenylethylene were the first hormonal compounds to be used in the clinic [1–3]. These compounds interacted with the ER and had efficacy in advanced breast cancer. Now, tamoxifen is the most widely used and tested drug in breast cancer [4]. It is recognized to significantly improve survival as adjuvant therapy in early breast cancer [5] as well as to reduce the incidence of breast cancer in healthy women at risk for the disease [6]. Despite concerns about unfavorable antiestrogenic effects on healthy tissues, it was paradoxically discovered that tamoxifen acted as an estrogen on bone, blood lipid, and the endometrium [7]. More recently the molecular structure and function of ER biology has been elucidated, revealing how tamoxifen and related drugs act as ligands to differentially switch on or off gene expression in specific tissues. However, the mechanism of the antiestrogenic effects of high-dose estrogens is still not clear [8,9]. The ability of separate antiestrogens to have alternative effects on various estrogen-regulated targets led to the term *selective estrogen receptor modulators* (SERMs). Until recently, high-dose estrogens have not been considered as SERMs, but it is clear that these agents also have antiestrogenic effects on tumors and estrogenic effects on the breast and endometrium. It is now possible to develop SERMs that range from full estrogen agonists to pure antagonists with different effects in separate target tissues. As such, SERMs offer the potential to treat and prevent a number of conditions including from osteoporosis, menopausal symptoms, cardiovascular disease, and breast/endometrial cancer. This article reviews the development of SERMs in breast cancer, addressing in particular tamoxifen's limitations, which SERMs have attempted to overcome, and the clinical data available to date with each of the SERM compounds.

III. TAMOXIFEN—THE MOST WIDELY USED SERM

The triphenylethylene nonsteroidal antiestrogen tamoxifen was first synthesized in the 1960s and found to have clinical activity in postmenopausal women with advanced breast cancer [4]. It gained rapid acceptance because of a more favorable side-effect profile compared with the high-dose estrogens and androgens used for treatment [4]. Tamoxifen antagonizes the effects of estrogen in breast cancer cells by binding ER, inducing G1 cell-cycle arrest, and inhibiting tumor growth. Tamoxifen prevented growth of ER-positive breast tumor xenografts in vivo [10] and, at the same time, stimulated uterine growth [11] and supported the growth of endometrial xenografts in vivo [12]. A similar spectrum of estrogenic and antiestrogenic effects emerged in patients. An increase in vaginal secretions, vaginal dryness, and hot flushes were the most frequently reported antiestrogenic toxicities [13]. Owing to the estrogenic activity of tamoxifen in the liver, total serum cholesterol levels were reduced by 10 to 15% [14]. Likewise, bone mineral density was preserved in tamoxifen-treated postmenopausal women, although this effect was not apparent in premenopausal women [15,16]. In patients, tamoxifen functioned as an estrogen on the endometrium, with thickening and hyperplasia, together and a reportedly increased risk of endometrial cancer [17]. While some of these additional properties of tamoxifen are of potential benefit for women, SERMs were developed for breast cancer with the aim of reducing some of tamoxifen's toxicities. In terms of breast cancer therapy, a meta-analysis of all clinical trials found that 5 years of tamoxifen treatment significantly reduced the risk of recurrence (47% reduction in annual odds) and death (26% reduction in annual odds) in women with early-stage ER-positive breast cancer [5]. This benefit was greatest in women with ER-rich tumors and occurred across all age groups irrespective of nodal involvement. In addition tamoxifen's antiestrogenic effects on normal breast epithelial cells resulted in a 50% reduction in new contralateral breast cancers, evidence that provided much of the impetus to develop tamoxifen in chemoprevention. At the same time, the estrogenic effects of tamoxifen therapy on bone and cholesterol are of clinical benefit for these women, reducing the risk of osteoporosis and cardiovascular disease [14,15]. In the adjuvant setting, the increased risk of endometrial cancer posed by tamoxifen has been perceived as small in relation to the substantial benefit from reduction in breast cancer–related events [17]. However, in adjuvant and metastatic therapy with tamoxifen, breast epithelial cells and established tumors develop resistance to treatment. This may relate to the partial agonist effect of tamoxifen in stimulating tumor growth [8,19]. Experimental models have shown that novel antiestrogens devoid of agonist effects can antagonize tamoxifen-stimulated growth [12], and when used in treatment of hormone-sensitive tumors, may delay the emergence of resistance [20]. This generated hope that better SERMs with an improved antiestrogen/estrogen profile may overcome this form of resistance and improve further on the efficacy of tamoxifen in treating breast cancer.

IV. HIGH-DOSE ESTROGENS—THE FIRST SERMs

Testosterone was the first additive systemic therapy for breast cancer. This was rapidly followed by high-dose estrogens, particularly diethylstilbestrol [1–3] and ethinylestradiol [21]. Several other estrogens have been used, including dienestrol [22] and conjugated equine estrogens [23–25].

In randomized trials, DES or ethinylestradiol was generally equivalent to triphenylethylene antiestrogens. However, the studies were very small by modern standards [21] (Table 1). The 20-year results of the largest study were recently reported [26]. The response rates were not significantly higher for DES than for tamoxifen, and there was a survival advantage for the patients treated

Table 1 Summary of Clinical Trials Comparing Estrogen and Antiestrogen Therapy for Advanced Breast Cancer

Treatment	No. of Patients	Antiestrogen (%)	Estrogen (%)
Tam vs. EE$_2$ (Beex, 1981)	63	10/33 (33)	9/29 (31)
Naf vs. EE$_2$ (Heuson, 1975)	98	15/49 (31)	7/49 (14)
Tam vs. DES (Ingle, 1981)	143	23/69 (33)	30/74 (41)
Tam vs. DES (Paschold, 1981)	37	3/16 (19)	4/11 (36)
Tam vs. DES (Stewart, 1980)	72	9/29 (31)	6/27 (22)
Tam vs. EE$_2$ (Matelski, 1985)	43	10/19 (53)	6/24 (25)

Key: EE$_2$ = ethinylestradiol; Naf= nafoxidine; DES=diethylstilbestrol.

with DES. More important responses to both agents were seen at crossover, suggesting a degree of non–cross resistance between these two classes of SERMs (Table 2). We have studied the effectiveness of DES in a group of 30 patients with advanced breast cancer after a median of four previous endocrine therapies [27]. Of these, 29% obtained clinical benefit for a median duration of 49 weeks, indicating the usefulness of this "old" type of SERM treatment. In general, large doses of DES (5 mg tds) and ethinylestradiol (3 mg od) have been used, leading to greater toxicity compared with triphenylethylenes. Although serum "estrogen"

Table 2 Diethylstilbestrol (5 mg tds) Versus Tamoxifen (20 mg od) First-Line Treatment for Advanced Disease

	Tamoxifen (N=69)	Diethylstilbestrol (N=74)
CR	6 (9%)	8 (11%)
PR	17 (25%)	23 (31%)
CR + PR	23 (34%)	31 (42%)
MDR	9.9	11.8
5-year survival	16%	35%
Median	2.4 yrs	3.0 yrs
2nd response	5/16 (31%)	6/28 (21%)

Key: CR=complete response; PR=partial response; MDR=median duration of response; withdrawal response with diethylstilbestrol 5/18 (28%).

concentration has not been measured in any of these studies, it is likely to be very high (estimated at 10^{-7} to 10^{-6} M).

In Figure 1, we show the range of concentrations of serum estradiol that breast tumors, in vivo or in vitro, can respond to, and the changes that result in regressions. Relatively small changes induced by aromatase inhibitors result in regression. It is not clear why such large doses of estrogens have been used. It might be possible to use treatments to give serum concentrations of about 10^{-9} to 10^{-7} M. These treatments may be less toxic and lead to the reestablishment of this type of SERM therapy, giving added choice of treatment. In this regard, Stoll showed that responses in advanced breast cancer could be obtained by the use of doses of hormones as provided by the contraceptive pill [28].

V. NOVEL SERMs—POTENTIAL ADVANTAGES FOR BREAST CANCER

An understanding of how the triphenylethylene antiestrogen tamoxifen interacts with ER has allowed novel SERMs to be synthesized that possess an improved antiestrogenic/estrogenic profile. These drugs have been developed with the aim of retaining both the antagonist activity of tamoxifen within the breast and the agonist profile in bone and the cardiovascular system yet at the same time eliminating unwanted agonist effects on the gynecological tract and, in particu-

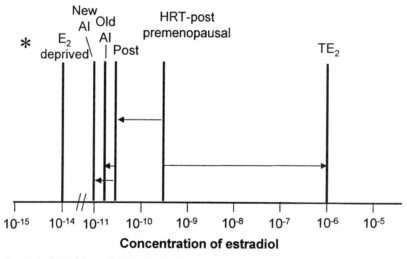

Arrows indicate [change] during endocrine therapy

Figure 1   Range of concentrations of serum estrogen during endocrine therapy.

lar, the uterus. Nonsteroidal SERMs fall into two broad categories—those that are structurally similar to the triphenylethylene structure of tamoxifen (Fig. 2) and those that are structurally different and more related to the benzothiophene structure of raloxifene (Fig. 3). A third class of antiestrogens includes the steroidal antiestrogen ICI-182,780 (fulvestrant), which is a structural derivative of estradiol with a long hydrophobic side chain at the 7 alpha position (Fig. 3) [29]. Pharmacologically, these latter compounds are pure antiestrogens that not only impair ER dimerization but also induce ER degradation [30,31]. These compounds act as potent antiestrogens in all tissues including the breast, uterus, and probably bone. Some may argue that fulvestrant is not a true SERM because it lacks selective agonist/antagonist effects in different tissues and acts through a fundamentally different mechanism of action. Others have suggested that it represents one end (i.e., a pure antiestrogen) of the SERM spectrum, with estrogen as a pure agonist at the other end and all other SERMs falling somewhere in between [8].

Each of the SERMs has demonstrated pharmacological or pharmacodynamic benefit over tamoxifen in various preclinical studies and as a consequence had a profile that supported clinical development in women with advanced breast cancer. The potential preclinical advantage for these SERMs included either greater potency due to enhanced affinity for ER, greater efficacy compared with tamoxifen against breast cancer in vitro or in vivo, and reduced risk of toxicity compared with tamoxifen on end organs (Table 3). If resistance to tamoxifen occurs in part due to the agonist effects of the drug in stimulating tumor regrowth [18,19,32], SERMs would be expected to either be active against tamoxifen-resistant tumor or to delay the emergence of resistance. In the clinic, this profile would manifest either as a superior response rate or delay the emergence of resistance during long-term therapy. As such, one might expect to see evidence of activity for SERMs in phase II studies in tamoxifen-resistant breast cancer, offering an increased duration of clinical response or time to disease progression compared with tamoxifen in randomized phase III trials or even as an alternative first-line therapy for ER-positive hormone-sensitive breast cancer (Table 3). The progress to date with each SERM compound is reviewed, in particular recent data from clinical trials of SERMs in women with either tamoxifen-resistant or hormone-sensitive breast cancer.

A.   Tamoxifen-Like Triphenylethylene SERMs

Of the triphenylethylene derivatives, clinical data from phase II/III clinical trials in women with advanced breast cancer have been published with four triphenylethylene tamoxifen-like compounds (toremifene, droloxifene, idoxifene, and TAT-59). For each one, preclinical data suggested an improved SERM profile compared with tamoxifen and led to their clinical development.

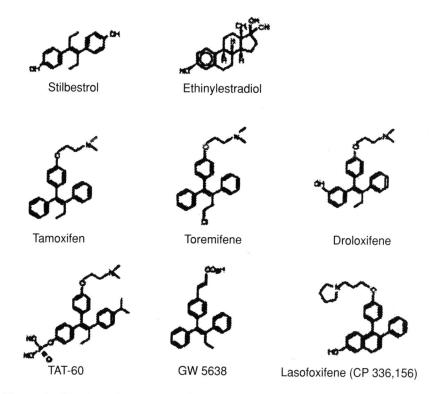

Figure 2   Structure of estrogen and tamoxifen-like SERMs.

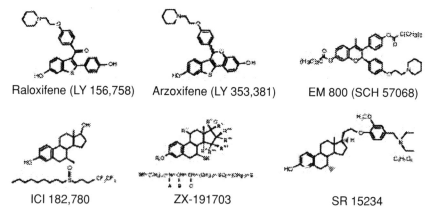

Figure 3   Structure of fixed-ring SERMs and ICI 182780 (fulvestrant).

Table 3 The Ideal Profile of a Novel SERM in Comparison with Tamoxifen

Preclinical
Greater binding affinity for ER
Ability to antagonize estrogen-dependent growth factor of breast cancer cells in
  vitro
Equal or greater inhibition of hormone-dependent xenograft growth in vivo
Activity against tamoxifen-dependent (resistant) tumors
Delayed emergence of antiestrogen resistance in vivo
Reduced agonist effects in uterotrophic assays
Lack of stimulation of endometrial cancer cells in vitro/in vivo
Lack of DNA adduct formation
Prevention of bone loss in ovariectomized animals

Clinical
Activity in hormone-sensitive breast cancer at least equivalent to tamoxifen
Increase in time to disease progression compared to tamoxifen
Activity in tamoxifen-resistant breast cancer
Improved side-effect profile (i.e., less hot flashes)
No endometrial thickening/hyperplasia/cancer risk
Preservation of bone mineral density
Reduction in serum cholesterol

1. Toremifene

Toremifene's only structural difference compared with tamoxifen relates to a single chlorine atom at position 4 (Fig. 2). The pharmacological profile of both drugs is similar [33,34]. Unlike tamoxifen, toremifene was not found to be hepatocarcinogenic in preclinical models [35,36]. This may relate to an inability of toremifene to induce DNA adducts in the rat liver [37]. Toremifene had a similar relative binding affinity (RBA) for ER compared with tamoxifen and inhibited the growth of ER-positive breast cancer cells in vitro [38] and hormone-dependent breast cancer xenograft growth in vivo [39]. However, like tamoxifen, toremifene had estrogenic effects on both endometrial cells and the uterus in vivo [40,41], although it had slightly reduced estrogenic effects on bone [42]. Toremifene was developed as a triphenyl-ethylene derivative of tamoxifen that may have less genotoxic potential; it could be a safer antiestrogen for breast cancer treatment.

High-dose toremifene (120 to 240 mg) has been investigated in five phase II studies as second-line therapy in 260 patients with tamoxifen-resistant breast cancer. These patients had failed either to respond to tamoxifen for advanced disease, progressed after an initial response, or had relapsed on adjuvant tamoxifen. In the largest study, 102 patients were treated with 200 mg of toremifene daily. The overall objective response rate was only 5% [95% confidence interval (CI) 3 to 7%], with an additional 23% of patients who had stable disease for a median of 7.8 months. However, the authors felt that the latter could relate to slow progression of an intrinsically indolent tumor [43]. Responses were more likely in those patients who had previously responded to tamoxifen for advanced disease. In the second study, 56 patients with tamoxifen-refractory breast cancer were treated with toremifene 240 mg daily [44]. Objective responses were seen in only 2 patients (4%, 95% CI 0.5 to 1.4%) with stable disease for > 5 months in 9 patients, with activity again more likely in previous tamoxifen responders. In the third study in 51 patients with tamoxifen-refractory disease, a higher objective response rate of 14% was seen, with an additional 19% of patients having stable disease for > 6 months [45]. However, the two other smaller studies found no responders to 240 mg of toremifene in tamoxifen-refractory patients, including a randomized study against tamoxifen with prospective crossover at progression on each antiestrogen [46,47]. Thus, while occasional tamoxifen-refractory patients may have an objective response to toremifene, especially if they had responded to tamoxifen previously, cross-resistance probably exists between the two drugs [48].

As first-line therapy in hormone-sensitive advanced breast cancer, five phase II studies in 175 patients showed objective response rates of 48 to 68%, with toremifene in doses of 60 to 240 mg daily suggesting that higher response rates occurred with the 240-mg dose [36]. Low-dose (20 mg) toremifene was associated with a response rate of only 21% in an additional small study and was not investigated further [49]. Subsequently, five large phase III randomized controlled trials have been published that have compared toremifene (40 to 60 mg) with tamoxifen (20 to 40 mg) as first-line endocrine therapy in advanced breast cancer (Table 4) [50–54]. The response rate to toremifene in these larger multicenter studies was lower than that in the phase II studies and ranged from 21 to 38%. In all these studies, toremifene showed equivalent efficacy to tamoxifen for objective response rate, stable disease, time to disease progression, and overall survival (Table 4). In addition, two of these studies randomized patients between 60 mg toremifene and higher doses (200/240 mg) and found no significant difference in efficacy [51,53]. There was no difference in drug-related toxicities, and both toremifene and tamoxifen were well tolerated. A recent meta-analysis of 1421 patients from these trials showed a similar response rate for toremifene compared with tamoxifen (24 vs. 25.3%), with no significant difference in time to disease progression (hazard ratio 0.98, 95% CI 0.87 to 1.11) or overall survival (hazard ratio 0.98, 95% CI 0.83 to 1.15) [55]. Any potential difference in carcinogenicity that had been identified in preclinical studies was not evaluated in any of these studies. However, at least two adjuvant studies were subsequently initiated to compare efficacy and long-term tolerability and safety in early breast cancer patients. Preliminary data from approximately 900 postmenopausal, node-positive patients after a median follow-up of 3.4 years has been reported, and there were no significant differences in efficacy or tolerability compared with tamox-

Table 4 Summary of Clinical Efficacy Data from the Randomized Phase III Trials of Toremifene (40–60 mg/day) Versus Tamoxifen (20–40 mg/day) as First-Line Endocrine Treatment of Advanced Breast Cancer in Postmenopausal Women (ER status positive or unknown)

Study	Toremifene			Tamoxifen		
	n	ORR (%)	TTP(mo)	n	ORR (%)	TTP (mo)
Hayes et al. (51)	221	21	5.6	215	19	5.8
Pyrhonen et al. (52)	214	31	7.3	201	37	10.2
Gershanovich et al. [53]	157	21	4.9	149	21	5.0
Nomura et al. (50)	62	24	5.1	60	27	5.1
Milla-Santos et al. [54]	106	38	11.9	111	32	9.2
Meta-analysis[a] (55)	**725**	**24.0**	**4.9**	**696**	**25.3**	**5.3**

Key: ORR=objective response rate, including complete response and partial response: TTP=median time to disease progression.
[a]The meta-analysis [55] was published in 1999 and includes data from the first four trials along with a small unpublished German study but did not include the Spanish study [54], which was published in 2001.

ifen [56]. In particular, the number of subsequent second cancers was similar, although longer follow-up will be needed to see whether any differences emerge.

2. Droloxifene

Structurally, droloxifene is 3-hydroxytamoxifen and has a tenfold higher RBA for ER compared with tamoxifen [57]. In preclinical studies, droloxifene had several potential advantages over tamoxifen, including a shorter half-life [58], greater growth inhibition of breast cancer cells and reduced estrogenicity in the rat uterus [59], and absence of DNA adduct formation or carcinogenicity [60]. However, like tamoxifen, it also behaved as an estrogen in bone, preserving bone mineral density [61].

Early phase I/II studies suggested some efficacy in patients who had previously received tamoxifen [62,63]. A phase II study of droloxifene 100 mg daily in 26 patients who had received previous tamoxifen found a response rate of 15%, with stable disease > 6 months in a further 5 (19%) patients [64]. A large randomized dose-finding study of 20, 40, or 100 mg droloxifene in 369 patients as first-line therapy showed objective response rates of 30, 47, and 44%, respectively [65,66]. Better response duration and time to disease progression were seen with the two higher doses, and there were no significant drug-related toxicities. Other first-line phase II studies were undertaken, including one study in 39 patients that showed a response rate of 51% (95% CI 35 to 67%) and a median time to progression of 8 months [67]. These first-line data suggested a level of efficacy comparable to that of tamoxifen, and randomized phase III studies comparing droloxifene versus tamoxifen were initiated. However, droloxifene was found to be less active than tamoxifen and further development was stopped [68,69].

3. Idoxifene

Idoxifene is a SERM that is metabolically more stable than tamoxifen. It has a pyrrolidine side chain with an iodine atom at the 4 position. This confers increased binding affinity for ER [70]. Idoxifene inhibited hormone-dependent breast cancer growth and was more effective than tamoxifen at inhibiting both MCF-7 cell growth in vitro and rat mammary tumor growth in vivo [71]. As a SERM, idoxifene had estrogenic agonist effects on bone [72]. However, MCF-7 xenograft growth in the absence of estradiol was more inhibited for idoxifene than for tamoxifen in vivo, suggesting a reduced agonist activity on cancer cells [73]. Likewise, reduced stimulation of uterine weight was seen in various uterotrophic assays [71,72]. Thus, idoxifene was developed in the hope that the reduced agonist profile in breast and gynecological tissues would be an advantage over tamoxifen for breast cancer patients.

In a phase I study of idoxifene, 14 patients previously treated with tamoxifen, 2 patients had a partial response and 3 had disease stabilization for > 6 months [74]. Results from a randomized phase II study showed little evidence of significant clinical activity for idoxifene in tamoxifen-resistant breast cancer [75]. A total of 56 postmenopausal patients with progressive locally advanced/metastatic breast cancer previously treated with tamoxifen 20 mg/day were randomized to idoxifene 40 mg/day or tamoxifen 40 mg/day. With idoxifene, 2 patients with partial (objective response rate 9%) and 2 with stable disease were seen. In contrast, no objective responses were seen with higher-dose tamoxifen; however, 2 patients had stable disease. In a phase III trial, 220 postmenopausal women with metastatic breast cancer were randomized to receive either idoxifene 40 mg/day or tamoxifen 20 mg/day as first-line endocrine therapy [76]. Prior adjuvant tamoxifen had been stopped at least 12 months previously and been received by 21 and 14% of the patients, respectively. The objective response rate (CR+PR) was 20% (95% CI 12.7 to 28.2%) for idoxifene and 19% (95% CI 12.5 to 28.2%) for tamoxifen, with a median duration of objective response of 8.1 months for idoxifene and 7.3 months for tamoxifen. In addition, stable disease for ≥ 6 months was observed in 19% of idoxifene- and 29% of tamoxifen-treated patients. Overall, there was no significant difference in time to disease progression or overall survival. Possible drug-related side effects (i.e., hot flushes) were infrequent (<5%) and similar in incidence between both groups. There was no difference in gynecological adverse events between idoxifene and tamoxifen. However, in a parallel osteoporosis program, an increased incidence of uterine prolapse and polyps was reported in idoxifene-treated women. Despite a reduced agonist profile for idoxifene seen in preclinical studies, there appears to be no major difference in terms of clinical efficacy or safety profile between idoxifene and tamoxifen. Further development of the drug was stopped.

Other structural analogues of tamoxifen (Fig. 2) have been synthesized, including TAT-59, which has a tenfold higher affinity for ER than tamoxifen and has been shown to be more effective at inhibiting human breast cancer xenograft growth in vivo [77,78]. However, it was equivalent to tamoxifen in a phase III trial, and further development has been abandoned [79].

4. Other Tamoxifen-Like Derivatives in Development

GW5638 is a carboxylic derivative in early clinical development that demonstrated significantly reduced agonist activity on the uterus in ovariectomized rats. However, it remained a full agonist in reducing cholesterol and maintaining bone mineral density [80]. CGP 336,156 (lasofoxifene) is a derivative of tetrahydronapthalene. In animal studies, it maintained bone mineral density [81] and therefore may find an application for the prevention of osteoporosis [9]. There are few (if any) published clinical data for these compounds in advanced breast cancer.

5. Clinical Efficacy of Tamoxifen-Like SERMs

From the clinical data following failure of tamoxifen in advanced breast cancer, overall little significant activity has been observed with the first-generation tamoxifen-like SERMs (toremifene, droloxifene, and idoxifene), with a median response rate from all studies of only 5% (range 0 to 15%) (Table 5). The reduced agonist profile seen with droloxifene and idoxifene in preclinical studies may have been tissue or cell-specific and did not appear to manifest itself in any improved efficacy in treating or preventing tamoxifen resistance in patients with breast cancer. If the agonist activity of tamoxifen were a major mechanism for

Table 5 Overall Efficacy of Tamoxifen-Like SERMs in Advanced Breast Cancer[a]

| | Tamoxifen-resistant | | Hormone-sensitive | | |
	Phase II ORR (%)	SD	Phase II ORR (%)	Phase III ORR (%)	TTP
Toremifene	0–14	16–30	21–68	21–38	4.9–11
Droloxifene	15	19	30–51		
Idoxifene	9	9		20	6.5
Median	**5**	**18**		**31**	**6.9**

Key: ORR=% patients with an objective response, including complete response and partial response; SD=% patients with stable disease for ≥ 6 months; TTP=median time to disease progression in months.
[a]Response rate ranges from clinical trial results from phase II studies of toremifene and droloxifene in tamoxifen-resistant or hormone-sensitive patients and phase III trials in first-line versus tamoxifen.

the development of resistance, one might have hoped that SERMs with reduced agonist activity might have resulted in a longer response duration or time to progression. The fact that they did not implies that unlike the steroidal antiestrogen ICI 182,780 (fulvestrant), these drugs are probably completely cross-resistant with tamoxifen. Perhaps this is not surprising, given the similar tamoxifen-like mechanism of action and structure-function interaction with ER for these triphenylethylene compounds. In contrast, fulvestrant acts by downregulating ER expression [30,31]. This may explain why the drug appears to have much better activity in tamoxifen-resistant breast cancer than toremifene or idoxifene [83,82]. The definitive test of this hypothesis will be the results of the current first-line trials of fulvestrant, where one may anticipate that time to progression could be prolonged compared with tamoxifen, as has been demonstrated in xenograft models [20].

As first-line therapy, the combined phase II/III clinical trial data for tamoxifen-like SERMs (toremiphene, droloxifene, and idoxifene) suggest a median response rate of 31% (range 20 to 68%), with a median time to disease progression of 6.9 months (Table 5). In the randomized first-line trials in hormone-sensitive advanced breast cancer, both toremifene and idoxifene were shown to be very similar to tamoxifen in terms of clinical efficacy and toxicity [50–54,76], while droloxifene appeared to be inferior [68]. The toxicity profile was the same, including gynecological effects seen with idoxifene. On the basis of these current data, it is unlikely that the first-generation triphenylethylene SERMs will replace tamoxifen for advanced breast cancer.

B. Fixed-Ring SERMs

Greater optimism has surrounded the profile of fixed-ring SERMs (Fig. 3). This may translate into an improved clinical benefit for breast cancer patients. Much of the enthusiasm relates to the fact that these drugs appear devoid of any agonist activity in the endometrium while at the same time appearing to be potent antiestrogens in the breast and retaining agonist activity in bone. Structurally, most of these drugs resemble the benzothiophene raloxifene, which is the most extensively studied SERM in this class.

1. Raloxifene

The binding affinity of raloxifene for ERs is similar to that of tamoxifen [84]. Most of the pharmacological data showed similar activity to tamoxifen in terms of inhibiting breast cancer cells in vitro and rat mammary tumor growth in vivo [85,86]. In preclinical models, the drug maintained bone mineral density [87] and reduced total cholesterol [88], but it had significantly less estrogenic activity on endometial cells compared with tamoxifen and could inhibit tamoxifen-stimulated endometrial cancer growth in vivo [12]. Raloxifene was developed and is indicated for osteoporosis based on clinical trials that showed prevention of bone loss in postmenopausal women [89]. While raloxifene was not developed as an antiestrogen for breast cancer, these are limited data on the activity of raloxifene in patients with advanced breast cancer. In a small study, of 14 patients resistant to tamoxifen therapy following an initial response, only 1 had a minor response when treated with 200 mg of raloxifene [90]. In 21 patients with ER-positive metastatic breast cancer treated with raloxifene 150 mg bid as first-line therapy, 4 (19%) had a partial response for a median duration of 22 months, with an additional 3 (14%) patients showing stable disease [91]. Raloxifene does not appear to relieve vasomotor symptoms such as hot flashes. However, during raloxifene's development for osteoporosis, it was found to significantly reduce the incidence of breast cancer (in particular ER-positive tumors) in postmenopausal women by 76% (95% CI 56 to 87%), without any increase in endometrial thickening or risk to the gynecological tract [92,93]. Because tamoxifen may also reduce the incidence of breast cancer, albeit despite an increased risk of endometrial cancer and thromboembolic events [6], it is being compared to raloxifene as a chemopreventive in the current Study of Tamoxifen and Raloxifene (STAR) trial. The potential exists that as a SERM raloxifene may reduce breast cancer incidence with a better safety profile compared with tamoxifen. It is hoped that this trial will clarify which patients (i.e., what level of breast cancer risk) derive benefit from chemoprevention.

2. Arzoxifene

LY 353381 (arzoxifene) is a benzothiophene analogue that is a more potent antiestrogen with an improved SERM profile compared with raloxifene [94]. In particular, arzoxifene was a more potent inhibitor of breast cancer cells in vitro than either tamoxifen or raloxifene, and it inhibited growth of mammary tumor xenografts in vivo [95,96]. As a SERM, arzoxifene in preclinical studies was a more potent agonist on bone and cholesterol metabolism than raloxifene [97,98], with no evidence of any estrogen-like agonist effects on uterine tissues [94]. In view of these promising data, arzoxifene has entered clinical development for the treatment of breast cancer.

In a phase I study, 32 patients who had received a median of two prior endocrine therapies were treated with arzoxifene in doses ranging from 10 to 100 mg daily [99]. No significant toxicities were seen, and transvaginal ultrasound showed no endometrial thickening following 3 months of therapy. Six patients had stable disease for a median of 7.7 months (range 6 to 33 months). In a phase II study as first-line therapy, 92 patients were randomized to either 20 mg or 50 mg arzoxifene daily [100]. Only 9% of patients had received tamoxifen previously in the adjuvant setting. There was no difference in response rate (36 vs. 34%), clinical benefit rate, which included stable disease (63 vs. 64%), or time to disease progression (10.4 vs. 8.9 months). Likewise, toxicities were minor, although 30% reported minor hot flashes. More recently, preliminary results were reported of a further phase II trial that compared both doses in 63 tamoxifen-resistant patients and separately in 49 patients with hormone-sensitive disease (i.e., first-line therapy) [101]. Response rates were low in the tamoxifen-resistant patients (10% for 20 mg, 3% for 50 mg), all of whom either had relapsed on adjuvant tamoxifen after at least 1 year of therapy or progressed on tamoxifen for advanced disease following an initial response. In contrast, a response rate of 30% was seen with 20 mg of arzoxifene in the hormone-sensitive group, with a further 17% having stable disease and an overall median time to progression of 8.3 months. The response rate for the 50-mg dose was somewhat lower (8%), although numbers are small (only 25 patients). Based on all the phase II data, 20 mg of arzoxifene has now been taken forward into a large multicenter phase III trial against tamoxifen as first-line therapy.

3. EM-800

This is an orally active so-called pure nonsteroidal antiestrogen that is a prodrug of the active benzopyrene derivative EM-652 (SCH 57068) [102]. The binding affinity of EM-652 for ER is significantly greater than that of estradiol, tamoxifen, raloxifene, or fulvestrant [103]. The prodrug EM-800 is a potent antiestrogen and was more effective than 4-hydroxytamoxifen and fulvestrant at inhibiting estradiol (E2)-induced cell proliferation in breast cancer cells in vitro. Furthermore, in the absence of E2, no agonist effects on growth were observed [104]. In ZR-75-1 xenografts, EM-800 was significantly more effective than tamoxifen at inducing tumor regressions in vivo, and in the absence of E2-antagonized tamoxifen-stimulated tumor growth [105]. In intact mice, EM-800 was 30-fold more potent than tamoxifen at inhibiting uterine weight and reducing uterine/vaginal ER expression [106]. Likewise, EM-800 was devoid of any stimulatory effect on alkaline phosphatase activity (a sensitive marker of estrogenic activity) in Ishikawa endometrial carcinoma cells [107], while EM-652 had no agonist activity in an immature rat uterotrophic assay [108]. In addition, studies have shown that EM-800 prevented bone loss in the ovariectomized rat [109] and lowered serum cholesterol levels [102]. Interestingly, EM-800 appears to significantly downregulate ER levels both in tumors and normal estrogen-sensitive tissues in a similar fashion to the steroidal antiestrogen fulvestrant [106]. Its specific agonist effects on bone differentiate it from fulvestrant, which has not been shown to prevent bone loss. As such, EM-800/EM-652 has a potentially promising SERM profile.

In terms of clinical development, a phase II study of EM-800 (20 or 40 mg) was undertaken in 43 postmenopausal women who had failed tamoxifen either in the metastatic or adjuvant setting [102,110]. There was one CR and 5 PRs (response rate 14%), with most of the responses occurring in those who had received at least 3 years adjuvant tamoxifen [110]. An additional 10 (23%) patients had stable disease for > 6 months. On the basis of these results, a randomized phase III study in patients who had failed tamoxifen was undertaken, comparing the efficacy of EM-800 (20 or 40 mg) with the third-generation aromatase inhibitor anastrozole. At the defined interim review, when over 300 patients had been entered, the efficacy was substantially less than that of anastrozole and the trial was terminated (C. Tendler, personal communication, 2001). There are no data at present on the activity of EM-800 in the first-line hormone-sensitive population.

4. ERA-923

This is a novel SERM that appears to have an improved preclinical profile. ERA-923 is now being evaluated in a randomized dose-finding phase II trial (25 mg vs. 100 mg) as second-line therapy in 100 ER-positive patients with tamoxifen-resistant metastatic breast cancer. A similar randomized phase II trial has been proposed in receptor-positive hormone-sensitive metastatic breast cancer as first-line therapy.

5. Clinical Efficacy of Fixed-Ring SERMs

In preclinical models, these new compounds appear to offer a greater increase in potency and tumor growth inhibition, with an improved SERM profile on other tissues, in comparison with the tamoxifen-like SERMs. Currently, there are too few clinical data to know whether these potential advantages will translate into beneficial effects for breast cancer patients. However, in tamoxifen-resistant patients, the levels of activity reported for raloxifene [90], arzoxifene [101], and EM-800 [102] are all low (Table 4), with a median response rate of 6.5%, which is very similar to that observed with the tamoxifen-like SERMs (Table 5). It is probable that its activity in first-line therapy will be similar to that of tamoxifen, as the only phase II data with raloxifene and arzoxifene give a median response rate of 30%, with a median time to progression of 9.4 months (Table 6). Results of ongoing phase II/III trials with arzoxifene and ERA-923 are awaited, but to

Table 6 Overall Efficacy of Second- and Third-Generation SERMs in Advanced Breast Cancer[a]

	Tamoxifen-resistant Phase II		Hormone-sensitive Phase II	
	ORR (%)	SD (%)	ORR (%)	TTP
Raloxifene	0		19	
Arzoxifene	3–10	3–7	30–36	8.3–10.4
EM-800	14	23		
Median	**6.5**	**7**	**30**	**9.4**

Key: ORR=% patients with an objective response, including complete response and partial response; SD=% patients with stable disease for ≥ 6 months; TTP=median time to disease progression in months.
[a]Response rate ranges from clinical trial results from phase II studies of raloxifene, arzoxifene, and EM-800 in tamoxifen-resistant or hormone-sensitive patients.

date there is little clinical evidence to suggest that, in advanced breast cancer, substantial improvements in efficacy will be made over tamoxifen.

C. "Pure" Antiestrogens

Another avenue of development of SERMs has been to produce steroidal analogues of estrogen with a bulky side chain at either the 7α [111–114] or the 11α positions of estradiol [115], which are completely lacking in agonist activity. These agents have been termed "pure" antiestrogens and include ICI 164,384, fulvestrant (Faslodex, formerly ICI 182,780), and RU 58668. The most advanced of these, in terms of both preclinical and clinical evaluation, is the steroidal compound fulvestrant [Fig. 3] [114].

1. Fulvestrant: Mode of Action

Fulvestrant is one of two steroidal antiestrogens with pure antiestrogenic activity developed from a series of 7α-alkyl analogues of estradiol [114]. ICI 164,384 has been studied extensively in a preclinical setting, but it is the more potent fulvestrant that is being actively studied in patients with breast cancer [111,112].

Fulvestrant is distinguishable from tamoxifen and the other SERMs both pharmacologically and by its molecular activity. Although both classes of agent mediate their effects through the ER, they differ significantly in their downstream effects.

The activity of the steroidal antiestrogens such as fulvestrant is very different from that of tamoxifen. The steroidal antiestrogens bind to the ER, but because of their long bulky side chains at the 7α and 11β positions, receptor dimerization appears to be sterically hindered [31]. There is evidence that ER turnover is increased and nuclear localization disrupted with a concomitant reduction in the number of detectable ER molecules in the cell both in vitro and in vivo [116]. This is in contrast to the stable or increased levels of ER expression associated with tamoxifen and its analogues. In vitro and in vivo studies suggest that because of ERs' "downregulation," ER-mediated transcription is completely attenuated as fulvestrant inactivates both AF-1 and AF-2. This completely suppresses the expression of estrogen-dependent genes. Thus, fulvestrant is not only described as a pure antiestrogen but also as an estrogen receptor downregulator.

a. Clinical Studies

The data surrounding the clinical potential of fulvestrant in patients with breast cancer are encouraging. Administration of a short-acting, propylene glycol–based formulation of fulvestrant at doses of 6 or 18 mg daily, by intramuscular injection for one week to postmenopausal breast cancer patients prior to surgery resulted in a reduction in proliferation as measured by Ki67-labeling index and a reduction or absence of expression of ER and progesterone receptors (PgR) in ER-positive tumors [112]. Treatment with fulvestrant also resulted in a clinically significant reduction in the expression of the estrogen-regulated gene pS2, but this was unrelated to tumor ER status. Similar experiments with tamoxifen had produced no change in ER expression, slightly increased PgR expression, and a reduction in the Ki67-labeling index after a median of 21 days of treatment.

Although fulvestrant reduced ER expression to almost undetectable levels, no other changes suggestive of an endocrine-insensitive phenotype were observed [111]. This coupled with the absence of changes in Ki67 in ER-negative tumors suggests that the effect is the result of antagonism of estrogen at the ER level. This antiestrogenic effect has been confirmed in a study in premenopausal patients scheduled for hysterectomy for benign gynecological disease who were randomized to receive either seven consecutive daily doses of the short-acting formulation of fulvestrant or observation prior to surgery. No increase in endometrial thickness and significantly lower ER expression in the myometrium was observed in the fulvestrant-treated patients [117,118].

In a much larger preoperative study, the antitumor effects of single-dose, long-acting fulvestrant have been compared with those of tamoxifen in postmenopausal primary breast cancer patients prior to surgery [119]. A total of 201 patients were randomized to receive either fulvestrant over a range of doses (50, 125, or 250 mg) administered intramuscularly or tamoxifen administered orally at a dose of 20 mg/day or matching tamoxifen placebo for 14 to 21 days prior to surgery. A dose-dependent reduction in the levels of ER expression was observed across all three doses of fulvestrant compared with placebo. Also, when the fulvestrant dose normally used clinically (250 mg) was compared with tamoxifen, there was a significantly greater reduction in ER index for fulvestrant. A dose-dependent reduction in PgR expression was observed following fulvestrant treatment, which was greater for all three doses of fulvestrant than for tamoxifen, which actually resulted in stimulation of PgR [119] expression. At all three doses, fulvestrant reduced proliferation. These data again provide evidence that fulvestrant acts as an ER downregulator with clear antiestrogenic and antiproliferative activity [119]. Furthermore, the effect on PgR provides evidence of a more complete blockade of this ER-dependent pathway compared with tamoxifen, which increases PgR levels because of its partial agonist activity [119].

The clinical efficacy of fulvestrant has also been demonstrated in a small phase II trial in 19 patients with tamoxifen-refractory disease who received a long-acting monthly intramuscular injection, starting with 100 mg in the first month and increasing to 250 mg for the second and subsequent months in the absence of local and systemic toxicity: 13 patients achieved a clinical benefit, with a median duration of 25 months, 7 demonstrated a partial response (PR), and 6 had stable disease [SD] [83,112]. These data clearly confirmed the lack of cross-resistance with tamoxifen observed in preclinical studies. Furthermore, luteinizing hormone and follicle-stimulating hormone levels rose after the patients were removed from tamoxifen but then plateaued, suggesting that there is no effect of fulvestrant on the pituitary-hypothalamic axis. Hot flashes and sweats were not induced. Negative effects were not observed on the liver, brain, or genital tract, suggesting that fulvestrant might have fewer side effects in terms of menopausal symptoms than tamoxifen. Thus, fulvestrant at the drug concentrations used in this study was effective as second-line antiestrogen therapy, supporting a mechanism of action distinct from tamoxifen's. In addition, this phase II study clearly indicated that fulvestrant was well tolerated. Also, comparison with a well-matched historical control group of patients treated with the progestin megestrol acetate suggested a longer duration of response for patients receiving fulvestrant (26 months versus 14 months (Fig. 4) [83].

b. Phase III Data

The phase II second-line and preoperative trials reported above provided the initiative for two phase III studies, one in North America and one in Europe, Australia, and South Africa (ROW). These studies compared the efficacy and tolerability of fulvestrant (250 mg) administered once monthly with the third-generation aromatase inhibitor anastrozole (Arimidex) (1 mg), administered orally once daily, in postmenopausal women whose disease had progressed on or

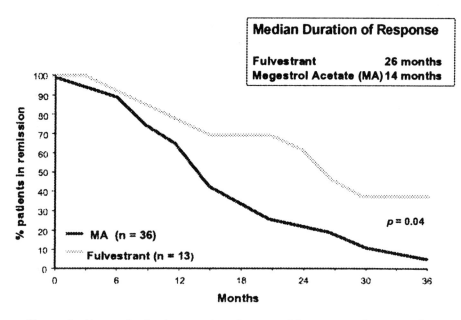

Figure 4 Nonrandomized comparison between fulvestrant and megestrol acetate as second-line therapy for advanced breast cancer.

after prior endocrine therapy [120,121]. The vast majority (>96%) of patients across both trials had received prior tamoxifen therapy. The North American trial was a double-blind trial and recruited patients from 83 centers in the United States and Canada, while the second trial was an open-label study conducted principally in Europe. It recruited patients from 82 centers. A total of 400 and 451 patients were analyzed for efficacy in the North American and ROW trials respectively. The primary endpoint in both trials was time to disease progression, with secondary endpoints including objective response, duration of response, time to death, tolerability, quality of life, and pharmacokinetics.

The median time to disease progression was numerically longer with fulvestrant than with anastrozole for both the North American (5.4 vs. 3.4 months) and ROW (5.5 vs. 5.1 months) trials but was not statistically significant in either trial. The objective response rates were not significantly different in either trial: 17.5% for both arms in the North American trial and 20.7 versus 15.7% for fulvestrant and anastrozole respectively in the ROW trial. In those patients who responded, median duration of response to fulvestrant and anastrozole was 19.3 and 10.5 months, respectively, in the North American trial and 14.3 months and 14.0 months, respectively, in the ROW trial. The clinical benefit rates (defined as complete and partial responses and disease stabilization lasting $\geq$ 24 weeks) for fulvestrant versus anastrozole were 42.2 versus 36.1% for the North American trial and 44.6 versus 45.0% for the ROW trial. In both trials, the most frequently reported adverse events were gastrointestinal disturbances (e.g., nausea, vomiting, constipation, diarrhea); 53.4 and 39.7% of patients suffered from at least one gastrointestinal disturbance in the North American and ROW trials, respectively. Overall, the incidence of adverse events was similar for the recipients of anastrozole and fulvestrant in both trials. The withdrawal rates in the fulvestrant and anastrozole groups were low in both trials, with 2.5 versus 2.6% of patients withdrawing due to an adverse event in the North American trial and 3.2 versus 2.2% of patients withdrawing due to an adverse event in the ROW trial [119,120]. In both studies, fulvestrant was at least as effective as the aromatase inhibitor anastrozole, with a longer duration of response in the North American trial, confirming fulvestrant as an effective treatment in postmenopausal patients with advanced breast cancer recurring or progressing even after tamoxifen therapy. Fulvestrant was also well tolerated and is the first antiestrogen reported to be at least as effectiveas a new-generation aromatase inhibitor. This is of particular significance in light of the fact that two trials comparing anastrozole with tamoxifen in the first-line treatment of breast cancer have shown anastrozole to be superior to tamoxifen, both in terms of time to progression and of a lower incidence of thromboembolic events and vaginal bleeding [121,122].

VI. CONCLUSION—FUTURE ROLE FOR SERMs IN BREAST CANCER

It is unclear to what extent any preclinical advantages that have been observed for each of these SERMs over tamoxifen may be predictive for clinical outcome in the treatment of advanced breast cancer. So far, the clinical data in advanced breast cancer summarized above are somewhat disappointing for the tamoxifen-like SERMs. Instead, much greater potential may exist either in the adjuvant or chemopreventive setting, where an improved SERM profile on bone, lipid metabolism, and the endometrium will be of maximum benefit. It remains to be seen whether vasomotor symptoms associated with both tamoxifen and raloxifene are any less frequent. The dilemma faced by those developing these therapies, however, is the need to demonstrate clinical activity against breast cancer that is at least equivalent to that of tamoxifen. The clinical data outlined above suggest that while there is probably little role for other triphenylethylenes and fixed-ring SERMS following failure of tamoxifen, their efficacy and tolerability in hormone-sensitive advanced breast cancer is probably equivalent to that of tamoxifen. It is possible that fulvestrant will prove superior to tamoxifen in the first-line comparative phase III trial to be reported in late 2001. Further studies will be needed to determine how it should be integrated into the treatment of advanced breast cancer with the new aromatase inhibitors. It is now clear that the third-generation aromatase inhibitors (i.e., letrozole, anastrozole) are superior and better tolerated than tamoxifen [121–123]. Fulvestrant is at least equivalent to anastrozole in tamoxifen failures and could be superior in patients with advanced breast cancer not previously treated with tamoxifen. It also remains to be seen whether the new orally bioavailable pure antiestrogens SR16234 and ZK 191703 will have equivalent or superior potency to the intramuscularly given fulvestrant. It is known that breast cancer cells adapt in vitro when subjected to long-term estrogen deprivation, remaining ER-positive and becoming hypersensitive to very low concentrations of E2 [124]. It is conceivable that potent antiestrogens, including SERMs, could be active in this setting, and clinical trials with fulvestrant following aromatase inhibitor failure are in progress.

An alternative role for SERMs could be as adjuvant therapy, either alone or in combination with aromatase inhibitors, thus providing protection to the bone and cardiovascular system while enhancing antitumor efficacy. While it has always been thought that endocrine therapies are better given in sequence rather than in combination, this has been challenged recently by data in premenopausal ER-positive advanced breast cancer, where combined estrogen deprivation with an LH-RH agonist and an antiestrogen was superior to either therapy alone, including overall survival [125]. However, in the development of SERMs as adjuvant therapy, there seems to be no shortcut to performing some form of clinical efficacy/safety study in advanced breast cancer. Additional evidence of a SERM's biological activity and clinical efficacy could be ascertained from short-term randomized neoadjuvant studies as undertaken for idoxifene [126], raloxifene [127], and fulvestrant [128]. The next 5 years will be crucial to see whether the latest generations of SERMs have a significant role in breast cancer therapy and what that role might be.

REFERENCES

1. Haddow A, Watkinson JM, Paterson E. Influence of synthetic oestrogens upon advanced malignant disease. Br Med J 1944; 2:393–398.
2. Binnie GG. Regression of tumours following treatment with stilboestrol and x-ray therapy with notes on cases of breast tumour which regressed on stilboestrol alone. Br J Radiol 1944; 17:42–45.
3. Stilboestrol for advanced breast cancer. A combined investigation. R Soc Medicine. Br Med J 1944; 2:20–21.
4. Cole MP, Jones CTA, Todd IDH, et al. A new antiestrogenic agent for breast cancer. An early appraisal of ICI 46,474. Br J Cancer 1971; 25:270–275.
5. Collaborative Early Breast Cancer Trialists Group. Tamoxifen for Early Breast Cancer: An overview of the randomized trials. Lancet 1998; 351:451–1467.
6. Fisher B, Costantino JP, Wickerham DL, et al. Tamoxifen for the prevention of breast cancer, Report of the National Surgical Adjuvant Breast and Bowel Project P-1 study. J Natl Cancer Inst 1998; 90:1371–1388.
7. Jordan VC. The development of tamoxifen for breast cancer therapy. In Jordan VC, ed. Long-Term Tamoxifen Treatment for Breast Cancer. Madison, WI: University of Wisconsin Press, 1994: 3–26.
8. Osborne CK, Zhao H, Fuqua SAW. Selective estrogen receptor modulators; Structure, function, and clinical use. J Clin Oncol 2000; 8:3172–3186.
9. Levenson AS, Jordan VC. Selective oestrogen receptor modulation; molecular pharmacology for the new millennium. Eur J Cancer 1999; 35:1628–1639.
10. Osborne CK, Hobbs K, Clark GM. Effects of estrogens and antiestrogens on growth of human breast cancer cells in athymic nude mice. Cancer Res 1985; 45:584–590.
11. Jordan VC, Robinson SP. Species specific pharmacology of antiestrogens: Role of metabolism. Fed Proc 1987; 46:1870–1874.
12. Gottardis MM, Ricchio MD, Satyaswaroop PG, Jordan VC. Effect of steroidal and nonsteroidal antiestrogens on the growth of a tamoxifen-stimulated human endometrial carcinoma (EnCa101) in athymic mice. Cancer Res 1990; 50:3189–3192.
13. Love RR, Cameron L, Connell BL, et al. Symptoms associated with tamoxifen treatment in post-menopausal women. Arch Intern Med 1991; 151:1842–1847.
14. Rutquivst LE, Mattsson A. Cardiac and thrombembolic morbidity among post-menopausal women with early-stage breast cancer in randomized trials of adjuvant tamoxifen. J Natl Cancer Inst 1993; 85:1398–1406.
15. Love RR, Mazess RB, Barden HS, et al. Effects of tamoxifen on bone mineral density in post-menopausal women with breast cancer. N Engl J Med 1992; 326:852–856.

16. Powles TJ, Hickish T, Kanis JA, et al. Effect of tamoxifen on bone mineral density measured by dual-energy x-ray absorptiometry in healthy pre-menopausal and post-menopausal women. J Clin Oncol 1996; 14:78–84.

17. Fisher B, Costantino JP, Redmond CK, et al. Endometrial cancer in tamoxifen-treated breast cancer patients; Findings from the National Surgical Adjuvant Breast and Bowel Project (NSABP) B-14. J Natl Cancer Inst 1994; 86:527–537.

18. Osborne CK, Fuqua SAW. Mechanisms of tamoxifen resistance. Breast Cancer Res Treat 1994; 32:49–55.

19. Johnston SRD. Acquired tamoxifen resistance in human breast cancer: Potential mechanisms and clinical implications. Anticancer Drugs 1997; 8:911–930.

20. Osborne CK, Coronado-Heinsohn EB, Hilsenbeck SG, et al. Comparison of the effects of a pure steroidal antioestrogen with those of tamoxifen in a model of human breast cancer. J Natl Cancer Inst 1995; 87:746–750.

21. Matelskie H, Huberman M, Zipoli T, et al. Randomized trial of estrogen vs tamoxifen therapy for advanced breast cancer. Am J Clin Oncol 1985; 8:128–133.

22. Walpole AL, Paterson E. Synthetic oestrogens in mammary cancer. Lancet 1949; 2:783.

23. Androgens and estrogens in the treatment of disseminated mammary carcinoma. Retrospective study of 1944 patients. Council on Drugs. JAMA 1960; 172:1271–1283.

24. Segaloff A, Gordon D, Carabasi RA, et al. Hormonal therapy of cancer of the breast. VII: Effect of conjugated oestrogens (equine) on clinical course and hormone secretion. Cancer 1954; 7:758–763.

25. Taylor SG III, Slaughter DP, Smejkal W, et al. The effects of sex hormones on advanced carcinoma of the breast. J Cancer 1948; 1:4.

26. Peethambaram PP, Ingle JN, Suman VJ, et al. Randomized trial of diethylstilboestrol vs tamoxifen in post-menopausal women with metastatic breast cancer. An updated analysis. Breast Cancer Res Treat 1999; 54:117.

27. Lonning PE, Taylor PD, Anker G, et al. High-dose estrogen treatment in post-menopausal breast cancer patients heavily exposed to endocrine therapy. Breast Cancer Res Treat 2001; 67:111–116.

28. Stoll BA. Effect of Lyndiol, an oral contraceptive, on breast cancer. Br Med J 1967; 1:150–153.

29. Wakeling AE. Similarities and distinctions in the mode of action of different classes of antioestrogens. Endocr Rel Cancer 2000; 7:17–28.

30. Dauvois S, Daniellan PS, White R, Parker ML. Antiestrogen ICI 164,384 reduces cellular estrogen content by increasing its turnover. Proc Natl Acad Sci USA 1992; 89:4037–4041.

31. Parker MG. Action of pure antiestrogens in inhibiting estrogen receptor function. Breast Cancer Res Treat 1993; 26:131–137.

32. Howell A, Dodwell DJ, Anderson H, Redford J. Response after withdrawal of tamoxifen and progestagens in advanced breast cancer. Ann Oncol 1992; 3:611–617.

33. Robinson SP, Parker CJ, Jordan VC. Preclinical studies with toremiphene as an antitumour agent. Breast Cancer Res Treat 1990; 16:9–17.

34. DiSalle E, Zaccheo T, Ornati G. Antiestrogenic and antitumour properties of the

new triphenylethylene derivative toremiphene in the rat. J Steroid Biochem 1990; 36:203–206.

35. Hard GC, Latropoulos MJ, Jordan K, et al. Major differences in the hepatocarcino-genicity and DNA adduct forming ability between toremiphene and tamoxifen in female Crl;CD (BR) rats. Cancer Res 1993; 53:4534–4541.

36. Karlsson S, Hirsimaki Y, Mantyla E, et al. A two-year dietary carcinogenicity study of the antiestrogen toremiphene in Sprague-Dawley rats. Drug Chem Toxicol 1996; 19:245–266.

37. White IN, DeMatteis F, Davies A, et al. Genotoxic potential of tamoxifen and anologues in female Fischer F344/n rats, DBA/2 and C57BL/6 mice and in human MCL-5 cells. Carcinogenesis 1992; 13:2197–2203.

38. Kangas L, Nieminen AL, Blanco G, et al. A new triphenylethylene compound, Fc-1157a. II. antitumour effects. Cancer Chemother Pharmacol 1986; 17:109–113.

39. Robinson SP, Jordan VC. Antiestrogenic action of toremiphene on hormone-de-pendent, -independent, and heterogenous breast tumour growth in the athymic mouse. Cancer Res 1989; 49:1758–1762.

40. O'Regan RM, Cisneros A, England GM, et al. Effects of the antiestrogens tamox-ifen, toremifene, and ICI 182,780 on endometrial cancer growth. J Natl Cancer Inst 1998; 90:1552–1558.

41. Tomas E, Kauppila A, Blanco G, et al. Comparison between the effects of tamox-ifen and toremifene on the uterus in post-menopausal breast cancer patients. Gy-necol Oncol 1995; 59:241–266.

42. Marttunen MB, Hietanen P, Tiitinen A, Ylikorkala O. Comparison of effects of ta-moxifen and toremiphene on bone biochemistry and bone mineral density in post-menopausal breast cancer patients. J Clin Endocrinol Metab 1998; 83:1158–1162.

43. Vogel CL, Shemano I, Schoenfelder J, et al. Multicenter phase II efficacy trial of toremiphene in tamoxifen-refractory patients with advanced breast cancer. J Clin Oncol 1993; 11:345–350.

44. Pyrhonen S, Valavaara R, Vuorinen J, Hajba A. High dose toremifene in advanced breast cancer resistant to or relapsed during tamoxifen treatment. Breast Cancer Res Treat 1994; 29:223–228.

45. Asaishi K, Tominaga T, Abe O, et al. Efficacy and safety of high-dose NK 622 (toremifene citrate) in tamoxifen failed patients with breast cancer. Gan To Kagaku Ryoho 1993; 20:91–99.

46. Jonsson PE, Malmberg M, Bergljung L, et al. Phase II study of high dose toremifene in advanced breast cancer progressing during tamoxifen treatment. An-ticancer Res 1991; 11:873–876.

47. Stenbygaard LE, Herrstedt J, Thomsen JF, et al. Toremifene and tamoxifen in ad-vanced breast cancer—A double-blind cross-over trial. Breast Cancer Res Treat 1993; 25:57–63.

48. Wiseman LR, Goa KL. Toremifene; a review of its pharmacological properties and clinical efficacy in the management of advanced breast cancer. Drugs 1997; 54:141–160.

49. Valavaara R, Pyrhonen S. Low dose toremifene in the treatment of estrogen

receptor positive advanced breast cancer in post-menopausal women. Curr Ther Res 1989; 46:966–973.

50. Nomura Y, Tominaga T, Abe O, et al. Clinical evaluation of NK 622 (toremifene citrate) in advanced or recurrent breast cancer—A comparative study by a double-blind method with tamoxifen. Gan To Kagaku Ryoho 1993; 20: 247–258.

51. Hayes DF, Van Zyl JA, Hacking A, et al. Randomized comparison of tamoxifen and two separate doses of toremifene in post-menopausal patients with metastatic breast cancer. J Clin Oncol 1995; 13:2556–2566.

52. Pyrhonen S, Valavaara R, Modig H, et al. Comparison of toremifene and tamoxifen in post-menopausal patients with advanced breast cancer: A randomised double-blind, the "Nordic" phase III study. Br J Cancer 1997; 76:270–277.

53. Gershanovich M, Garin A, Baltina D, et al. A phase III comparison of two toremifene doses to tamoxifen in post-menopausal women with advanced breast cancer. Breast Cancer Res Treat 1997; 45:251–262.

54. Milla-Santos A, Milla L, Rallo L, Solano V. Phase III trial of toremifene vs tamoxifen in hormonodependent advanced breast cancer. Breast Cancer Res Treat 2001; 65:119–124.

55. Pyrhonen S, Ellman J, Vuorinen J, et al. Meta-analysis of trials comparing toremiphene with tamoxifen and factors predicting outcome of antiestrogen therapy in post-menopausal women with breast cancer. Breast Cancer Res Treat 1999; 56:133–143.

56. Holli K, Valvaara R, Blanco G, et al. Toxicity and early survival results of a prospective randomized adjuvant trial comparing toremifene and tamoxifen in node-positive breast cancer. Proc Am Soc Clin Oncol 2000; 19:87a.

57. Roos WK, Oeze L, Loser R, Eppenberger U, et al. Antiestrogen action of 3-hydroxy-tamoxifen in the human breast cancer cell line MCF-7. J Natl Cancer Inst 1983; 71:55–59.

58. Eppenberger U, Wosikowski K, Kung W. Pharmacologic and biologic properties of droloxifene, a new antiestrogen. Am J Clin Oncol 1991; 141:S5–S14.

59. Loser R, Seibel K, Roos W, Eppenberger U. In vivo and in vitro antiestrogenic action of 3-hydroxytamoxifen, tamoxifen and 4-hydroxytamoxifen. Eur J Cancer Clin Oncol 1985; 21:985–990.

60. Hasmann M, Rattel B, Loser, R. Preclinical data for droloxifene. Cancer Lett 1994; 84:89–95.

61. Ke H, Simmons HA, Pierie CM, et al. Droloxifene, a new estrogen antagonist/agonist, prevents bone loss in ovariectomised rats. Endocrinology 1995; 136:2435–2441.

62. Stamm H, Roth R, Almendral A, et al. Tolerance and efficacy of the antiestrogen droloxifene in patients with advanced breast cancer. J Steroid Biochem 1987; 28(suppl):1085.

63. Brietbach GP, Moous V, Bastert G, et al. Droloxifene: Efficacy and endocrine effects in treatment of metastatic breast cancer. J Steroid Biochem 1987; 28(suppl):1095.

64. Haarstad H, Gundersen S, Wist E, Raabe N, Mella O, Kvinnsland S. Droloxifene—A new antiestrogen. Acta Oncol 1992; 31:425–428.

65. Bruning PF. Droloxifene, a new antioestrogen in post-menopausal advanced breast cancer: Preliminary results of a double-blind dose-finding phase II trial. Eur J Cancer 1992; 28A:1404–1407.

66. Rausching W, Pritchard KI. Droloxifene, a new antiestrogen: Its role in metastatic breast cancer. Breast Cancer Res Treat 1994; 31:83–94.

67. Haarstad H, Lonning P, Gundersen S, et al. Influence of droloxifene on metastatic breast cancer as first-line endocrine treatment. Acta Oncol 1998; 37:365–368.

68. Dhingra K. Antiestrogens; tamoxifen, SERMs and beyond. Invest New Drugs 1999; 17:285–311.

69. Lien EA, Lonning PE. Selective oestrogen receptor modifiers (SERMs) and breast cancer therapy. Cancer Treat Rev 2000; 26:205–227.

70. McCague R, Leclerq G, Legros N, et al. Derivatives of tamoxifen: Dependence of antiestrogenicity on the 4-substituent. J Med Chem 1980; 32:2527–2533.

71. Chander SK, McCague R, Luqmani Y, et al. Pyrrolidino-4-iodotamoxifen and 4-iodotamoxifen, new analogues of the antiestrogen tamoxifen for the treatment of breast cancer. Cancer Res 1991; 51:5851–5858.

72. Nuttall ME, Bradbeer JN, Stroup GB, et al. A novel selective estrogen receptor modulator prevents bone loss and lowers cholesterol in ovariectomised rats and decreases uterine weight in intact rats. Endocrinology 1998; 139:5224–5234.

73. Johnston SRD, Riddler S, Haynes BP, et al. The novel antioestrogen idoxifene inhibits the growth of human MCF-7 breast cancer xenografts and reduces the frequency of acquired antiestrogen resistance. Br J Cancer 1997; 75:804–809.

74. Coombes RC, Haynes BP, Dowsett M, et al. Idoxifene: Report of a phase I study in patients with metastatic breast cancer. Cancer Res 1995; 55:1070–1074.

75. Johnston SRD, Gumbrell L, Evans TRJ, et al. A phase II randomized double-blind study of idoxifene (40 mg/d) vs. tamoxifen (40 mg/d) in patients with locally advanced/metastatic breast cancer resistant to tamoxifen (20 mg/d). Proc Am Soc Clin Oncol 1999; 18:109 (abstr 413).

76. Johnston SRD, Gorbunova V, Lichinister M, et al. A multicentre double-blind randomized phase III trial of idoxifene versus tamoxifen as first-line endocrine therapy for metastatic breast cancer. Proc Am Soc Clin Oncol 2001; 20:A113.

77. Toko T, Sugimoto Y, Matsuo E, et al. TAT-59, a new triphenylethylene derivative with antitumour activity against hormone-dependent tumors. Eur J Cancer 1990; 26:397–404.

78. Lino Y, Takai Y, Ando T, et al. A new triphenylethylene derivative TAT-59: Hormone receptors, insulin-like growth factor 1 and growth suppression of hormone dependent MCF-7 tumours in athymic mice. Cancer Chemother Pharmacol 1994; 34:372–376.

79. Nomura Y, Nakajima M, Tominaga, Abe O. Late phase II study of TAT-59 (miproxifene phosphate) in advanced or recurrent breast cancer patients (a double blind comparative study with tamoxifen citrate). Gan To Kagaku Ryoho 1998; 25:1045–1063.

80. Wilson TM, Norris JD, Wagner BL, et al. Dissection of the molecular mechanism of action of GW5638, a novel estrogen receptor ligand, provides insights into the role of estrogen receptor in bone. Endocrinology 1997; 138:3901–3911.

81. Ke HZ, Paralkar VM, Grasser WA, et al. Effects of CP-336,156, a new non-steroidal estrogen agonist/antagonist, on bone, serum cholesterol, uterus and body composition in rat models. Endocrinology 1998; 139:2068–2076.

82. Howell A, DeFriend D, Robertson J, et al. Response to a specific antiestrogen (ICI182,780) in tamoxifen-resistant breast cancer. Lancet 1995; 345:29–30.

83. Robertson JFR, Howell A, DeFriend D, et al. Duration of remission to ICI182,780 compared to megestrol acetate in tamoxifen-resistant breast cancer. Breast 1997; 6:186–189.

84. Black LJ, Jones CD, Folcone JF. Antagonism of estrogen action with a new benzothiophene-derived antiestrogen. Life Sci 1983; 32:1031–1036.

85. Moulin R, Merand Y, Poirier D. Antiestrogenic properties of keoxifene, trans-4-hydroxytamoxifen and ICI 164,384, a new steroidal antiestrogen in ZR-75-1 human breast cancer cells. Breast Cancer Res Treat 1989; 14:65–76.

86. Gottardis MM, Jordan VC. The antitumor action of keoxifene (raloxifene) and tamoxifen in the N-nitromethylurea-induce rat mammary carcinoma model. Cancer Res 1987; 47:4020–4024.

87. Jordan VC, Robinson SP. Species specific pharmacology of antiestrogens: Role of metabolism. Fed Proc 1987; 46:1870–1874.

88. Balfour JA, Goa KL. Raloxifene. Drugs Aging 1998; 12:335–341.

89. Delmas PD, Bjarnason NH, Mitlak BH, et al. Effects of raloxifene on bone mineral density, serum cholesterol concentrations, and uterine endometrium in postmenopausal women. N Engl J Med 1997; 337:1641–1647.

90. Buzdar A, Marcus C, Holmes F, et al. Phase II evaluation of LY156758 in metastatic breast cancer. Oncology 1988; 45:344–345.

91. Gradishar WJ, Glusman JE, Vogel CL, et al. Raloxifene HCL, a new endocrine agent, is active in estrogen receptor positive (ER +) metastatic breast cancer. Breast Cancer Res Treat 1997; 46:53 (abstr 209).

92. Cummings SR, Eckert S, Krueger KA, et al. A, Jordan VC. The effect of raloxifene on risk of breast cancer in postmenopausal women: Results from the Multiple Outcomes of Raloxifene Evaluation (MORE) randomized trial. JAMA 1999; 281:2189–2197.

93. Cauley JA, Norton L, Lippman ME, et al. Continued breast cancer risk reduction in post-menopausal women treated with raloxifene: 4-year results from the MORE trial. Breast Cancer Res Treat 2001; 65:125–134.

94. Sato M, Turner CH, Wang TY, et al. A novel raloxifene analogue with improved SERM potency and efficacy in vivo. J Pharmacol Exp Ther 1998; 287:1–7.

95. Fuchs-Young R, Iversen P, Shelton P, et al. Preclinical demonstration of specific and potent inhibition of mammary tumour growth by new selective estrogen receptor modulators (SERMs). Proc Am Assoc Cancer Res 1997; 38:A3847.

96. Johnston SRD, Riddler S, Detre S, Dowsett M. Dose-dependent inhibition of MCF-7 breast cancer xenograft growth with LY353381, a novel selective estrogen receptor modulator (SERM). Proc Am Assoc Cancer Res 2000; 41:25 (abstr 164).

97. Sato M, Zeng GQ, Rowley E, et al. LY353381.HCL; an improved benzothiphene analogue with bone efficacy complimentary to parathyroid hormone-(1–34). Endocrinology 1998; 139:4642–4651.

98. Rowley E, Adrian MD, Bryant H, et al. The new SERM LY353381.HCL has advantages over estrogen, tamoxifen, and raloxifene in reproductive and nonreproductive tissues of aged ovariectomised rats. Proc Am Soc Bone Min Res 1997; A490.

99. Munster PN, Buzdar A, Dhingra K, et al. Phase I study of a third generation selective estrogen receptor modulator LY353381.HCL in metastatic breast cancer. J Clin Oncol 2001; 19:2002–2009.

100. Baselga J, Llombart-Cussat A, Bellet M, et al. Double-blind randomized phase II study of a selective estrogen receptor modulator in patients with I locally advanced or metastatic breast cancer. Breast Cancer Res Treat 1999; 57:A25.

101. Buzdar A, O'Shaughnessy J, Hudis C, et al. Preliminary results of a randomized double-blind phase II study of the selective estrogen receptor modulator (SERM) arzoxifene in patients with locally advanced or metastatic breast cancer. Proc Am Soc Clin Oncol 2001; 20:A178.

102. Labrie F, Labrie C, Belanger A, et al. EM-652 (SCH 57068), a third generation SERM acting as a pure antiestrogen in the mammary gland and endometrium. J Steroid Biochem Mol Biol 1999; 69:51–84.

103. Martel C, Provencher L, Li X, et al. Labrie F. Binding characteristics of novel antiestrogens to the rat uterine estrogen receptors. J Steroid Biochem Mol Biol 1998; 64:199–205.

104. Simard J, Labrie CL, Belanger A, et al. Characterisation of the effects of the novel non-steroidal antiestrogen EM-800 on basal and estrogen-induced proliferation of T47-D, ZR-75-1 and MCF-7 human breast cancer cells in vitro. Int J Cancer 1997; 73:104–112.

105. Couillard S, Gutman M, Labrie C, et al. Comparison of the effects of the antiestrogens EM-800 and tamoxifen on the growth of human breast ZR-75-1 cancer xenografts in nude mice. Cancer Res 1998; 58:60–64.

106. Luo S, Martel C, Sourla A, et al. Comparative effects of 28-day treatment with the new anti-estrogen EM-800 and tamoxifen on estrogen-sensitive parameters in intact mice. Int J Cancer 1997; 73:381–391.

107. Simard J, Sanchez R, Poirier D, et al. Blockade of the stimulatory effect of estrogens, OH-tamoxifen, OH-toremifene, andraloxifene on alkaline phosphatase activity by the antiestrogen EM-800 in human endometrial adenocarcinoma Ishikawa cells. Cancer Res 1997; 57:3494–3497.

108. Johnston SRD, Detre S, Riddler S, Dowsett M. SCH 57068 is a selective estrogen receptor modulator (SERM) without uterotrophic effects compared with either tamoxifen or raloxifene. Breast Cancer Res Treat 2000; 64:A163.

109. Martel C, Picard S, Richard V, et al. Prevention of bone loss by EM-800 and raloxifene in the ovariectomised rat. J Steroid Biochem Mol Biol 2000; 74:45–56.

110. Labrie F, Champagne P, Labrie C, et al. Response to the orally active specific antiestrogen EM-800 (SCH-57070) in tamoxifen-resistant breast cancer. Breast Cancer Res Treat 1997; 42:A211.

111. Howell A, DeFriend DJ, Robertson JF, et al. Pharmacokinetics, pharmacological and antitumour effects of the specific anti-oestrogen ICI 182780 in women with advanced breast cancer. Br J Cancer 1996; 4:300–308.

112. Wakeling AE, Dukes M, Bowler J. A potent specific pure antioestrogen with clinical potential. Cancer Res 1991; 51:3867–3873.
113. Wakeling AE, Bowler J. ICI 182,780, a new antioestrogen with clinical potential. J Steroid Biochem Mol Biol 1992; 43:173–177.
114. van de Velde P, Nique F, Planchon P, et al. RU 58668: a further in vitro and in vivo pharmacological data related to its antitumoral activity. J Steroid Biochem Mol Biol 1996; 59:449–457.
115. Pink JJ, Jordan VC. Models of estrogen receptor regulation by oestrogens and antioestrogens in breast cancer cell lines. Cancer Res 1996; 56:2321–2330.
116. Dukes M, Miller D, Wakeling AE, Waterton JC. Antiuterotrophic effects of a pure antioestrogen, ICI 182780: Magnetic resonance imaging of the uterus in ovariectomised monkeys. J Endocrinol 1992; 134:239–247.
117. Dowsett M, Howell R, Salter J, et al. Effects of the pure anti-estrogen ICI 182780 on estrogen receptors, progesterone receptors and Ki67 antigen in human endometrium in vivo. Hum Reprod 1995; 10:262–267.
118. Robertson JFR, Nicholson R, Anderson E, et al. The anti-tumour effects of single dose long acting faslodex (ICI182780) compared with tamoxifen in postmenopausal primary breast cancer patients treated before surgery. Breast Cancer Res Treat 2000; 59:99.
119. Howell A, Robertson JFR, Quaresma-Albano J, et al. Comparison of efficacy and tolerability of fulvestrant (Faslodex™) with anastrozole (Arimidex™) in post menopausal women with advanced breast cancer (ABC)-preliminary results. Breast Cancer Res Treat 2000; 64:A27.
120. Osborne CK, Pippen J, Jones SE, et al. Faslodex (ICI 182,780) shows longer duration of response compared with arimidex (anastrozole) in post-menopausal (PM) women with advanced breast cancer (ABC). Preliminary results of a phase III North American trial. Breast Cancer Res Treat 2001; 65:A261.
121. Nabholtz JM, Buzdar A, Pollack M, et al. Anastrozole is superior to tamoxifen as first-line therapy for advanced breast cancer in postmenopausal women: Results of a North American multicenter randomized trial. J Clin Oncol 2000; 18:3758–3767.
122. Bonneterre J, Thurlimann B, Robertson JFR, et al. Anastrozole versus tamoxifen as first-line therapy for advanced breast cancer in 688 postmenopausal women: Results of the tamoxifen or arimidex randomized group efficacy and tolerability study. J Clin Oncol 2000; 18:3748–3757.
123. Mouridsen H, Gershanovich M, Sun Y, et al. Superior efficacy of letrozole (femara) versus tamoxifen as first-line therapy for post-menopausal women with advanced breast cancer: Results of a phase III study of the International Letrozole Breast Cancer Group. J Clin Oncol 2001; 19:2596–2606, 2001.
124. Masamura S, Santner SJ, Heitjan DF, Santen RJ. Estrogen deprivation causes estradiol hypersensitivity in human breast cancer cells. J Clin Endocrinol Metab 1995; 80:2918–2925.
125. Klijn JGN, Blamey RW, Boccardo F, et al. Combined tamoxifen and luteinising hormone-releasing hormone (LHRH) agonist versus LHRH agonist alone in premenopausal advanced breast cancer: A meta-analysis of four randomized trials. J Clin Oncol 2001; 19:343–353.

126. Dowsett M, Dixon JM, Horgan K, et al. Antiproliferative effect of idoxifene in a placebo-controlled trial in primary human breast cancer. Clin Cancer Res 2000; 6:2260–2267.

127. Dowsett M, Lu Y, Hills M, et al. Effect of raloxifene on Ki67 and apoptosis. Breast Cancer Res Treat 1999; 57:31.

128. DeFriend D, Howell A, Nicholson RI, et al. Investigation of a new pure antiestrogen (ICI 182,780) in women with primary breast cancer. Cancer Res 1995; 54:408–414

5

Other Endocrine and Biological Agents in the Treatment of Advanced Breast Cancer

Jan G. M. Klijn, Els M. J. J. Berns, and John A. Foekens
Daniel den Hoed Cancer Center
Erasmus University Medical Center
Rotterdam, The Netherlands

I. ABSTRACT

Numerous factors such as oncogenes, tumor suppressor genes, hormones, growth factors and receptors, proteases, cytokines and others are involved in either malignant transformation, (de)differentiation, proliferation, tumor invasion, distant metastasis, neoangiogenesis, and/or development of therapy resistance. Modern cell biological parameters can be used for (a) determination of prognosis; (b) selection of (high-risk) patients for therapy; (c) selection of specific therapy, depending on tumor and patients characteristics; and (d) development of new treatment modalities using these biological parameters for molecular target-directed therapies. Modern molecular biological techniques are used for molecular profiling, molecular monitoring, and molecular targeting. In this chapter, we discuss several new developments in the endocrine and biological therapy of breast cancer. The development of an increasing number of new biologicals will make future research very exciting.

II. INTRODUCTION

Apart from antisteroidal agents—such as selective estrogen receptor modulators (SERMs) and estrogen receptor downregulators (for example, a pure antiestrogen such as Faslodex) as well as aromatase inhibitors—other endocrine and biological agents play an increasingly important role in the treatment of breast cancer. It will be difficult to review all these agents, because, as was highlighted in the abstracts of the last American Society of Clinical Oncology (ASCO) meeting in San Francisco, more than 300 agents are currently reported to be under investigation. The Pharmaceutical Research and Manufacturers of America, an organization representing the research-based pharmaceutical industry, has also conducted a recent survey, which concluded that more than 350 new medicines for the treatment of cancer are under development [1–3]. For this reason, this discussion focuses on our data; the reader is referred to the cited articles for more extensive reference lists on the various topics.

III. LH–RH AGONISTS

Since our first report [4] on the treatment of premenopausal metastatic breast cancer, the results of a series of phase II and phase III studies with different luteinizing hormone–releasing hormone (LH-RH) analogues have been published, showing an objective response in 161 (38%) of 419 patients [5]. There appeared to be no difference in efficacy between single LH-RH agonist treatment and surgical oophorectomy [6] or tamoxifen [7]. However, based on a pivotal three-arm trial, the treatment combination of a LH-RH agonist and tamoxifen was superior to treatment with either drug alone with respect to response rate, progression-free survival, and overall survival (Table 1) [7]. The plasma estradiol concentrations were strongly increased in those patients treated with long-term tamoxifen therapy only, but these were suppressed to postmenopausal values with the addition of the LH-RH agonist buserelin [7]. Most striking were the effects on overall survival, which showed a doubling of the actuarial 5-year survival percentages during combined treatment (34%) versus single treatment [15–18%). The results of this trial were confirmed by a recent meta-analysis (Table 2) and have consequences for the application in the adjuvant setting [7–10]. Two studies using surgical oophorectomy and two others using medical castration by goserelin and leuprolide, respectively, showed no difference in disease-free and overall survival in patients with ER-positive primary tumors when compared with standard cyclophosphamide/methotrexate/5-fluorouracil (CMF) chemotherapy [7,9,10]. Five other trials demonstrated that the combination of a LH-RH agonist and tamoxifen tended to be superior or substantially superior to standard chemotherapy with the CMF or cyclophosphamide/adriamycin/5-fluorouracil (CAF) regimens. The results of the intergroup study of Davidson et al. indicated that the effects of adjuvant treatment with tamoxifen after CAF chemotherapy

Table 1 Summary of Results EORTC Trial 10881

Parameter	LHRH agonist N=54	Tamoxifen N=54	LHRH agonist + tamoxifen N=53	p Value
CR + PR	34%	28%	48%	0.11
NR	36%	26%	31%	
PD	30%	46%	21%	
Not evaluable (n)	7	4	5	
CR + PR + NC >6 months	62%	44%	75%	0.007
Median PFS (months)	6.3	5.6	9.7	0.03
Median overall Survival (years)	2.5	2.9	3.7	0.01
Actuarial survival at 5 years	15%	19%	34%	
Actuarial survival at 7 years	5%	10%	30%	

Key: EORTC, European Organization for Research and Treatment of Cancer; *N,* number; CR, complete response; PR, partial response; NC, no change; PD, progressive disease; PFS, progression-free survival.

may be greater among women who have had cessation of ovarian function, either as a result of chemotherapy (in women above 40 years of age) or by the addition of goserelin (especially in women below 40 years) [9,10]. However, in contrast to metastatic disease [7], in the adjuvant setting, a randomized trial comparing combined LH-RH agonist plus tamoxifen treatment with tamoxifen treatment alone is lacking.

Table 2 Summary Results of a Meta-Analysis of Four Randomized Trials Comparing an LH-RH[a] Agonist Alone with the Combined Treatment of Tamoxifen Plus an LH-RH Agonist in Premenopausal Advanced Breast Cancer

Endpoint	LH-RH agonist alone N=256	LH-RH agonist plus tamoxifen N=250	Hazard ratio/ odds ratio (95% CI)	Log rank p value
Objective response	29.7%	38.8%	0.67 (0.46–0.96)	0.03
Median progression-free survival (months)	5.4	8.7	0.70 (0.58–0.85)	0.0003
Median overall survival (years)	2.5	2.9	0.78 (0.63–0.96)	0.02

[a]Luteinizing hormone–releasing hormone.
Source: Ref. 8.

In view of the greater efficacy of combined treatment in metastatic disease [7,8] and the fact that, in comparison with standard adjuvant chemotherapy, combined endocrine treatment is more effective than single-agent treatment [9,10] with surgical or medical castration in the adjuvant setting, it can be concluded that combined endocrine treatment must now be the standard endocrine therapy in premenopausal patients.

IV. OTHER ENDOCRINE AGENTS

Several other endocrine agents can be used in the treatment of breast cancer [11]. Of special interest are progesterone antagonists and progesterone receptor modulators (Table 3) [12,13]. Progesterone antagonists (antiprogestins) or progesterone receptor (PgR) modulators (PRMs) form an interesting category of new hormonal agents in the treatment of breast cancer. In vitro, the antiproliferative effects of different progesterone antagonists are mainly observed in estrogen-stimulated growth of PgR-positive tumor cell lines. Depending on the type of cell line, the culture medium, and the concentration of the agent used, the prog-

Table 3 Antitumor Effects of Single Treatment with Antiprogestins in Postmenopausal Patients with Metastatic Breast Cancer

Authors	Anti progestin	Dose (mg/day)	N	CR	PR	NC	PD
Pretreated patients							
Romieu et al. (1987)	Mifepristone (third-line)	200	22	0	3	9	10
Klijn et al. (1989)	Mifepristone (second-line)	200–400	11	0	1	6	4
Jonat et al. (1994)	Onapristone (second-line)	100	90	1	8	38	43
		TOTAL	123	1	12	53	57
				(1%)	(10%)	(43%)	(46%)
First-line patients							
Perrault et al. (1996)	Mifepristone (first-line)	200	28	0	3 (11%)	11 (39%)	14
Robertson et al. (1999)	Onapristone (first-line)	100	18	0	10 (56%)	2 (11%)	7
		TOTAL	46	0 (0%)	13 (28%)	13 (28%)	21 (46%)

Key: N, number; CR, complete response; PR, partial response; NC, no change; PD, progressive disease.
Source: Ref. 13.

esterone antagonists can be found to have stimulatory or inhibitory effects on the biological response measured [13]. In various experimental models involving tumors in animals, different progesterone antagonists showed greater antitumor activity than tamoxifen or high-dose progestins. Most interestingly, combination treatment of different progesterone antagonists (mifepristone, ORG 31710, onapristone) or PRMs with either different antiestrogens (tamoxifen, droloxifen, ICI 164384), or an aromatase inhibitor (atemestane), showed greater antitumor efficacy than treatment with each single type of drug alone [13,14]. These additive antiproliferative effects were demonstrated in various experimental in vitro and in vivo models. In some studies, these effects were accompanied by additive effects on several cell biological parameters. In pretreated postmenopausal patients with metastatic breast cancer, objective responses have been observed in 10–12%, and stable disease recorded for about 42–46% of patients (Table 3). In two trials of antiprogestins in previously untreated patients, on the other hand, objective response rates of 11% and 56% were reported (Table 3) [13]. The clinical development of onapristone has now been stopped because of liver toxicity. The development of potent new progesterone antagonists and further clinical investigation of combined therapy using progesterone antagonists with antiestrogens are therefore urgently needed.

V. THERAPIES DIRECTED AT MOLECULAR TARGETS

The development of tests for biological markers allows us to improve (a) determination of prognosis, (b) selection of (high-risk) patients for therapy, (c) selection of specific therapy depending on tumor and patient characteristics, and (d) development of new treatment modalities. Numerous markers such as oncogenes, tumor suppressor genes, hormones, growth factors and receptors, proteases, cytokines, and other factors are involved in malignant transformation, (de)differentiation, proliferation, tumor invasion, distant metastasis, neoangiogenesis, and/or development of therapy resistance. Many of these biological parameters have been investigated as prognostic factors in patients with breast cancer [15–17].

In the last decade, we have investigated a large series of these factors with respect to their value for prediction of prognosis and response to endocrine and systemic chemotherapy [15,16,18–36]. The best predictors for a good response to treatment with tamoxifen were found to be the estrogen receptor (ER), PgR, and PS2 [20], while TP53 mutations [32], p53 overexpression [26], HER2/neu amplification or overexpression [15,16,22], epidermal growth factor receptor (EGFR) [15,16], vascular endothelial growth factor (VEGF) [34], urokinase-type plasminogen activator (uPA) [21], and thymidine kinase (TK) [33] appeared to be strong predictors for a poor response to tamoxifen.

VEGF, in addition to being a potent angiogenic factor and an inducer of blood vessel hyperpermeability, has some interesting effects on endothelial cells. It stimulates proliferation and migration; stimulates the expression of adhesion molecules, uPA, uPA receptor (uPAR), and plasminogen activator inhibitor type 1 (PAI-1) as well as matrix metalloproteinase type 2 (MMP-2); and it decreases the expression of TIMP-1 and TIMP-2. In our recent study of 845 primary breast tumors, the cytosolic levels of VEGF were inversely related to those of ER and PgR [34]. Breast tumors with high levels of VEGF were more likely to metastasize to the viscera than to the bone and soft tissues. For patients with advanced breast cancer, the tumor VEGF level appeared to be an independent marker predicting a poor outcome on first-line tamoxifen or CMF/FAC chemotherapy [34].

Table 4 contains some examples of present therapies directed to molecular targets. Rituxan, a monoclonal antibody directed against the CD20 antigen of B cells, has induced remissions in approximately 50% of relapsed or refractory subtypes of malignant lymphoma. Recently the signal transduction inhibitor Gliveec (imatinib mesylate; ST1-571) appeared to induce spectacular remissions in patients with gastrointestinal stromal tumors (GIST-tumors) [37] and chronic myeloid leukemias [38]. The efficacy of this compound in targeting c-Kit mutations and platelet-derived growth factor (PDGF) receptors will be tested in patients with other tumor types in the near future.

Several matrix metalloproteinase inhibitors are in clinical development (Table 5), but more powerful and specific inhibitors are needed [39,40]. Endostatin and angiostatin are presently being tested in phase I studies. Another new

Table 4 Therapies Directed at Molecular Targets

Compound
Rituxan
Herceptin (anti-Her2/neu)
EGFR inhibitors:
C-225 (Cetuximab)
ZD-1839 (Iressa)
OSI-774
PKI-166
STI-571 (Gliveec)
Angiogenesis inhibitors:
Endostatin
Angiostatin
Anti-VEGF
Matrix metalloproteinase inhibitors
Farnesyl transferase inhibitors

Key: EGFR, epidermal growth factor receptor; VEGF, vascular endothelial growth factor.

Table 5   Matrix Metalloproteinase (MMP) Inhibitors in Clinical
Development

Compound	Company	Status
AG3340	Agouron Pharmaceuticals	Phase II/III
BAY 12-9566	Bayer Corporation	Development halted
BMS 275291	Bristol-Myers Squibb	Phase I
CGS 27023A	Novartis Pharma	Phase I
Batimastat	British Biotech	No further development
Marimastat	British Biotech	Phase II/III
Col-3 (metastat)	Collagenex	Phase I

Source: Ref 39.

and important class of anticancer drugs comprises farnesyl transferase inhibitors, which are active in tumor cells with and without oncogenic RAS mutations [41].

Currently growth factors and growth factor receptors (Table 6) seem to be the most suitable targets for monoclonal or polyclonal antibody therapy in breast cancer and other types of tumors, but tyrosine kinase and other signal transducing molecules could provide likely targets today and in the future. A good example of this recent work is the development of trastuzumab (Herceptin), a monoclonal antibody directed to the HER2/neu receptor [42–46], which was recently awarded the Galenus Award 2001 (in The Netherlands) as the most innovative medication. As single treatment Herceptin appeared effective in heavily pretreated patients with overexpression of HER2/neu in their breast tumors; but, most interestingly, it appeared to potentiate the efficacy of standard cytotoxic

Table 6   Growth Factors and Receptor
Targets in Breast Cancer

Compound
Epidermal growth factor receptor family
EGFR
HER2/neu
HER3
HER4
Insulin receptor
Insulin-like growth factor type I and II receptors
Fibroblast growth factor family receptors
Vascular endothelial growth factor receptors
Platelet-derived growth factor receptors
Transforming growth factor β receptors
Somatostatin receptors

chemotherapy [42–46], probably by preventing the recovery of damaged tumor cells. Also, in a recent Dutch study, the results of treatment with Herceptin were very promising both as single agent and in combination with chemotherapy (unpublished data). The first study with adjuvant Herceptin began in 2001. Antibodies against EGFR [47] and the VEGF receptor are also presently being tested in clinical trials, but these have shown some serious side effects.

An increasing number of pharmaceutical companies are developing specific tyrosine kinase inhibitors or other drugs interfering with different signal transduction pathways [3]. At the last ASCO meeting in San Francisco, data were presented on the EGFR-tyrosine kinase inhibitor Iressa, which showed it could inhibit estradiol-stimulated tumor cell growth and PgR-expression, that it decreased the proliferation index of ductal carcinomas in situ (DCIS) in xenografts (in contrast to Herceptin), was effective against Herceptin-resistant HER+ mammary tumor cells (MDA-361), and had a synergistic antiproliferative effect in combination with Herceptin in vitro on SK-Br-3 mammary tumor cells that were positive for both EGFR and HER2/neu (over)expression.

Manipulation of the GH-IGF1 axis is another approach for trying to induce tumor remission [15,16,27,48–50]. However, this is complicated owing to physiological functions of growth hormone, insulin-like growth factors, and the many binding proteins involved. Tumors containing high levels of somatostatin receptors can be successfully targeted by radioactive somatostatin analogues.

VI. FUTURE PROSPECTS

Molecular biological techniques will not be used only for molecular targeting for future medications but also for molecular profiling and molecular monitoring [51–54]. With respect to treatment, combined treatment modalities seem to be most promising at present (Table 7). However, the development of new biologi-

Table 7 Future Aspects

Combined treatment modalities that are most promising:
• Combined endocrine therapy
• Combined blockade of different signal transduction pathways
• Combination of growth factor antagonists and protease inhibitors (antimetastatic agents) or inhibitors of angiogenesis
• Standard systemic (antiproliferative) therapies in combination with new biological treatments

Problems:
• Rapidly growing (and already huge) number of biologicals
• Not enough patients for testing all potential combinations
• Need for preclinical testing
• Too much paperwork and bureaucracy

---

cal agents [1–3] will increase rapidly in the forthcoming decades, raising several problems. The addition of the usually expensive biological agents to the world market of oncology drugs will increase costs. Another problem will be the mounting difficulty of finding enough patients and monitoring facilities to carry out the trials required to test these compounds, both as single agents and in combination therapies. There will be increasing pressure to test possible combinations in preclinical experimental models to select the most effective ones. Nonetheless, in spite of the heavy burden of paperwork and bureaucracy, the prospect of all these scientific developments promises to make the next decade very exciting.

ACKNOWLEDGMENT

We thank Petra Bos for typing the manuscript.

REFERENCES

1. Schein PS. The case for a new national program for development of cancer therapeutics. J Clin Oncol 2001; 19:3142–3153.
2. Holmer AF. Survey: New medicines in development for cancer—354 new weapons are in development for the war on cancer. Washington, DC: Pharmaceutical Research and Manufacturers of America, 1999.
3. Sausville EA, Johnson JI. Molecules for the millennium: How will they look? New drug discovery year 2000. Br J Cancer 2000; 83:1401–1404.
4. Klijn JGM, de Jong FH. Treatment with a luteinising-hormone–releasing-hormone analogue (Buserelin) in premenopausal patients with metastatic breast cancer. Lancet 1982; 1:1213–1216.
5. Klijn JGM. LH-RH analogs in the treatment of metastatic breast cancer: Ten years experience. In: Höffken K, ed. Peptides in Oncology: LH-RH Agonists and Antagonists. Berlin: Springer-Verlag, 1992:75–90.
6. Taylor CW, Green S, Dalton WS, et al. Multicenter randomized clinical trial of goserelin versus surgical ovariectomy in premenopausal patients with receptor-positive metastatic breast cancer. An intergroup study. J Clin Oncol 1998; 16:994–999.
7. Klijn JGM, Beex LVAM, Mauriac L, et al. and members of the EORTC Breast Cancer Cooperative Group. Combined treatment with buserelin and tamoxifen in premenopausal metastatic breast cancer: a randomized study. J Natl Cancer Inst 2000; 92:903–911.
8. Klijn JGM, Blamey RW, Boccardo F, et al. for the Combined Hormone Agents Trialists' Group and the European Organization for Research and Treatment of Cancer. Combined tamoxifen and luteinizing hormone–releasing hormone (LHRH) agonist versus LHRH agonist alone in premenopausal advanced breast cancer: a meta-analysis of four randomized trials. J Clin Oncol 2001; 19:343–353.
9. Davidson NE. Combined endocrine therapy for breast cancer—New life for an old idea? J Natl Cancer Inst 2000; 92:859–860.

10. Henderson IC. Endocrine therapy, chemotherapy, or both as adjuvant systemic treatment of patients with early breast cancer. Educational Book ASCO, 2001:53–60.

11. Klijn JGM, Setyono-Han B, Bontenbal M, et al. Novel endocrine therapies in breast cancer. Acta Oncol 1996; 35:30–37.

12. Klijn JGM, de Jong FH, Bakker GH, et al. Antiprogestins, a new form of endocrine therapy for human breast cancer. Cancer Res 1989; 49:2851–2856.

13. Klijn JGM, Setyono-Han B, Foekens JA. Progesterone antagonists and progesterone receptor modulators in the treatment of breast cancer. Steroids 2000; 65:825–830.

14. Bakker GH, Setyono-Han B, Portengen H, et al. Endocrine and antitumor effects of combined treatment with an antiprogestin and antiestrogen or luteinizing hormone–releasing hormone agonist in female rats bearing mammary tumors. Endocrinology 1989; 125:1593–1598.

15. Klijn JGM, Berns EMJJ, Foekens JA. Prognostic factors and response to therapy in breast cancer. Cancer Surveys 1993; 18:165–198.

16. Klijn JGM, Berns EMJJ, Foekens JA. Prognostic and predictive factors in breast cancer. In: Manni A, ed. Contemporary Endocrinology: Endocrinology of Breast Cancer. Totowa, NJ: Humana Press, 1999:205–220.

17. Isaacs C, Stearns V, Hayes DF. New prognostic factors for breast cancer recurrence. Semin Oncol 2001; 28:53–67.

18. Foekens JA, Portengen H, van Putten WLJ, et al. Prognostic value of receptors for insulin-like growth factor 1, somatostatin, and epidermal growth factor in human breast cancer. Cancer Res 1989; 49:7002–7009.

19. Klijn JGM, Berns EMJJ, Schmitz PIM, Foekens JA. The clinical significance of epidermal growth factor receptor (EGF-R) in human breast cancer: A review on 5232 patients. Endocr Rev 1992; 13:3–18.

20. Foekens JA, Portengen H, Look MP, et al. Relationship of pS$_2$ with response to tamoxifen therapy in patients with recurrent breast cancer. Br J Cancer 1994; 70:1217–1223.

21. Foekens JA, Look MP, Peters HA, et al. Urokinase-type plasminogen activator (uPA) and its inhibitors PAI-1 predict poor response to tamoxifen therapy in recurrent breast cancer. J Natl Cancer Inst 1995; 87:751–756.

22. Berns EMJJ, Foekens JA, van Staveren IL, et al. Portengen H, Klijn JGM. Oncogene amplification and prognosis in breast cancer: Relationship with systemic treatment. Gene 1995; 159:11–18.

23. Foekens JA, Klijn JGM, Natoli C, et al. Expression of tumor-associated 90K-antigen in human breast cancer: No correlation with prognosis and response to first-line therapy with tamoxifen. Int J Cancer 1995; 64:130–134.

24. Nooter K, Brutel de la Rivière G, Klijn JGM, et al. Multidrug resistance protein in recurrent breast cancer. Lancet 1997; 349:1885–1886.

25. Nooter K, Brutel de la Riviere G, Look MP, et al. The prognostic significance of expression of the multidrug resistance-associated protein (MRP) in primary breast cancer. Br J Cancer 1997; 76:486–493.

26. Berns EMJJ, Klijn JGM, van Putten WLJ, et al. p53 Protein accumulation predicts poor response to tamoxifen therapy of patients with recurrent breast cancer. J Clin Oncol 1998; 16:121–127.

27. Bontenbal M, Foekens JA, Lamberts SWJ, et al. Feasibility, endocrine and anti-tumour effects of a triple endocrine therapy with tamoxifen, a somatostatin analogue and an antiprolactin in post-menopausal metastatic breast cancer: A randomized study with long-term follow-up. Br J Cancer 1998; 77:115–122.

28. Berns EMJJ, van Staveren IL, Klijn JGM, Foekens JA. Predictive value of SRC-1 for tamoxifen response of recurrent breast cancer. Breast Cancer Res Treat 1998; 48:87–92.

29. Foekens JA, Diamandis EP, Yu H, et al. Expression of prostate specific antigen (PSA) correlates with poor response to tamoxifen therapy in recurrent breast cancer. Br J Cancer 1999; 79:888–894.

30. van der Flier S, Brinkman A, Look MP, et al. Bcar1/p130Cas protein and primary breast cancer: Prognosis and response to tamoxifen treatment. J Natl Cancer Inst 2000, 92:120–127.

31. Foekens JA, Peters HA, Look MP, et al. The urokinase system of plasminogen activation and prognosis in 2780 breast cancer patients. Cancer Res 2000; 60:636–643.

32. Berns EMJJ, Foekens JA, Vossen R, et al. Complete sequencing of TP53 predicts poor response to systemic therapy of advanced breast cancer. Cancer Res 2000; 60:2155–2162.

33. Foekens JA, Romain S, Look MP, et al. Thymidine kinase and thymidylate synthase in advanced breast cancer: response to tamoxifen and chemotherapy. Cancer Res 2001; 61:1421–1425.

34. Foekens JA, Peters HA, Grebenchtchikov N, et al. Moespot A, van der Kwast TH, Sweep CG, Klijn JGM. High tumor levels of vascular endothelial growth factor predict poor response to systemic therapy in advanced breast cancer. Cancer Res 2001; 61:5407–5414.

35. van de Wetering M, Barker N, Harkes IC, et al. JGM, Clevers H, Schutte M. Mutant E-cadherin breast cancer cells do not display constitutive Wnt signaling. Cancer Res 2001; 61:1421–1425.

36. Dorssers LCJ, Veldscholte J, van der Flier S, Klijn JGM, Beex LVAM, Foekens JA. Tamoxifen resistance in breast cancer: elucidating mechanisms. Drug 2001; 61:1721–1733.

37. Joensuu H, Roberts PJ, Sarlomo-Rikala M, et al. Silberman SL, Capdeville R, Dimitrijevic S, Druker B, Demetri GD. Effect of the tyrosine kinease inhibitor STI571 in a patient with a metastatic gastrointestinal stromal tumor. N Engl J Med 2001; 344:1052–1056.

38. Druker BJ, Talpaz M, Resta DJ, et al. Efficacy and safety of a specific inhibitor of the BCR-ABL tyrosine kinase in chronic myeloid leukemia. N Engl J Med 2001; 344:1031–1037.

39. Hidalgo M, Eckhardt SG. Development of matrix metalloproteinase inhibitors in cancer therapy. J Natl Cancer Inst 2001; 93:178–193.

40. Hidalgo M, Eckhardt SG. Matrix metalloproteinase inhibitors: How can we optimize their development? Ann Oncol 2001; 12:285–287.

41. Johnston SRD. Farnesyl transferase inhibitors: a novel targeted therapy for cancer. Lancet Oncol 2001; 2:18–26.

42. Piccart MJ, Punt CJA, eds. Workshop proceedings: HER2 State-of-the-Art Confer-

ence November 21–23, 1999, Montreux, Switzerland. Ann Oncol 2001; 12(suppl 1):1–107.

43. Slamon DJ, Leyland-Jones, B, Shak S, et al. Eiermann W, Wolter J, Pegram M, Baselga J, Norton L. Use of chemotherapy plus a monoclonal antibody against HER2 for metastatic breast cancer that overexpresses HER2. N Engl J Med 2001; 344:783–792.

44. Eisenhauer EA. From the molecule to the clinic—Inhibiting HER2 to treat breast cancer (editorial). N Engl J Med 2001; 344:841–842.

45. Seidman AD, Fornier MN, Esteva FJ, et al. Weekly trastuzumab and paclitaxel therapy for metastatic breast cancer with analysis of efficacy by HER2 immunophenotype and gene amplification. J Clin Oncol 2001; 19:2587–2595.

46. Burstein HJ, Kuter I, Campos SM, et al. Clinical activity of trastuzumab and vinorelbine in women with HER2-overexpressing metastatic breast cancer. J Clin Oncol 2001; 19:2722–2730.

47. Woodburn JR. The epidermal growth factor receptor and its inhibition in cancer therapy. Pharmacol Ther 1999; 82:241–250.

48. Holly JMP, Gunnell DJ, Smith GD. Growth hormone, IGF-I and cancer. Less intervention to avoid cancer? More intervention to prevent cancer? J Endocrinol 1999; 162:321–330.

49. Dolan JT, Miltenburg DM, Granchi TS, et al. Treatment of metastatic breast cancer with somatostatin analogues—A meta-analysis. Ann Surg Oncol 2001; 8:227–233.

50. Helle SI. The insulin-linke growth factor system in breast cancer—Effects of endocrine treatment and alterations in tumor burden. Thesis. Bergen, Norway: Haukeland University Hospital, 2001.

51. Polyak K, Riggins GJ. Gene discovery using the serial analysis of gene expression technique: Implications for cancer research. J Clin Oncol 2001; 19:2948–2958.

52. Collins FS, McKusick VA. Implications of the human genome project for medical science. JAMA 2001; 285:540–544.

53. Perou CM, Sørlie T, Elsen MB, et al. Molecular portraits of human breast tumours. Nature 2000; 406:747–752.

54. Berns EMJJ, van Staveren IL, Verhoog L, et al. Molecular profiles of BRCA1-mutated and matched sporadic breast tumours: Relation with clinicopathological features. Br J Cancer 2001; 85:538–545

Panel Discussion 1

Advanced Breast Cancer

Manfred Kaufmann and Henning T. Mouridsen, *Chairmen*
Monday, June 25, 2001

M. Kaufmann: I would like to thank the organizers for inviting us to this marvelous site, here in Scotland, and also for the opportunity to chair this first session on advanced breast cancer. The audience of experts on the endocrine treatment of breast cancer gives us the opportunity to find some conclusions, guidelines, and recommendations in the treatment of metastatic breast disease. There have been some consensus conferences on adjuvant treatment, but there are no recent recommendations for the treatment of metastatic disease, especially in endocrine treatment. I think this is a chance to provide a consensus on this topic.

Let me just summarize the experience we have so far, in the treatment with tamoxifen. We all know that the clinical benefit for palliation is around 40% (range 30–50%) in endocrine-responsive tumors. This range holds true for all stages in the development of abnormal cells into breast cancer cells in the primary tumor. Take the reduction of breast cancer with tamoxifen over 5 years in the adjuvant setting, for example, there will be around 50% fewer recurrences, 50% less contralateral breast cancer, and there will be around 40% less invasive cancer for precursor lesions (e.g., DCIS).

If you look at the prevention of breast cancer, there will be about 50% less noninvasive and invasive beast cancer.

With this audience, we really have the chance to develop some recommendations or even guidelines for the endocrine treatment of advanced breast cancer with all the drugs that are now available to us in clinical practice. In particular, we have drugs with different mechanisms of action, like tamoxifen and the newer SERMs, aromatase inhibitors, aromatase inactivators, gestagens and luteinizing-hormone–releasing hormone (LH-RH) analogues. Tamoxifen started with the palliation of breast cancer in 1977 and its use has now expanded to the adjuvant setting, to precursor lesions and for prevention. For the third-generation aromatase inhibitors, we have enough information for palliation, and we are just starting to collect information in the adjuvant situation. We have lots of information on the gestagens and we have a lot of data on the LH-RH analogues even in the adjuvant setting. We also have information on Faslodex and information on the newer SERMs. Our goal now is to define what can be the standard endocrine treatment for metastatic disease and what is optional or experimental. I will now hand over the microphone to Henning Mouridsen and we will start with the discussion of what are the indications for endocrine therapy in metastatic disease.

H. Mouridsen: Let us try first to define which patients should be offered endocrine therapies. I will make some statements that may or may not be provocative to try and start the discussion. First I think it is generally accepted we should look at hormone receptor status. So far, in general terms, receptor-positive patients are those who are candidates for endocrine therapy. But, should we also be using other predictive factors or other predictors of response today? Should we use general markers for endocrine therapy or specific markers for specific endocrine therapies. Should we for instance use PS2? Should we measure aromatase in the tumor? Can we measure it today? These are our first questions. Would steroid receptors (estrogen and/or progesterone) be sufficient according to today's knowledge and technology to select patients for endocrine therapy?

M. Kaufmann: So the first question would be: "Should we have data on metastatic tissue or is it possible to have just information on the primary tumor?"

M. Dowsett: There is a very marked drop in the time to progression (TTP) that occurs in the first 3 months of all of these trials presented here despite the patients being, in general, estrogen receptor (ER)–or progesterone receptor (PgR)–positive: there appears to be about 40% of patients dropping out of these studies already. I don't think we are yet in a position to add molecular markers to identify these. The closest we have is perhaps with HER-2 and, given than Daniel Hayes has recently reviewed this, he might like to comment on that. I think we should all agree to retrieve as many of these blocks, tissues, etc., as we possibly can, so that studies can be done in a prospective sense, in the way that Matthew Ellis did in the neoadjuvant study with letrozole, such that we can begin to look for new markers and really begin to identify and differentiate those patients who will benefit from these treatments from those who won't. At the present time, I don't think we have markers that really add usefully to this, but we have enormous potential to determine that, if we set ourselves the task of collecting these materials.

W. Miller: Maybe I can make a general remark. Clearly we do need other predictors, but there is no doubt that the ER is a very powerful predictor. I wonder, given that we seem to have trials set up that are prepared to accept a substantial number of ER-unknown patients, whether we should address the situation (I thought Mitch Dowsett was going to allude to it). We really need to make every possible endeavor to ensure that ER measurements are made in patients who have been recruited to trials of endocrine therapy (particularly when it is a new endocrine therapy) before we are to go on to look at other predictors which might be more difficult to measure.

M. Dowsett: Just to respond, there is a particular reason why I didn't allude to that, Bill (Miller). The letrozole-versus-tamoxifen trial does not illustrate that well. If you look at the receptor-unknown group in that study, they separate letrozole and tamoxifen just as well as the receptor-positive group. All the same, I agree that we don't want that receptor-unknown group and we should exclude it from our trials in general. However, I think it is more significant in the adjuvant trials where the ER-negative group are not just nonresponsive but have actually more aggressive tumors that relapse earlier and drive the event rate so markedly that even if you have a small ER-unknown group, it can really make a major difference to the outcome of the study. I think in advanced disease it is not quite so important, but we should exclude patients whose ER status is unknown.

C. Benz: I see the issue dividing into those markers necessary for enrolment into a trial versus those markers to be studied in a correlative manner. As Mitch Dowsett pointed out, you would not want ER-negative tumors in an endocrine therapy trial unless you had some novel hypothesis to test. I also see Bill Miller's point that we need tissue access for marker studies that can be done in a correlative or belated fashion to explore new hypotheses. For instance, we've seen endocrine trials where ER/PgR unknown tumors constituted nearly 50% of the total treatment population. I would like to see not only ER but also PgR assays performed, since Bill McGuire first showed that PgR alone appears to be very predictive of endocrine response. However, that also introduces the question of assay validity. The validation of new marker assays is critical and the only way we can move forward is if we archive tissue, both in paraffin blocks as well as in a cryopreserved state, since many new marker assays cannot be done on paraffin-archived material.

C. Rose: I think we have to scrutinize the response data a little bit in these last trials comparing specific aromatase inhibitors with tamoxifen, because what we are seeing are response rates in the order 20–30%. This is for first-line endocrine therapy in a population that is predominantly steroid receptor–positive. Even if you have 50% of patients who are receptor–unknown, 70–80% will be receptor–positive if you analyze it. So in large cohorts of patients we are seeing response rates around 20–30% in various studies, where we know what is going on regarding response rates. Mentioning Bill McGuire, in the early days we thought that 60% of ER–positive patients would actually respond to endocrine therapy. Now we are seeing response rates down to 20–30%. This is of importance in our decision of whether to choose cytotoxic or endocrine therapy up front.

M. Ellis: We tend to assume that in a pure hormone receptor–positive population we would not see any patients with rapid disease progression on endocrine therapy, but I have a horrible suspicion that the population of patients with hormone receptor–positive but endocrine therapy–resistant disease is quite large. These tumors express ER but some somehow have bypassed the requirement for estrogen for growth.

P. Lønning: This is a comment on what Carsten Rose said. He is completely right that response rates have gone dramatically down, but if we look at the reason for this, it is because the group of durable, stable disease has gone up similarly. If we look at what is happening, a lot of patients are moved from the group of responders into the group with durable, stable disease because of the much more stringent criteria in modern studies. The change is not as dramatic as it would at first appear.

C. Rose: Yes, but we haven't seen that in trials of cytotoxic therapy. There you still see higher rates of response, even higher than we would have thought about 10 years ago. So, I don't think that that is the full explanation, Per (Lønning), i.e., that we are more concerned about response rate and its definition. I think that something else is going on here. It could also relate to the assay performed. The earlier data, to quote Bill McGuire again, were based on the dextran-coated charcoal (DCC) assay, whereas now patients are recruited on the basis of an immunohistochemical assay and in many instances unfortunately without good quality control. That applies also and maybe especially when you are performing the PgR assay.

W. Eiermann: This is a very academic discussion. It would perhaps be easier to formulate the question from a clinical point of view the other way around: "Who are the patients who should not receive endocrine therapy?" This is much easier to define because, if we are talking about ER- and/or PgR-unknown patients, often old blocks are not available and not every institution is able to perform receptor assays again and so on. It may be much easier to formulate the question the other way around: "Which patients should not receive endocrine therapy?"

The answer is that every patient should receive endocrine therapy apart from (a) the clinical situation where there is rapid remission and (b) the tumor is receptor–negative in actual tumor material.

J. Forbes: I have a similar concern that it is not quite as neat as that a high level of ER corresponds to perfect response. Some of the ER-positive patients may be nonresponders for a number of reasons. The prior tamoxifen treatment that many of them have received in current studies is different to the earlier studies with the charcoal assay, when tamoxifen was not used. There is a keenness to put patients into trials, and perhaps even a very low level of ER in an IHC assay gets patients into trials. There are other gray areas; for example, the difference between the ER status of the primary tumor and the metastatic tumor. Is the tumor at distal metastatic sites necessarily the same? If you sample a skin nodule, is that perhaps the same as disease in the liver or bone? These tumor cells may grow at different sites preferentially depending on their endocrine sensitivity.

M. Dowsett: I just wonder whether Dan Hayes would be prepared to make a comment on a study that I know he was involved with, which he presented at the AACR this year. One of the problems we clearly have with patients presenting with advanced breast cancer is that they don't always have blocks available for us to go back and get sections from, although we'd like to be able to do that wherever possible. There are more and more people taking an interest in the possibility of characterizing the breast cancer cells that circulate in the blood of metastatic breast cancer patients. The data that Dan Hayes showed were the first I've seen where the cells have been separated out and quantified and there was actually an attempt to measure HER-2 in those cells. That would appear to be a great move forward if it could be generally successful, and it would be particularly useful in relation to the sort of biological agents that Jan Klijn was talking about if we could get these cells out and do functional assays. I would like Dan Hayes to comment on whether this is realistic. Are we in the near future going to be able to do this on most of our metastatic breast cancer patients?

D. Hayes: I agree with some of the earlier comments. The issue is not who should receive endocrine therapy but who should *not* receive it, since it has such low toxicity. One is hard pressed not to treat someone unless there is absolutely no chance of benefit. So far the only thing we have found with that kind of predictive strength is ER and PgR. We had hoped earlier on that HER-2 would be a very strong predictive factor. All of you know Adrian Harris's original publication. We published data on circulating ErbB2 suggesting that there was a dramatic difference in response to droloxifene between those who were Erb-2–positive and negative. However, subsequent studies haven't really supported this. I'm convinced that ErbB2 does decrease the odds of response but doesn't wipe them out. I personally feel that if you are ER–positive and HER-2–positive, you still have a fairly good chance of benefiting. I think it is less than if you are ER–positive and HER-2–negative. I believe that most of these predictive factors are principally important for giving us insights into the biology that stimulates smart people (like in this room) to figure out ways to modulate those coexisting factors, whether it is ErbB2 or other things that might make hormone therapy work better. For example, Matthew Ellis has an ongoing study right now with aromatase inhibitors and Herceptin to which we have recruited. That is the right way to proceed.

The concept of detection of circulating cancer cells has been around for 50 or 60 years. However, the technology to do so has been troublesome. In the last 5 years, two or three different companies have come up with relatively easy assays. We are involved with one such company called Immunicon, which has identified so-called ferrous solutions that stay in suspension, rather than using magnetic beads, which drop to the bottom of the suspension. The particles in the solution are coated with antiepithelial antibodies. Fundamentally the assay is a simple blood test. They are working on a completely automated system, so that one can stick the tube in one end and at the other end you get a computer readout that quantitates circulating epithelial cells. It is actually not that easy, but it is getting there. The technology has changed in the last 18 months. We are particularly interested in being able to phenotype, genotype, and "biologically" type these cells when we isolate them. That is where I believe the field is going to go. The paper we had at AACR is very much a preliminary one, saying that once we find these cells, we can actually phenotype them and determine whether they are HER-2–positive or not. It is a long way from clinical utility, but I believe that it may be a very powerful tool to use in our phase II trials to get fairly rapid information in terms of modulation.

My two comments are related. I think in the next 3–5 years we will move in this direction. For example, Matthew Ellis has included this assay in his trial already and we are part of that. I recommend that you keep an eye on our work and that of other companies like BIS, who have a similar system and are trying to do this too.

R. Nicholson: It may be worth bearing in mind here that when we mention ERs and breast cancer, we are still only measuring the total protein levels within the cancer cells. We are not monitoring whether they are activated or not. As such, the current ER assays can only be an imprecise indicator of therapeutic response to anti-hormonal drugs. Importantly this also applies to HER-2 and EGFR and their downstream signaling components, which are also factors that can modify ER signaling.

H.-J. Senn: I would like to try to reconcile these questions concerning who should receive endocrine therapy for metastatic breast cancer (or not). Which way round should the question be? I think most of us, like the Swiss Group for Clinical Cancer Research, are used to dividing metastatic breast cancer populations into low- and high-risk disease. Receptor positivity is one of the factors that guide the therapeutic approach. Besides receptor positivity, about which we could discuss what is positive and what is negative for hours without agreement, there are other factors that guide us in treating patients with primary endocrine therapy: the tumor-free interval, the extent of metastatic disease, the type of metastatic disease (bone, soft tissue, or visceral disease), the patient's age, menopause, and so on. This would make it easier. Since we have already gone this way in adjuvant therapy, having had several consensus meetings, we have decided to group the patients as endocrine-responsive and endocrine-nonresponsive, as well as low and high risk of disease. I think that such an approach would be appropriate for your endeavor of trying to have a consensus in the treatment of metastatic breast cancer.

M. Ellis: There was an abstract presented by Schmid et al. at ASCO 2000 (number 398) in which the authors attempted to identify clinical factors associated with a favorable outcome on letrozole therapy. This analysis suggested that, in addition to factors we all recognize—such as visceral versus nonvisceral and short versus long disease-free interval—a body-mass index greater than 30 kg/m^2 was associated with a poor outcome. One possible explanation for this is that overweight patients have more aromatase activity and may need higher doses of aromatase inhibitor.

W. Miller: I would like to come back to your basic question Henning (Mouridsen) ("Which patients should be offered endocrine therapy?") and maybe be a little more provocative. I think the question should be subdivided into "who should receive endocrine therapy inside and outside trials?" My point would be that if you are intending, by means of a trial, to compare the efficacy of two agents, and maybe one is a novel endocrine agent, I don't know how you can afford to have studies with a substantial number of ER-unknown patients in them. If you do, you potentially dilute out the differences between arms when every power is needed. I can think of two trials involving anastrozole and tamoxifen, one of which had 40% or more of ER-unknown patients in it, and showed no difference between the drugs. The other, which was of the same design, but with fewer ER-positive patients, did show a difference. ER status has been used to try to explain the differences between the trials. I think, therefore, that one could avoid this, especially in a trial situation. If you put a lot of resources into these trials, you should not be wasting those resources by including a large number of ER-unknown patients. In contrast, I wonder if, outside a trial, this audience would be prepared to accept the philosophy that if endocrine therapy is associated with a lack of toxicity, we should use it (particularly in advanced disease). Of course if we accept this nondiscriminatory philosophy, we might be wasting our time doing these sophisticated assays to try to distinguish those tumors that which are more likely to respond from those that are not.

H. Sasano: I would like to comment on the quality of specimens from the standpoint of pathologists who have been asked to respond to questions regarding the efficacy of a possible therapy from a clinician. I have three comments. First, regarding the circulating cells, we have performed extensive studies on the detection of circulating carcinoma cells, not in breast cancer but in esophageal squamous cancer, which is very prevalent in Japan. One can detect the presence of circulating cells using a cytokeratine immunostain. However, it is important to note that almost all of these circulating cells are undergoing apoptosis and by no means is there a direct correlation with the presence of foci of metastasis. It is very difficult to detect nuclear antigens, including P53 and MYB-1, at this juncture. It is, especially in these circulating tumor cells, rather premature to determine the presence or absence of ER-alpha. We recommend that pleural cell effusion cytology or FNA is performed, in which more viable cells are available for examination. Second, cryogenic preservation was mentioned earlier. In our experience, the quality of cryogenic specimens is markedly variable among institutions, so we should stick to markers which can be examined in 10% formalin fixed or in paraffin embedded tissue specimens. Finally, I think that it is also important to standardize the method of estrogen receptor measurement. So far, the best is the combination of immunohisto-chemistry and image analysis.

H. Mouridsen: Maybe we should move on to another topic. In brief conclusion, steroid receptors are still the best predictors of response. Although not optimal, they are the best we have today. We should select patients for endocrine therapy according to their receptor status (i.e., tumors which are ER- and/or PgR-positive). We should make every effort to do translational research to try and understand why receptor-positive cases do not respond to endocrine therapy and thus improve the prediction and selection of patients for endocrine therapy.

J. Forbes: I would make a plea that we prospectively collect information about prior endocrine treatment, which may be ovarian ablation and variations of that, in premenopausal patients and tamoxifen in post-menopausal patients. We really do need to learn what the influence of prior tamoxifen is and when the recurrence takes place with respect to subsequent responses. At the present time we just have conjecture.

I. Smith: I guess scientifically it is important to identify your best markers and so on to understand what is going on. But from the point of view of the clinician, the best way is, and always has been, just to give the drug. These are safe, nontoxic drugs and the thera-peutic trial is the way of being 100% certain whether your patient is going to respond or not. We know from many trials in the past that patients do not lose out clinically by being on an endocrine agent to which they do not respond before they go onto chemotherapy pro-vided that they do not have life-threatening disease. I think we need to keep this pragmatic point in mind.

M. Ellis: I think that is an important point when you are looking at the first-line data of tamoxifen vs. letrozole, because if you think about which drug you should use as a clinical test to distinguish between estrogen-dependent breast cancer and estrogen-independent disease it makes sense to use letrozole because the response rate to it is higher than that to tamoxifen. This choice could prove critical for the palliative management of some patients, because tumors that progress rapidly on tamoxifen are often not offered further endocrine management on the assumption that tumors that exhibit intrinsic tamoxifen resistance never respond to further endocrine management. In fact, data from the second-line trials suggested that the response rate to letrozole in this situation is around 15%.

A. Howell: I agree totally (with M. Ellis, I. Smith, and W. Miller) that a pragmatic test is fine for women in the clinic and you don't need to know the ER status. What we need is a very thorough research study with biopsy of lesions at relapse to get a good indication of what happens to ER status between the primary tumor and relapse. We have some data, but we need to do that again properly. As Rob Nicholson said, we have several mechanisms of resistance. It is not beyond the wit of the clever biologists to try to look for activated ER. How you do that, I'm not sure, but we really need it, because these are women who have metastatic tumors where the ER is not working by the assay you have just developed, and they need to go on to probably something like endocrine therapy plus a receptor tyrosine kinase inhibitor (RS) or endocrine therapy plus a demethylating agent, or some other experimental treatment. It is the people in this room who have to do these studies to try to get an indication of whether the ER that doesn't seem to be working can in some way be reactivated.

P. Lønning: First, I'd like to address what Carsten (Rose) said about deeper understanding. If you look at the papers that have compared the two techniques, like the paper from the Baylor group, it actually suggests the opposite, that immunostaining could be better. What this and other papers raise is the problem of what should be the detection limit when you call it positivity. Should it be 1%, 5%, or 10% of the cells? Listening to my British colleagues here recommending performing tests, let me ask you this provocative question: Do any of you recommend that we stop using the ER? I'm not talking about which sensitivity limit we should use or which techniques. Do any of you recommend that we should treat patients without looking at ER status?

A. Howell: Well, yes is the short answer, for the reasons that Ian Smith gave and others have given. Of course we should measure receptors and I think what you're saying is that the British don't do it enough (and you're right), but if you have a patient who has relapsed after 15 years and you can't find the block, she is an old lady, and you don't want to subject her to a bone biopsy, you try endocrine therapy. There are several clinical scenarios here.

P. Lønning: I accept there are situations where you cannot retrieve the blocks and there are reasons why you can't measure it, but that was not my question. My question was whether we should stop measuring it.

A. Howell: If you had something better then you could stop measuring it, but I think that you should start measuring PgR.

I. Smith: Per (Lønning), it is a completely redundant question because we measure ER in new patients for endocrine therapy. The cohort of older patients when we didn't measure estrogen receptors is going away.

W. Miller: Would you put your patient into a trial of letrozole vs. tamoxifen without being able to retrieve the block and know the ER status?

A. Howell: That is a different issue completely. I agree with what everyone has been saying, that these trials are precious. We have this problem when the trial in Europe provides one answer and the trial in North America provides a different answer. In the future (Kent Osborne made this point at a meeting recently held in Boston), nobody should get into an endocrine trial, adjuvant or advanced, without us knowing the ER status, because we waste patients. On that issue I am totally firm. On the other issue, I am wobbly.

M. Kaufmann: We have to stop the discussion to try to summarize. It is difficult to find final conclusions. I think we should divide low- and high-risk patients and the major factor for making endocrine treatment decisions is still ER and PgR receptor status. If possible the measurements should be done on biopsies of the metastatic lesion. In the adjuvant setting, we come to the conclusion that immunohistochemistry will be superior to the biochemical assay. But besides receptor status, other factors are relevant for treatment decisions. I would conclude that the high-risk situation (i.e., life-threatening disease with pathological liver enzyme levels) is not an indication for starting endocrine treatment. Also, if there is no endocrine response with previous treatment, this is also an indication for chemotherapy. Today we have to get more information on how effective endocrine treatment is, because we have data from the old trials where clinical benefit was around 50%, but in the new trials it is only around 20%.

J. Klijn: I have a comment on your statement regarding liver metastases. The reason that liver metastases do not respond very well to endocrine treatment is the negative correlation between site of metastases and ER status. Most patients with liver metastasis are ER-negative, but in our experience with LH-RH agonists combined with tamoxifen, it appeared that patients with ER-positive liver metastasis did very well with endocrine treatment. So in principle, the presence of liver metastases is not a contraindication for endocrine treatment.

M. Kaufmann: I agree, that is the same observation as we have seen, for example, using exemestane. Therefore, I think that pathological liver enzymes are no indication for endocrine treatment.

A. Howell: What do you mean by pathological liver enzymes?

M. Kaufmann: For example, sixfold over the normal range.

A. Howell: I agree with Jan (Klijn) entirely. I think the old data we have, that livers don't respond, are in women who present with massive liver disease. It is important, as Jan Klijn said, to realize that liver does respond, and we mustn't exclude those from these trials.

M. Kaufmann: Sorry, I already excluded liver metastases as an absolute contraindication for endocrine therapies.

W. Eiermann: We should clearly define liver enzyme increase. If you have a threefold liver enzyme increase, that is a life-threatening disease, and then you should use a therapy that induces a very rapid remission. Liver metastases respond to endocrine therapy also. All the Zoladex trials and others showed that endocrine drugs work in patients with DFS less than 2 years.

M. Kaufmann: Can you live with threefold and 12 months?

W. Eiermann: Yes.

A. Bhatnagar: The discussion today has been proceeding in a way that has not focused on differentiating between two clear situations. The clinical trials that should be done in the future are going to have to be much more tightly controlled. Thus we should define very clearly the parameters to be measured in a clinical trial and then quite separately discuss whether these same parameters need to be measured in clinical practice before initiating therapy. That applies not only to the advanced breast cancer situation but also to early breast cancers and all of the other situations where results from a clinical trial may become standard clinical practice.

M. Kaufmann: Can we have some more comments on what will be necessary for future trials and their design? Is it PgR, HER-2, tumor aromatase, or E2 levels we should be looking at?

M. Dowsett: In terms of the studies to do in relation to the new endocrine trials, I couldn't agree more with Tony (Howell) regarding doing biopsies on the metastases. At the present time, in advanced breast cancer, we are going to be almost always be dealing with patients who have received endocrine therapy in the adjuvant situation. We know very little at the moment about what that initial endocrine therapy does to the biochemistry of the tumors and molecular determinants of response to the second agent. There are some opportunities for us to do studies of that type at the present time, with the very large adjuvant trials that are ongoing. I don't know of any of those trials that are comprehensively collecting tissue from the pretreatment blocks, but perhaps the focus should be those patients who are having their first local relapse where, in about 50% of cases, there will be further surgery. In these circumstances we can get paired biopsies from the pretreatment and relapsed situation. This will not just give us information on the mechanisms of resistance but can begin to allow us to think more about how we deliver these new biological therapies. For example, can it be that the patients now are overexpressing EGF receptor and HER-2, when they weren't before? These would then be a target, whereas if we just look at the pretreatment situation, we might reject that patient as a target for our therapy. These sorts of studies are extremely important and there is a real opportunity for us to do those studies now.

J. Forbes: The considerations about future trials are very important. The more precisely the study population is defined, the less representative it is of the general population. That means that the result may not necessarily be transferable very widely, but it does allow us to get closer to reality with answers about biological questions. We need to understand this in advance. The wider we make the eligibility requirements, e.g., for ER positivity, the less precise the answer obtained and paradoxically the wider the results might be applied. We have to consider the biological questions in advance, and that may be the only information that comes out of the trial, not necessarily a therapeutic advantage.

J. Ingle: I have several suggestions. Adherence to better standards for future trials will serve everybody better. We've talked about ER positivity. A patient who is ER-negative should never be let into a study. Patients who are ER-unknown should not go into clinical trials. Patients who do not conform to a measurable category (e.g., RECIST: Response Evaluation Criteria in Solid Tumors, JNCI 2000; 92:205–216) should not be included because this unmeasurable, amorphous category causes problems. Double-blind trials should be done. Those simple criteria would serve the science much better and in the long run would allow you to be more efficient with the use of your patients.

M. Ellis: One thing I would add to that list is mandatory block collection. This is controversial, but we were able to achieve mandatory correlative science in the preoperative Letrozole 024 study—i.e., the patients could not enter study unless they agreed to a biopsy. The consent for this investigation worked in 15 countries in 55 centers.

M. Kaufmann: We should now leave this topic and come to the next point, which is the recommendation of endocrine sequences and combinations. It is open to question which will be the first-choice endocrine treatment, especially considering that many patients will have had tamoxifen as adjuvant treatment. In this context we have to discuss the results of aromatase inhibitors in advanced breast cancer.

So far there are three drugs available: letrozole, anastrozole, and exemestane. How do you rate the percentage response rates for these drugs? We have seen there is some advantage for letrozole in in vitro studies of aromatase inhibition. Is this also true in the clinical situation, in first-line treatment?

J. Ingle: I think it is very tough to make a judgment on which is the best aromatase inhibitor in this day and age. We all have biases. Henning Mouridsen's study, which was just recently published, makes many of us choose letrozole for use in the clinic. However, if someone challenged me to use evidence-based medicine to show that letrozole is unequivocally better than anastrozole, I don't think anyone here could provide that evidence. Exemestane is a little bit less of a problem, at least in the United States, because it is not approved as first-line treatment and the phase II/III study of exemestane vs. tamoxifen is still being done.

M. Kaufmann: The question is not "Which is the best drug?" The question is which data do we have so far and which are the *key studies* for these three drugs?

P. Lønning: If we look at exemestane, the first-line results are promising, but the numbers of observations are too small to allow any conclusions at this stage. I think we all accept that the letrozole study is very convincing with respect to the very careful way they have analyzed the data with respect to previous exposure to tamoxifen as well as ER status. We can't say that letrozole is better than anastrozole, but what we can say is that critical data are missing for anastrozole. If you are to claim that anastrozole is better than tamoxifen, as was shown in one trial (although they were comparable in the other trial), we need more details to pool the analysis and use the argument of looking only at ER-positive patients. You can't just discharge 55% of the patients enrolled in a trial.

M. Ellis: I think there are obvious weaknesses and scientific problems associated with retrospective unplanned subset analysis of the type used to interpret the anastrozole vs. tamoxifen data. In general, trials of endocrine therapy in metastatic breast cancer have tended to show that ER-unknown and ER-known populations behave in a similar way clinically, presumably because the vast majority of the "unknowns" are ER-positive anyway. The letrozole vs. tamoxifen trial illustrates this principle nicely, since in both receptor-known and receptor-unknown populations, letrozole was found to be superior to tamoxifen. For the European anastrozole trial, the population "known to be receptor-positive" has been presented separately, because doing this shows more of an advantage for anastrozole in terms of time to progression. There was no difference between the two drugs in patients with hormone receptor–unknown disease. This conclusion could be a statistical artifact, and there remains a question mark over whether anastrozole truly has shown a clear clinical advantage over tamoxifen.

W. Eiermann: I am reluctant to compare the letrozole study to the anastrozole study. Per Lønning clearly showed this morning the disadvantage of the anastrozole study. There are some questions that have not been answered. From a clinical point of view, it is a close race between letrozole and anastrozole, and it will be very difficult to find an advantage for one of these drugs. Also, it is not worth a study, as you would need thousands of patients to show a difference in the advanced disease. This would be expensive and makes no sense.

Another point is side effects. In the anastrozole study (tamoxifen arm) you see thromboembolic events in 7.5% of patients, whereas you see thromboembolic events in only 2% of patients in the letrozole study (tamoxifen arm), which is 3 times less in efficacy and side effects. You can't compare studies with each other.

M. Ellis: My point wasn't whether you can use the data to say one is better than the other. Obviously you can't. You need a double-blind randomized comparison between the two. My point is simply that the hormone receptor subset analysis conducted for anastrozole studies can be questioned from the viewpoint of scientific purity.

P. Lønning: I outlined this earlier on my slide. If they are going to pool the data, why don't they look at the response rates in the European study in the subgroup of receptor-positive patients? As far as I could understand from the paper, this information was not given. We also have to remember that the time to progression became slightly better for anastrozole compared to tamoxifen in the European study when they looked at only the receptor-positive patients. This was not statistically significant unless it was pooled with the North American data. They did not separately analyze those not previously exposed to tamoxifen in either study, and there were twice as many patients who got adjuvant tamoxifen in the North American study than in the European study. I am not saying that this is the reason for the difference, but it surprises me that they have not come up with any of these data, particularly because they may potentially be beneficial and supporting their claims. We don't know the answer. At the same time, as long as we do not have these answers, we can only say that anastrozole is similar to tamoxifen. We cannot say that anastrozole is superior to tamoxifen based on the data we have in hand.

A. Howell: I don't think we can say that it is not superior. I think we have already talked about this. If you do a relatively dirty study, you get an answer which doesn't help us. That is the argument for doing studies that are very precise. One other comment that may be important: Kent Osborne presented more data on Suzanne Fuqua's 303 mutation in the ER, which makes cells exquisitely sensitive in terms of proliferation to low levels of estradiol. We have data supporting that. It may be that this very neat study from Mitch Dowsett and Per Lønning, which showed that letrozole was superior to anastrozole in terms of total body aromatase inhibitory activity, may well be important in the future, given that at least 60% of ER-positive breast cancers have this mutation and letrozole may be superior in this situation.

M. Gnant: I believe it is not that important which one of these aromatase inhibitors is superior to the other in current treatment. The most important question concerns their interaction and sequence. In a patient failing on a steroidal aromatase inhibitor, does it make sense to treat with a nonsteroidal? Pretty soon we will see data from patients who received aromatase inhibitors in the adjuvant phase. Is it reasonable to use letrozole for a woman who failed on anastrozole? I believe that by numbers, these questions are far more important than whether you have a 5% greater reduction of estrogen sulfate in the serum.

M. Kaufmann: I think this was an important comment for the discussion and for guidelines.

J. Forbes: The only conclusion at the moment is that there is no clear evidence of difference. There is clear evidence that there is a very similar efficacy. The longer-term use will depend on tolerance and side effects, including the effects on bone in the long term, and on the uncommon but serious side effects. We don't have sufficient data as yet. I would predict that a direct comparison of letrozole and anastrozole would be very similar to a direct comparison of tamoxifen and toremifene. They are very similar agents, a similar class of drug, and are likely to have similar breast cancer efficacy. It would need a very large study to establish this. I think the focus should be on sequences as well, and we shouldn't discard tamoxifen. If patients have an aromatase inhibitor as an adjuvant treatment, they may well be responsive to some type of SERM (including tamoxifen) for recurrence of breast cancer.

H. Mouridsen: I think in the long run the most critical issue is time to second progression. When the patients are crossed over, do we lose what we gained first-line in terms of superiority of aromatase inhibitor over tamoxifen? Unfortunately, we will never get valid second-line data from the anastrozole study, because there was no planned crossover. Thus data to be provided will be from highly selected patients.

M. Kaufmann: Can the audience accept that there is no clear difference between these three agents?

J. Ingle: Unfortunately we all live in a period of relative uncertainty and we do not have level-one evidence. However, when you don't have level-one evidence, you get into expert opinion. I think that based on two pieces of information—the recently published phase III study of letrozole vs. tamoxifen, which had a superior outcome (a better outcome for the aromatase inhibitor than in the anastrozole study) and the crossover data (although small) showing that there appears to be superior aromatase inhibition with letrozole than with anastrozole—

I. Smith: What we do know is that anastrozole is not better than letrozole. We know that from the two areas of evidence the Jim Ingle has just mentioned. I don't think it matters very much whether they are equally good, because all the time we are building our knowledge base. So the common sense, pragmatic, current "gold standard" is letrozole, because it is at least as good (it doesn't matter if it's better) as anastrozole. So we go on with letrozole and that is the target for the next endocrine agent to beat.

M. Kaufmann: This was a good point.

J. Klijn: I would like to ask Jim Ingle what is the hard proof that letrozole is better than anastrozole? When you look at the data, although the study with letrozole was more detailed, when you look at the main parameter, time to progression, there is clearly no difference in months gained with anastrozole and letrozole. The difference in p values is dictated mainly by the number of patients in the trial. There are no hard data that one of these compounds is better than the other before we have a comparative study.

A. Howell: I agree with Jan Klijn entirely. We just have to be very careful about comparing studies. Jim Ingle knows this as well as anyone else. You can bring out a study of letrozole vs. megestrol acetate in the United States and letrozole doesn't work against megestrol acetate in the United States. It appears to be just as good or slightly inferior to megestrol acetate in this study. You just have to be careful about making those comments, because comparing between studies is fraught with difficulties.

P. Lønning: I agree with what you say Tony (Howell), but there are two issues here. The first is the biochemical evidence that, in vivo, there is no doubt that letrozole is a much better suppressor of estrogen levels. Whether that translates into clinical effects, we don't know yet. What I was questioning in my talk was that a lot of the parameters we are presented with from the letrozole study are not shown with anastrozole. They started doing the subgroup analysis by pooling the ER-positive patients from the two studies, but if you are going to do subgroup analysis, we like to see all the details, like the effects in those who were not exposed to tamoxifen in both anastrozole studies and all of these other issues that were very carefully addressed in the letrozole study. Obviously, AstraZeneca has the data for these trials on file so why can't they release them?

M. Kaufmann: Can we conclude from this discussion that there is no clear difference between letrozole, anastrozole, and exemestane? Anastrozole is not better than letrozole. There are fewer data on exemestane in comparison to letrozole and anastrozole.

J. Forbes: But that is not quite correct in terms of the data. We cannot conclude that it is either better or worse. We only have indirect comparisons, and it may be misleading to base conclusions on indirect comparisons. These comparisons are hypothesis-generating. They do not answer the questions we want answers to at the moment. It may also be misleading to do subgroup analyses in this, and it is even more misleading to do cross-trial comparisons.

M. Kaufmann: Can we conclude that there are no clear differences between the three drugs?

H. Mouridsen: We have to exclude exemestane in the first-line situation. We don't have sufficient data.

A. Bhatnagar: I think we are once again moving away from clinical trials leading to clinical practice.

M. Kaufmann: This was my next question. If a patient comes in to your office, which of these drugs would you give her for first-line treatment of metastatic disease?

D. Hayes: I don't think we're ready to ask that question, let alone answer it. Given the conversation we have just had, I think that it is very fair, at least in the United States, that both of these drugs are approved. It very much depends on how you, as a clinician, practice. For us as a group of so-called experts to try to give such an opinion I think is wrong. We should say that these are interesting drugs and that the data are out there and we can say that they are both as good as or better than tamoxifen as first-line therapy in the metastatic setting.

M. Kaufmann: But there was a clear basis for this question from one of our experts, James Ingle. I would like to get an impression of the general thoughts and what people really do today in clinical practice.

H. Mouridsen: Could I rephrase the question? Which is the first-line endocrine therapy today: should it be tamoxifen or should it be an aromatase inhibitor? Also, should it be so in patients with no prior endocrine therapy or in patients with prior adjuvant tamoxifen? This might be another way of putting the question. What is the optimal first-line therapy in a postmenopausal woman with advanced breast cancer?

M. Kaufmann: I think it is clear that second-line treatment is either an aromatase inhibitor or tamoxifen. Is it aromatase inhibitors instead of gestagens? Do you all agree we can skip this sequence? Today the sequence is tamoxifen, aromatase inhibitors, and then gestagens as a third-line treatment.

M. Gnant: Is this in patients who have been exposed to tamoxifen?

M. Kaufmann: That is the next topic.

M. Dowsett: The data so far are pretty compelling for the aromatase inhibitors being better than tamoxifen as first-line agents. However, their overall success could still depend on what the outcome of the crossover, particularly in the letrozole study; as this was a prospective part after failure to the first agent, we may in fact have elicited resistance to tamoxifen in the aromatase inhibitor group. That may reverse one's position, but at the present time, we would select the aromatase inhibitor as more effective first-line treatment.

K. Tonkin: It is very unusual for us to see patients who have metastatic breast cancer who we think are candidates for endocrine therapy (in this day and age) and who have not had adjuvant tamoxifen. There are going to be a few coming through, because they are going to be diagnosed as metastatic disease up front or whatever, but the vast majority of women we're going to see with metastatic breast cancer who we think are candidates for endocrine therapy have had tamoxifen. Not only that, more and more of them have had tamoxifen not just for 1 or 2 years but for 5 years. That's the second point. The third point is that it is going to make a tremendous difference, as we have said before, whether these patients have relapsed on tamoxifen or whether they have relapsed within 12 months of tamoxifen or longer, and added to that you've got the kind of issue now with respect to the chemotherapy they have had. If you're talking about someone who has had six cycles of taxane-based chemotherapy and she has now relapsed within a year of being on tamoxifen, I don't care what you give her, she's going to do very badly. So we're in a completely different era now than with patients who might have had CMF and a year of tamoxifen. We are extremely fortunate to have the aromatase inhibitors, because I think the vast majority of women that we're going to see with metastatic disease have had treatment with tamoxifen in the adjuvant setting.

M. Kaufmann: This is clinical reality.

C. Rose: I think we need to put this in perspective. If we go back to how we actually introduced tamoxifen for first-line metastatic disease, we had no trial whatever at that time that showed any benefit for tamoxifen except that the side effects were very modest compared with other endocrine therapies. Still, we had indications that castration in premenopausal and high doses of estrogens might be even better as first-line therapy for postmenopausal patients. So now we are discussing if we should take issue with very large, well-conducted trials where we know exactly what was going on and where, if we pool all the data comparing specific aromatase inhibitors with tamoxifen, they all show that there is a superiority of the specific aromatase inhibitors over tamoxifen. I think for patients who have been treated adjuvantly with tamoxifen, there is no doubt that specific aromatase inhibitors should be first-line therapy. In the few cases where patients have not seen tamoxifen first, we do have very good evidence now that aromatase inhibitors are doing better than tamoxifen. So for that reason I see no compelling reason not to start out treating these patients first-line with aromatase inhibitors.

M. Kaufmann: We couldn't find a clear answer as to which drug is superior over the other. So are dramatically different side effects seen with these three drugs? I would say no.

W. Eiermann: I pointed out before that we have to look, for example, at thromboembolic events in the anastrozole study (where the incidence was 7.5%) and in the letrozole study (where it was 2% or so). Thus I say that you can't compare the studies with one another—neither the efficacy nor side effects—but if you look at the advantages of the aromatase inhibitors, you have to look at the endometrial cancer. This is a strong argument from the patient's side to favor first-line use of aromatase inhibitors for metastatic disease.

A. Brodie: In lieu of the fact that we do not have a lot of clinical information at the present time on sequencing, I would just like to mention a preclinical model that we have used. It's an intratumoral aromatase model with human breast cancer cells that are ER-positive. We have looked at the effects of sequencing and the model has been accurate at predicting the clinical response. Letrozole certainly was better that tamoxifen. However, an aromatase inhibitor alone is always superior to combining any aromatase inhibitor with tamoxifen. Although the combination is somewhat better than tamoxifen alone, it is never better than the aromatase inhibitor alone, and that goes for letrozole and anastrozole. As far a sequencing them, whether you start with tamoxifen first or letrozole first, the result is equivalent, but it is not as good as if you started and continued treatment with letrozole all the time. The tamoxifen response duration is quite a bit shorter alone than it is with letrozole.

H. Mouridsen: Can we just come back to the very important issue of the sequence and also prior therapy? I don't think it's true that the majority of patients who have developed metastases today have received adjuvant tamoxifen. In the two recently published trials of anastrozole and letrozole versus tamoxifen, 20% of the patients had received adjuvant tamoxifen. In 5 or 10 years, the majority of patients developing metastases will have had adjuvant tamoxifen. Today this is no more than 50%. So I think it's very important to define also, for those who have not had adjuvant tamoxifen, which is the proper sequence. I would agree with Carsten (Rose), that even for those subjects who have not had adjuvant tamoxifen, the proper sequence would be aromatase inhibitor first.

M. Gnant: There is absolutely no reason in my opinion not to give first-line aromatase inhibitors even if these patients have not been exposed to tamoxifen, since all the evidence we have was derived from cohorts where the majority of patients (as you pointed out) did not see tamoxifen. There is no longer a reason for giving tamoxifen as first-line treatment irrespective of prior endocrine therapy. Keep it for second-line therapy or whatever.

A. Howell: I would agree with that. I think that possibly the reason why we're seeing these differences between tamoxifen and aromatase inhibitors as first-line therapy is that there is a small group of patients who see tamoxifen as an estrogen de novo, because about 10% of those patients who haven't responded to tamoxifen, will respond to second-line treatment. So I think there is a strong argument for putting patients on aromatase inhibitors first. The second argument is that thromboembolic events are higher with tamoxifen than we think they are with aromatase inhibitors; therefore the latter may be the safer and (as the studies suggest) more active drugs. I can see no indication for giving tamoxifen first.

M. Kaufmann: To keep to our timing, I would like now to switch to the premenopausal situation.

P. Lønning: I would just like to comment that if you are going to treat patients who have not been exposed to tamoxifen with an aromatase inhibitor as first-line therapy, the only study that has reported the results for this subgroup separately is the letrozole study. Such a subgroup analysis has not been reported in the anastrozole studies. So you don't have the evidence to say that anastrozole is superior to tamoxifen in tamoxifen-naïve patients.

M. Kaufmann: Are there any comments for the first-line treatment in premenopausal patients with endocrine-responsive tumors and a low-risk situation?

J. Klijn: By treatment with LH-RH agonists, you make premenopausal women postmenopausal, so then we can restart the discussion of the last hour.

H. Mouridsen: Could I just ask John (Forbes), from your presentation of tamoxifen, I think you indicated, that we know tamoxifen and ovarian ablation to be equally effective for the premenopausal patients. My question is where we know that from. There are only two very, very small trials, as far as I know. From these studies you can conclude whatever you want to.

J. Forbes: Even the small overview that was done on the available data failed to show any advantage for either, but they are very small studies, I agree. Certainly the response rates are comparable, but these at least were direct comparisons where one was looking at response rates. It's not the same as comparing the aromatase inhibitors across trials, which is the basis for saying that there appears to be no difference between them. There is very substantial evidence from the EBCTCG overview that there is a comparable rate of relapse reduction with tamoxifen as with ovarian ablation (in the adjuvant setting). But we do need to remember that the early ovarian ablation studies were done on patients without any knowledge at all of estrogen receptors, and at least 20% and possibly as many as 50% might have been ER-negative in those studies, so the benefit of the ovarian ablation could be very substantially diluted.

J. Ingle: You're absolutely right. If you look at the history of metastasis in premenopausal patients, it's unbelievable how low the sample sizes are. The metanalysis of the four studies in the oophorectomy versus tamoxifen had, I think, 220 patients. In the goserelin versus oophorectomy study, I think it was 136. The meta-analysis of the LH-RH plus tamoxifen vs. LH-RH had 500.

H. Mouridsen: What about LH-RH analogues compared to ablation? Are there any studies to indicate any difference? (I would not expect any.) If not, then why not use ablation? Because we need persistently to keep these patients postmenopausal and it is cheaper.

J. Klijn: It is not cheaper, it is roughly equivalent with respect to cost of surgical oophorectomy and LH-RH agonist treatment in metastatic disease. I agree that in principle there is no difference in efficacy between these two treatment modalities. There was the Taylor's study of the SWOG with Kent Osborne as last author, showing that the curves are completely superimposable. The only potential advantage of the LH-RH agonist is the possible direct antitumor effects that these compounds have on the 50% or so of tumors that contain LH-RH receptors. But their affinity is very low and their clinical relevance is questionable. But the point is also that most trials are now done using LH-RH agonists. So if you base your clinical practice on trials, then, in principle, you have to use the drugs applied in trials.

M. Kaufmann: So this means that for all the further endocrine or chemotherapeutic treatment steps, if you do not use surgical castration, you must continue treatment with LH-RH analogues.

J. Forbes: There are other data, Mr. Chairman—your own on bone density reduction and then reversal on cessation of 2 years of LH-RH agonist. This may turn out to be an important advantage.

M. Kaufmann: Also, I think that from a psychological point of view, there is a real advantage for LH-RH analogues over surgical castration.

D. Hayes: I think part of the discussion here is lost. Most of our patients in the United States, even premenopausal women now, are already on tamoxifen when they relapse. Therefore, apropos of recommendations like this, does one take such a patient and ablate her ovaries, either by surgery or by agonists, and keep her on tamoxifen as well, or does one stop tamoxifen and both ablate her ovaries and then add an aromatase inhibitor? I would be very interested in hearing what one would do in the situation where a premenopausal ER-positive woman is on tamoxifen when she relapses.

A. Howell: Well, you have your own data in the United States. When you keep her on tamoxifen, then an LH-RH agonist doesn't work because of the agonist effect of tamoxifen, presumably. That has been done.

D. Hayes: Whose data are those?

A. Howell: There have been data reporting that an LH-RH agonist was not effective when tamoxifen was continued. Ask Kent Osborne.

D. Hayes: So it's ongoing tamoxifen, and then?

A. Howell: Well, the woman is on tamoxifen, you give her ablation, you keep her on tamoxifen, and you don't get a response. Whereas another study, by Kathy Pritchard, showed that if you take them off tamoxifen, then you do get a response. Those data are out there.

W. Miller: I wonder if I could just take up Jan Klijn's point. I agree with him that LH-RH analogue treatment makes premenopausal women postmenopausal. But John Forbes showed some data that, after 2 years, many women are no longer amenorrheic. Is this is true? You may give an aromatase inhibitor to women who may not be fully postmenopausal, and aromatase inhibitors in cycling women are not as effective as in postmenopausal women. I was wondering, there-fore, if Jan (Klijn) and John (Forbes) might like to clarify this point.

J. Forbes: We need to add a question as well. For what time period do you need to treat patients? Adjuvant cytotoxic chemotherapy, which produces advantages, is given for fairly short periods of time. Ta-moxifen is given for perhaps 5 years. The LH-RH agonist has an ef-fect for maybe 2 years. My opinion is that you'll get benefit with these endocrine agents with short treatment (e.g., 2 years) while presumably tumor cells are still present. So I don't think it is so im-portant to necessarily continue that for a longer period of time. Ta-moxifen also has another role: prevention. Maybe the other agents do, but we don't know that yet.

M. Dowsett: Bill (Miller), I think you might have misinterpreted John's slide there. I think the data from the adjuvant trial showed just 2 years usage of Zoladex. These weren't patients who were es-caping from suppression but actually patients who had been re-moved from suppression. Perhaps a wider comment concerns the question you (H. Mouridsen) put about castration versus LH-RH agonist. This seems to be more frequently asked when men are discussing breast cancer than when men are discussing prostate cancer.

K. Tonkin: In our province of Alberta, of our $34 million (CND) budget, $7 million goes on LH-RH agonists, which agrees with your point. I don't understand why, we don't talk about castrating the men with prostate cancer but glibly talk about castrating women with breast cancer. Someone mentioned cost. I can't believe that the cost of surgical castration is anywhere near the cost of putting someone on goserelin. Two months of treatment would surely be about the same as surgical castration. The only reason LH-RH agonists and surgery can cost the same is that, in the metastatic situation, we use the drugs for only a short time before progression.

D. Hayes: In a cost-effective analysis, they're about the same because you don't use it for very long in the metastatic setting.

K. Tonkin: In the real world, the number of women that I have actually treated who might be of premenopausal age but remain post-menopausal after they have had their adjuvant chemotherapy and are hormonal candidates is very small. The numbers in studies are quite low. I have given these women the LH-RH agonists for 3 months and, if they are genuine responders, I then send them for surgery. In my experience, this is a handful of people. This is a select population because most of these premenopausal women have been rendered postmenopausal by chemotherapy and/or they have visceral disease that you want to treat with chemotherapy.

J. Ingle: Henning (Mouridsen), with respect to your question of oophorectomy vs. LH-RH agonists, I think that at this point in time our knowledge base suggests they should be considered comparable. With respect to patients, when you present the options to a woman, some will choose the surgical approach, some will choose the nonsurgical approach. It is a very personal thing. I don't think that we have a basis for mandating one ovarian suppression approach at this time.

A. Howell: I would like to make a point, which may at first seem theoretical, but on further inspection may not be. In the ZEBRA trial, 2 years of ovarian suppression was equivalent to chemotherapy where there was partial ovarian suppression. One interpretation of why ovarian suppression for 2 years was "so good" was that these women had two endocrine therapies. First, they had suppression and the cells are gradually adapted to that low level, and then estrogen was given (relatively high dose estrogen to them), another endocrine therapy. In the future, in advanced disease, we may use LH-RH analogues in that way. So it may be better for those women who are going to have long-term endocrine responses in advanced disease, when we have more data, to give LH-RH analogues instead of oophorectomy.

M. Ellis: I was going to make a very practical point that we all appreciate but many general oncologists don't, that the aromatase inhibitors don't work in premenopausal women. I've seen a few women who were premenopausal and were given an aromatase inhibitor and came to me for a second opinion. I measured their estradiol on the inhibitor and it was not suppressed. The estrogen level in one premenopausal woman on letrozole was over 100. An important point to make here is that aromatase inhibitors do not suppress estrogen in premenopausal women and have to be combined with ovarian suppression or ablation.

M. Dowsett: Jim Ingle made a very reasonable point that the current knowledge base is that the LH-RH agonists are equivalent to oophorectomy, at least as far the woman's steroidal milieu is concerned. But that isn't quite correct. We did some work several years ago showing that there is still an underlying folliculogenesis in patients who are on the LH-RH agonists; the estrogen levels fluctuate and are somewhat higher than in postmenopausal women. Some work that was done in the benign gynecological field by David Baird and Steve Hillier in Edinburgh confirmed this but also showed that when you give tamoxifen to patients on LH-RH agonists, it suppressed the fluctuation. So the interaction at the pituitary/hypothalamic axis reduced those estrogen levels to postmenopausal levels. This is a subtle difference between postmenopausal/oophorectomized women and LH-RH agonist–treated patients and it probably doesn't matter a great deal, but they are not quite the same.

J. Ingle: That was from the standpoint of efficacy. There are subtle differences that may need to be exploited.

H. Mouridsen: I would like to conclude on sequencing in post- and premenopausal patients. Most of us agree that in postmenopausal patients, the first choice should be an aromatase inhibitor. Tamoxifen could be a second choice if the patients haven't had that previously. For the premenopausal patients who develop advanced breast cancer, it should probably be a combination of tamoxifen and ovarian suppression or ablation. If patients are on tamoxifen already, we don't know whether to continue with tamoxifen or discontinue. In premenopausal patients, by combining an LH-RH agonist and tamoxifen, we have for the first time seen a combined endocrine therapy that is superior to single-agent treatment. That leads to the question of the relevance of studies of complete estrogenic suppression (in premenopausal women to combine LH-RH agonists with an aromatase inhibitor and in postmenopausal women to combine an aromatase inhibitor with tamoxifen).

A. Howell: The EORTC study is a beautiful one and you are right, with an overview of those four studies, LH-RH plus tamoxifen might be the treatment of choice is premenopausal women. So what is the next trial? The next trial is LH-RH plus tamoxifen vs. LH-RH plus aromatase inhibition. I don't know if any companies would be interested in this. It would have to be a worldwide trial.

We'll have some information on tamoxifen plus aromatase inhibitor from the results of the ATAC trial later this year in San Antonio, albeit getting the answer in the adjuvant situation before you get it in the advanced situation. I wouldn't plan anything along those lines until we see the results of the ATAC trial.

M. Dowsett: I would like to ask one question relating to this. When Faslodex came through as a pure antiestrogen, which essentially degraded the estrogen receptor as well, we felt this would be the ultimate in terms of estrogen deprivation. With the aromatase inhibitors now, particularly with letrozole, we have almost got the ultimate in aromatase inhibition. I feel concerned that with the once-monthly dosing of Faslodex we might not have the ultimate in terms of pure antiestrogen. Are any of the newer agents that have been discussed bringing us closer to the ultimate, which might allow us to get closer to what Henning Mouridsen was asking for (complete estrogen deprivation) in one drug?

A. Howell: I take your point. When there is a phase III study, as was started with 182 (Faslodex) vs. anastrozole, there was 125-mg arm in there and there were responses, the odd response and some stabilizations. However, that arm was dropped fairly quickly. Faslodex was as good as anastrozole after tamoxifen, but there are questions about getting enough in. It is cumulative, as we showed in the first paper. Kent Osborne would like us to do a study of 2×50-mg injections vs. 500 mg, but that would need a huge study. As far as the other drugs are concerned, Schering AG had another 7-alpha, which they say is already active. It looks very active in premenopausal models of tamoxifen stimulated MCF-7 cells. It may be that is better and they may be able to get more in, but we don't have enough data on that. The other one was the Taiho compound, which also looks very good in the preclinical models, but it has agonist activity on bone and cholesterol. So you may think that it might not be as active as those 2,7-alpha drugs that we already have or are going to have.

M. Kaufmann: Are there any final comments from the audience that we have missed?

W. Eiermann: What is the answer for second-line treatment? No one has told us until now.

C. Benz: Let me refine my earlier question, because it is an important issue that was missed earlier. It seems to me that, as we switch from tamoxifen to aromatase inhibitors and progress sequentially in our endocrine therapies, we have to consider two classes of aromatase inhibitors and inactivators with potentially different mechanisms. Clinically and practically speaking, we would like to know whether we can use these different classes of antiaromatase agents sequentially. I would like to know if there is any evidence today in preclinical models about sequential use of antiaromatase agents.

M. Kaufmann: This is just a feeling: there are some data suggesting that sequencing is possible, but there are only scant crossover data on nonsteroidal and steroidal aromatase inhibitors.

A. Brodie: In the preclinical models, we made letrozole-resistant animals and the nonsteroidals (like anastrozole) did not work, although we didn't test exemestane. However, fadrozole was much better and did work very well on the letrozole-resistant tumors.

M. Kaufmann: Concerning Wolfgang Eiermann's question on sequencing, it depends which drug you start first.

I think we had an excellent session, where we drew conclusions on which patients should receive endocrine treatment, and we had some consensus on the sequence of the endocrine treatment for metastatic breast cancer. Dear colleagues, let me just close the session with a quote from the German poet Goethe: "The more we know, the more we doubt."

Part III

EARLY BREAST CANCER

6

Early Breast Cancer: Tamoxifen Overview

Carsten Rose
Lund University Hospital
Lund, Sweden

I. ABSTRACT

Tamoxifen has been used in the treatment of breast cancer since the 1970s, when it became the treatment of choice. Despite other endocrine breast cancer therapy options, tamoxifen remains the most widely used endocrine agent for treatment of both primary and metastatic disease.

This chapter reviews data on adjuvant tamoxifen therapy in patients according to nodal, menopausal, and steroid receptor status as well as summarizing data on the duration of tamoxifen therapy and the potential for tamoxifen as a replacement to cytotoxic therapy. In addition, the possibility of tamoxifen used concomitantly with chemotherapy or other endocrine therapies is briefly reviewed.

II. INTRODUCTION

Tamoxifen is a selective estrogen-receptor modulator and as such has dual properties, acting as both estrogen receptor (ER) agonist and antagonist [1]. The dominant effect of tamoxifen in breast tumors is caused by its antiestrogenic effect. This is mediated through competitive ER blockade, resulting in reduced transcription of estrogen-regulated genes. The cell cycle is thereby halted, inhibiting subsequent tumor growth. Tamoxifen was first introduced as a breast cancer treatment in the metastatic setting. It soon replaced diethylstilbestrol as a treatment of choice in postmenopausal women after tamoxifen was found to be as effective and to have fewer side effects, with withdrawal rates due to adverse events below 5% [2]. Owing to its efficacy and few side effects, tamoxifen was soon introduced in experimental trials evaluating its potential as adjuvant therapy for early breast cancer. Already, in an analysis of the first adjuvant tamoxifen study, The Copenhagen Breast Cancer Trials, tamoxifen showed superiority to placebo therapy in both pre- and postmenopausal patients with stages I, II, and III disease. Owing to the small number of patients, the trend in favor of tamoxifen was not significant at the latest published analysis in 1987, neither regarding recurrence-free survival or overall survival (OS) [Torben Palshf: Adjuvant endocrine therapy in pre- and postmenopausal women with breast cancer: Thesis, University of Copenhagen, Denmark]. In the postmenopausal patient group, one-third were randomized to diethylstilbestrol 1 mg three times a day. It is noteworthy that diethylstilbestrol also extended both recurrence-free and overall survival to the same extent as tamoxifen 10 mg three times a day. Subsequently, results from the Early Breast Cancer Trialists' Collaborative Group demonstrated beyond a doubt that adjuvant endocrine therapy with tamoxifen prolonged both recurrence-free and overall survival in both pre- and postmenopausal women provided that the tumors expressed steroid hormone receptors.

III. TAMOXIFEN IN PRE- AND POSTMENOPAUSAL WOMEN

Data from early trials suggest that younger women below age 50 do not benefit from tamoxifen therapy. Furthermore, a meta-analysis in 1988 of 28 tamoxifen and 40 chemotherapy trials concluded that treatment with tamoxifen resulted in a clear reduction in mortality only among women of age 50 and above [3]. Conversely, chemotherapy significantly reduced mortality only in premenopausal women. However, a meta-analysis carried out 10 years later gathered new data from 55 randomized tamoxifen trials enrolling more than 37,000 women in total [4]. When the data for 5 years' adjuvant tamoxifen were stratified by pre- and postmenopausal status, a difference was seen between the different age groups. In postmenopausal women, disease-free survival (DFS) and OS were reduced by 37% in women aged 50–59 years, while a greater reduction of 54% was seen in women aged 60 and above (Table 1). In premenopausal women, a substantial benefit was also seen in women treated with tamoxifen for 5 years. In the subgroup of ER-positive and ER-unknown patients, there was a substantial risk reduction in DFS and OS of 45% and 32%, respectively. In those premenopausal women treated with tamoxifen for 1 or 2 years, only a small benefit was seen.

Table 1   Risk Reductions in Disease-Free
Survival (DFS) and Overall Survival (OS) for
Postmenopausal Women, Stratified by Age,
Comparing Tamoxifen 5 Years Versus Placebo

Age (years)	DFS% (SD%)	OS% (SD%)
50–59	37% (6%)	11% (8%)
60–69	54% (5%)	33% (6%)
70	54% (15%)	34% (13%)

IV.   TAMOXIFEN IN RELATION TO NODAL AND STEROID RECEPTOR STATUS

A.   Node-Positive and Node-Negative Tumors

The 1998 meta-analysis confirmed the positive effect of tamoxifen, with reductions in the annual odds of recurrence occurring in both the node-positive (46% reduction) and node-negative (43% reduction) patients [4]. Furthermore, the annual odds of death from any cause were also reduced in the tamoxifen-treated groups (by 25 and 28%, respectively). Likewise, the absolute improvement in recurrence rate at 10 years was 14.9% among node-negative women; the corresponding figure among women with node-positive disease was an absolute improvement of 15.2%. The absolute improvement in survival at 10 years was 5.6% in node-negative, ER-positive patients treated for 5 years with tamoxifen. In node-positive, ER-positive patients, the absolute reduction in mortality was 10.9% at 10 years.

One of the largest trials included in the meta-analysis was the National Surgical Adjuvant Breast and Bowel Project (NSABP) trial B14 in 2844 node-negative, ER-positive breast cancer patients [5]. Patients treated in NSABP-B14 received placebo or tamoxifen for 5 years, with those receiving tamoxifen further randomized at 5 years to placebo or a further 5 years of tamoxifen. In the initial 5-year period, significantly fewer recurrences and deaths occurred in the tamoxifen group. At 10 years of follow-up, both DFS and OS were significantly greater in the tamoxifen-treated group compared with placebo. For DFS, the figures were 69% versus 57% ($p < 0.00001$) and 80% versus 76% for OS ($p < 0.2$), respectively. The benefit was seen in patients both under and over 50 years of age [6].

B.   ER-Positive and ER-Negative Tumors

The ER status of tumors has played an increasingly important role in the evaluation of outcome when patients are being treated with endocrine therapy. Although many trials have collected data on ER status, it is hard to analyze them together, as the methodology used and the definitions of ER status have varied depending on the protocol used. However, despite the fact that many of the early trials included ER-negative tumors with an average treatment period of only 1–2 years, a clear reduction in 5-year mortality has been shown with tamoxifen [7].

In the 1998 meta-analysis, the effect of tamoxifen in ER-negative tumors (~20% of the population) were confirmed to be poor. However, in the remaining ER-positive and so-called ER-unknown population (~48 and ~32%, respectively) recurrence and mortality rates were both increasingly and significantly reduced as the treatment period lengthened from 1 to 2 to 5 years (Table 2). Overall relative reductions in recurrence compared with placebo were reported as 18% (SD 3), 24% (SD 2), and 43% (SD 3) for 1, 2, and 5 years, respectively [4]. This was mirrored by reductions in mortality of 11% (SD 3), 14% (SD 2), and 23% (SD 4) for 1, 2, and 5 years, respectively. The greatest reductions were in ER-positive tumors after 5 years of tamoxifen with highly significant ($p<0.00001$) relative reductions in recurrence (50%) and mortality (28%) (Table 3) [4]. For patients with unknown ER status, the reductions were slightly lower although still significantly greater than for those with ER-negative tumors.

The effects in ER-negative tumors are less clear-cut. Although acting pri-

Table 2 Proportional Reductions in Recurrence and Mortality in ER-Positive Tumors During Approximately 10 Years of Follow-Up in Patients Treated with Tamoxifen for Early Breast Cancer Versus No Tamoxifen

Tamoxifen therapy duration (years)	Proportional reduction in recurrence (SD)		Proportional reduction in mortality (SD)	
1	21%[a]	(3%)	12%[b]	(3%)
2	29%[a]	(2%)	17%[a]	(3%)
5	47%[a]	(3%)	26%[a]	(4%)

[a]$p<0.00001$; [b]$p=0.0003$.

Table 3 Effect of 5 Years of Tamoxifen Therapy on Recurrence and Death Rates in ER-Status-Assessed Tumors

Estrogen-receptor level		Reduction in annual odds (SD)	
Class	Concentration (fmol/mg)	Recurrence	Death
Negative	<10	6% (11%)	−3% (11%)
Unknown	—	37% (8%)	21% (9%)
Positive	10	50% (4%)	28% (5%)
	10–99	43% (5%)	23% (6%)
	100	60% (6%)	36% (7%)

marily through the ER, tamoxifen has a number of other inhibitory effects on cell growth that are not mediated primarily through the ER [7]. Accordingly, several trials have also shown that ER-negative or ER-poor tumors may benefit slightly from tamoxifen treatment [8,9]. However, other trials have not confirmed these findings, showing either no effect or a detrimental effect of giving tamoxifen to patients with ER-negative tumors [10,11]. Indeed, the latter view is strongly supported by the findings of the 1998 meta-analysis, in which little or no benefit from tamoxifen was found in ER-negative tumors (Table 3) [4].

V. TAMOXIFEN VERSUS CHEMOTHERAPY

Although most data comparing tamoxifen with chemotherapy show chemotherapy to be more effective than tamoxifen, there are enough data to throw some doubt on this conclusion. One of the key trials comparing tamoxifen with chemotherapy was Study 01 by the Adjuvant Chemo-hormone Therapy Breast Cancer Study Group (GROCTA). In this trial, tamoxifen was compared with chemotherapy [six cycles of cyclophosphamide/methotrexate/fluorouracil (CMF) followed by four cycles of epirubicin]. The overall results indicated that tamoxifen-treated patients showed risks of relapse and death that were 36 and 32% lower, respectively, than with chemotherapy (p=0.001 and p=0.01, respectively) [12]. In the ensuing subgroup analyses, it was found that tamoxifen equaled chemotherapy in ER- and node-positive premenopausal women (n=237) with respect to DFS and OS. In contrast to this, in a subset of ER- and node-positive premenopausal patients (n=331) from a trial performed by the German Adjuvant Breast Cancer Group [13], CMF was found to be superior to 2 years of tamoxifen, both in DFS (84 vs. 49%, respectively) and OS (96 vs. 80%, respectively).

VI. DURATION OF TAMOXIFEN

Both meta-analyses from 1980 and 1999 have shown that currently 5 years of tamoxifen therapy can be recommended as the optimal treatment length. A Swedish study compared 5 years versus 2 years of tamoxifen treatment in 3887 postmenopausal women below age 75 with node-negative/positive tumors [14]. Those patients receiving 5 years of tamoxifen had statistically significant improvements in DFS and OS, with a relative reduction of 18% for both endpoints.

The 1998 meta-analysis found that after the exclusion of women with ER-negative tumors, the difference between 5 years and 1 or 2 years of adjuvant tamoxifen was large and independent of nodal status, dose, concurrent chemotherapy, age, or menopausal status [4]. The benefits of 5 years of adjuvant tamoxifen have been found in several direct comparative trials [15,16].

In an extension to the NSABP-B14 trial, 10 years of tamoxifen treatment was evaluated versus placebo. Following the initial 5 years of tamoxifen treatment, 1172 progression-free patients were rerandomized to either placebo or a further 5 years of tamoxifen therapy [17]. The main conclusion was that after 7 years of follow-up, there remained no benefit to extending tamoxifen beyond the initial 5 years of treatment (Table 4). Moreover, a slight advantage was observed in patients who discontinued therapy after 5 years with respect to those who continued tamoxifen (Table 4). In a further two trials, no benefit of 10 years of adjuvant tamoxifen has been found [18,19]. However, the follow-up may be too short to allow any conclusion other than that there are currently no data to suggest that extending adjuvant tamoxifen beyond 5 years is beneficial.

VII. TAMOXIFEN AS CONCOMITANT THERAPY

A. With Chemotherapy

Regardless of the outcomes of trials comparing chemotherapy vs. tamoxifen, all trials reviewed in the 1998 meta-analysis comparing concomitant chemoendocrine therapy with either treatment alone have shown benefits in recurrence and mortality favoring the combined treatment approach [4,20,21].

The NSABP B-20 trial compared tamoxifen alone with tamoxifen combined with MF (methotrexate/fluorouracil) or CMF (cyclophosphamide/MF) [20]. A total of 2306 breast cancer patients with node-negative and ER-positive tumors were randomized to one of the three treatment regimens and followed up for 5 years. The data showed that no subgroup of patients failed to benefit from chemotherapy, with both forms of combined therapy improving treatment outcomes more than tamoxifen alone (Table 5). Importantly, data from the International Breast Cancer Study Group (IBCSG) Trial VII indicate that tamoxifen should not be initiated before CMF, as this could be detrimental to the patient [22]. This conclusion came from a trial in 1266 node-positive postmenopausal breast cancer patients who received tamoxifen for 5 years or combined tamoxifen for 5 years with CMF cycles given early (months 1, 2, and 3), delayed (months 9, 12, and 15), or both (months 1, 2, 3, 9, 12, and 15).

Table 4 5-Year Versus 10-Year Tamoxifen Treatment

	Tamoxifen (5 years) $n=579$	Tamoxifen (10 years) $n=593$	p Value
Relapse-free survival	82%	78%	0.03
Disease-free survival	94%	92%	0.13
Overall survival	94%	91%	0.07

Table 5 Tamoxifen Monotherapy for 5 Years Versus
Tamoxifen for 5 Years Combined with CMF or MF[a,b]

	MFT $n=767$	Tamoxifen $n=771$	CMFT $n=768$
Relapse-free survival	90%*	85%	89%‡
Disease-free survival	92%§	87%	91%**
Overall survival	97%†	94%	96%

Key: M, methotrexate; F, fluorouracil; C, cyclophosphamide; T, tamoxifen.
[a]Patients receiving the combined chemoendocrine treatment benefited more
than those receiving tamoxifen alone.
[b]Compared with tamoxifen: *$p=0.01$; §$p<0.01$; †$p=0.05$; ‡$p=0.001$;
**$p<0.001$.

The key findings were that early CMF added to tamoxifen significantly increased 5-year DFS (21% relative risk reduction, $p=0.01$), while delayed CMF did not (3% relative risk reduction, $p=0.77$). Contrastingly, delayed CMF was associated with an increased risk of relapse in patients with ER-negative tumors, though this was not significant (27% relative risk increase, $p=0.15$).

B. With Other Endocrine Agents

In addition to combining tamoxifen with chemotherapy, new data are emerging on trials that combine endocrine agents like tamoxifen with goserelin, the LH-RH agonist, with or without chemotherapy. The Eastern Co-operative Oncology Group (ECOG) study has 6 years of follow-up data on 1504 premenopausal, node- and ER-positive patients. These patients were randomized to cyclophosphamide/adriamycin/fluorouracil (CAF) or CAF/goserelin or CAF/goserelin/tamoxifen [23]. The data from the trial suggest that there is a clear trend favoring the triple combination, with 78% of these patients experiencing DFS at 6 years vs. 70% for CAF/goserelin and 67% for CAF alone.

In one Austrian study, 1045 patients were randomized to either combined tamoxifen/goserelin or CMF [24]. After 4 years of follow-up, data would seem to indicate that the combined endocrine therapy is at least as effective as—if not better than—chemotherapy alone in terms of DFS.

Premenopausal patients with ER-positive tumors who are treated with endocrine drug combinations like tamoxifen and goserelin are effectively made postmenopausal, thereby increasing tamoxifen's efficacy. It would therefore seem prudent to suggest that, given the right combination of drugs and tumor type, most patients could benefit from endocrine therapy.

VIII. PROGNOSTIC AND PREDICTIVE FACTORS

From the 1998 meta-analysis, it has been shown that ER-negative tumors respond poorly to tamoxifen, while tumors with increasing levels of ER show a trend toward a better response to 5 years of adjuvant tamoxifen [4]. This trend becomes even more significant in ER-positive tumors (Table 3).

Furthermore, data from a trial by the Danish Breast Cancer Group investigated the concentrations of the progesterone receptor (PgR) [25,26]. The group found that at levels between 10 and 100 fmol/mg cytosolic protein, there was no benefit to being PgR-positive with respect to prognosis. However, at levels above 100 fmol/mg, there was a substantial prognostic benefit to being PgR-positive ($p=0.01$).

Data regarding ER and PgR status suggest that a quantitative assay might be a suitable tool for prognosis in early breast cancer. As yet the immunohistological assays performed in most situations today are not quantitative by any means.

IX. SUMMARY

Without a doubt, tamoxifen has been one of the most successful endocrine agents seen and used in breast cancer patients over the past 30 years. Although some might say that by today's evidence-based standards, tamoxifen would never have been approved, its lack of serious side effects was deemed enough of a benefit to ensure its approval for use as a cancer therapy.

Since the 1970s, a number of trials and meta-analyses have investigated tamoxifen's efficacy both in the primary and the metastatic disease setting. More recently, data have shown that 5 years of adjuvant tamoxifen therapy provides substantial benefits in ER-positive patients, with reductions in DFS and OS of up to 50 and 30%, respectively, thus beating the effects obtained by adjuvant cytotoxic therapy. In addition to prolonging and probably saving many lives, tamoxifen's introduction into the treatment of breast cancer has led to a better understanding of its mode of action, an extension of our knowledge about tumor endocrinology, and increased interest in discovering other endocrine drugs, thereby opening the doors to newer, safer, and more effective endocrine breast cancer therapies.

REFERENCES

1. Osborne CK. Steroid hormone receptors in breast cancer management. Breast Cancer Res Treat 1998; 51:227–238.
2. Baum M. Tamoxifen—The treatment of choice. Why look for alternatives? Br J Cancer 1998; 78(suppl 4):1–4.
3. Early Breast Cancer Trialists' Collaborative Group. Effects of adjuvant tamoxifen and of cytotoxic therapy on mortality in early breast cancer. An overview of 61 randomized trials among 28,896 women. N Engl J Med 1988; 319:1681–1692.

4. Early Breast Cancer Trialists' Collaborative Group. Tamoxifen for early breast cancer: An overview of the randomised trials. Lancet 1998; 351:1451–1467.

5. Fisher B, Costantino J, Redmond C, et al. A randomized clinical trial evaluating tamoxifen in the treatment of patients with node-negative breast cancer who have estrogen-receptor–positive tumors. N Engl J Med 1989; 320:479–484.

6. Fisher B, Dignam J, Bryant J, et al: Five versus more than five years of tamoxifen therapy for breast cancer patients with negative lymph nodes and estrogen receptor-positive tumors. J Natl Cancer Inst 1996; 88:1529–1542.

7. Osborne CK, Ravdin PM. Adjuvant systemic therapy of primary breast cancer. In: Harris JR, Lippman ME, Morrow M, Osborne CK eds. Diseases of the Breast. Philadelphia: Lippincott, 2000:599–632.

8. NATO Steering Committee. Controlled trial of tamoxifen as a single adjuvant agent in the management of early breast cancer. Br J Cancer 1988; 57:608–611.

9. Report from the Breast Cancer Trials Committee, Scottish Cancer Trials Office (MRC), Edinburgh. Adjuvant tamoxifen in the management of operable breast cancer: the Scottish Trial. Lancet 1987; 2:171–175.

10. Fisher B, Redmond C, Brown A, et al. Adjuvant chemotherapy with and without tamoxifen in the treatment of primary breast cancer: 5-year results from the National Surgical Adjuvant Breast and Bowel Project Trial. J Clin Oncol 1986; 4:459–471.

11. Hutchins L, Green S, Ravdin P, et al. CMF versus CAF with and without tamoxifen in high-risk node-negative breast cancer patients and a natural history follow-up study in low-risk node-negative patients: First results of intergroup trial INT 0102 (abstr). Proc ASCO 1998; 17:1a.

12. Boccardo F, Rubagotti A, Amoroso D, et al. Italian Breast Cancer Adjuvant Chemo-Hormone Therapy Cooperative Group Trials. GROCTA Trials. Recent Results Cancer Res 1998; 152:453–470.

13. Jonat W, Kaufmann M, Abel U. Chemo- or endocrine adjuvant therapy alone or combined in post-menopausal patients (GABG Trial 1). Recent Results Cancer Res 1989; 115:163–169.

14. Swedish Breast Cancer Cooperative Group. Randomized trial of two versus five years of adjuvant tamoxifen for post-menopausal early stage breast cancer. J Natl Cancer Inst 1996; 88:1543–1549.

15. Current Trials working Party of the Cancer Research Campaign Breast Cancer Trials Group. Preliminary results from the cancer research campaign trial evaluating tamoxifen duration in women aged fifty years or older with breast cancer. J Natl Cancer Inst 1996; 88:1834–1839.

16. Delozier T, Spielmann M, Macé-Lesec'h J, et al. Tamoxifen adjuvant treatment duration in early breast cancer: Initial results of a randomized study comparing short-term treatment with long-term treatment. Federation Nationale des Centres de Lutte Contre le Cancer Breast Group. J Clin Oncol 2000; 18:3507–3512.

17. Fisher B, Dignam J, Bryant J, Wolmark N. Five versus more than five years of tamoxifen for lymph node-negative breast cancer: Updated findings from the National Surgical Adjuvant Breast and Bowel Project B-14 randomized trial. J Natl Cancer Inst 2001; 93:684–690.

18. Stewart HJ, Forrest AP, Everington D, et al. Randomised comparison of 5 years of

adjuvant tamoxifen with continuous therapy for operable breast cancer. The Scottish Cancer Trials Breast Group. Br J Cancer 1996; 74:297–299.

19. Tormey DC, Gray R, Falkson HC (for the Eastern Cooperative Oncology Group). Postchemotherapy adjuvant tamoxifen therapy beyond five years in patients with lymph node-positive breast cancer. J Natl Cancer Inst 1996; 88:1828–1833.

20. Fisher B, Dignam J, Wolmark N, et al. Tamoxifen and chemotherapy for lymph node-negative, estrogen receptor-positive breast cancer. J Natl Cancer Inst 1997; 89:1673–1682.

21. Fisher B, Redmond C, Legault-Poisson S, et al. Postoperative chemotherapy and tamoxifen compared with tamoxifen alone in the treatment of positive-node breast cancer patients aged 50 years and older with tumors responsive to tamoxifen: Results from the National Surgical Adjuvant Breast and Bowel Project B-16. J Clin Oncol 1990; 8:1005–1018.

22. International Breast Cancer Study Group. Effectiveness of adjuvant chemotherapy in combination with tamoxifen for node-positive post-menopausal breast cancer patients. J Clin Oncol 1997; 15:1385–1394.

23. Davidson N, O'Neil A, Vukov A, et al. Effect of chemohormonal therapy in premenopausal node +, receptor + breast cancer: An Eastern Cooperative Oncology Group Phase III Intergroup trial. Proc Am Soc Clin Oncol 1999; 18:249a.

24. Jakesz H, Hausmaninger H, Samonigg H, et al. Comparison of adjuvant therapy with tamoxifen and goserelin vs CMF in premenopausal stage I and II hormone-responsive breast cancer patients: Four year results of Austrian Breast Cancer Study Group Trial 5. Proc Am Soc Clin Oncol 1999; 18:250a.

25. Rose C, Andersen JA, Andersen KW, et al. Adjuvant endocrine treatment of postmenopausal patients with breast cancer with high risk of recurrence. 5. Results from the DBCG (Danish Breast Cancer Cooperative Group) 77C randomized trial. Ugeskr Laeger 1991; 153:2283–2287.

26. Rose C, Thorpe SM, Andersen KW, et al. Beneficial effect of adjuvant tamoxifen therapy in primary breast cancer patients with high estrogen receptor values. Lancet 1985; 1(9419):16–19.

7

Aromatase Inhibitors and Early Breast Cancer

Paul E. Goss
University of Toronto
Princess Margaret Hospital
University Health Network
Toronto, Ontario, Canada

I. ABSTRACT

The management of early breast cancer (EBC) is critical in defining the long-term outcome of the disease. This period is a window of opportunity that can allow us to manipulate micrometastatic tumor cells (if present) when they may be sensitive to endocrine therapy.

Current clinical management of receptor-positive EBC in postmenopausal women is 5 years of systemic adjuvant tamoxifen therapy (and, depending on circumstances, multiagent chemotherapy), but the development of the third generation of aromatase inhibitors (AIs) necessitates a re-evaluation of this treatment paradigm. This article describes the ongoing clinical trials of these promising compounds and outlines how the trials will provide us with substantial new data. This information will help us to establish future treatment decisions, to reassess our preclinical models, and to define the direction of our future research in the endocrine treatment of breast cancer.

II. CURRENT TREATMENT AND ITS LIMITATIONS

Tamoxifen is one of the most successful anticancer drugs ever discovered in terms of lives saved. The Oxford Review group (EBCTCG) [1] recently estimated that, during the 1990s, about 20,000 U.K. deaths and 40,000 U.S. deaths were avoided, largely through the use of adjuvant tamoxifen therapy. The fact that we now have a new class of drugs, the aromatase inhibitors, that appear to be set to displace such an important lead drug, is truly remarkable and makes this an exciting time for us as well as for our patients.

Despite its success, tamoxifen does have limitations. An increased risk of four serious side effects has been linked to its use, including endometrial cancer, deep venous thrombosis, pulmonary embolism, and stroke. Furthermore, it is not always successful in preventing the growth of estrogen-dependent tumors, leading to what is known as tamoxifen "resistance." We are now beginning to recognize that long-term treatment with this compound may alter tumor cell biology and/or sensitivity to estrogens.

A. The Effects of Long-Term Tamoxifen and Possible Mechanisms of "Resistance"

Tamoxifen was one of the first of a group of drugs known as selective estrogen-receptor modulators (SERMs). It has primarily an antiestrogenic effect but also acts in some tissues as a weak estrogen. It has a very long half-life—at least several months and perhaps as much as a year [2]. This is an important consideration for the combination trials that are switching to another endocrine therapy after long-term treatment with tamoxifen. The timing of the start of the new treatment after the cessation of tamoxifen may be important for the therapeutic cytotoxic or cytocidal effect of the latter. Other SERMs might potentially be better than tamoxifen in this kind of trial design, and it is possible that a drug that destroys the ER, such as faslodex, might overcome such problems [3].

1. Mutations and Changes in the Estrogen Receptor

From the work of McGuire and colleagues, it has been suspected for some time that mutations in the estrogen receptor (ER) could play a role in tumor progression [4]. How much of a role is still not clear, since these mutations are found typically in mRNA and the physiological effects of ER mutations are unknown [5]. More recently, however, it has been proposed that a mutation in the ER protein may play a role in promoting the estrogen agonist action of tamoxifen [6].

In addition, through the work of Santen and others, it seems likely that tumor cells can develop hypersensitivity to estrogen in situ [7]. Their work, using MCF-7 cells, has shown that if tumor cells are deprived of estrogen in long-term culture, they can then be maximally stimulated by estradiol at a concentration four orders of magnitude lower than the optimal dose for control cells. Thus it is possible, in a scenario of estrogen inhibition by long-term tamoxifen treatment, that exogenous estrogens from the diet or estrogen synthesized by large bowel clostridia, for example, could provide sufficient stimulation for the continued growth of ER-positive tumors [7a].

2. Upregulation of Aromatase Expression and/or Activity

Transcription of the aromatase enzyme is regulated by a wide variety of enhancers, including cyclic AMP, phorbol esters, dexamethasone, prostaglandin E2, transforming growth factor B, and gamma interferon [8]. However, it remains to be shown that any of these have a direct effect on tumor progression. Overexpression of the aromatase gene is seen in some mouse mammary tumors, and in these cases it may be the result of a genetic mutation [9]. It is important to bear in mind, however, that the carcinoma cells are not the only source of aromatase in the tumor and that the expression of this enzyme by invasive macrophage cells may well be important in stimulating tumor growth and perhaps in tamoxifen "resistance" [10].

III. RATIONALE FOR UTILIZING AIs FOR THE TREATMENT OF EBC

There are a number of reasons why one should consider using AIs for the management of EBC, including possible failure on tamoxifen therapy; failure on other SERMs; and favorable comparisons of AIs with tamoxifen in the metastatic setting.

Failure with tamoxifen is quite frequent, and published work from the EBCTCG has shown that by 15 years after surgery, as many as two-thirds of "at risk" patients have died despite receiving adjuvant tamoxifen [1]. This is an improvement on not having any adjuvant therapy but demonstrates that the risk is still considerable. Saphner and coworkers (1996) [11] have calculated that the risk of recurrence up until 12 years after the start of therapy was also dependent on the number of positive nodes removed at surgery. They found that the lowest risk (maximal hazard rate 0.07 at 2–3 years) existed for node-negative patients, that it increased for women with up to three positive nodes, and was highest at all time points for women with four more positive nodes (maximally 0.23 at 2 years). The NSABP has demonstrated no improvement or a worsening of patient outcome if tamoxifen is given for longer than 5 years after surgery [12]. The ongoing trials, ATTOM (Adjuvant Tamoxifen Treatment—Offer More) and ATLAS (Adjuvant Tamoxifen: Long Against Shorter), are addressing this question further and the results will begin to be released over the next few years.

Alternative SERMs, such as raloxifene and faslodex, have to date not replaced tamoxifen as first-line treatment (see Chap. 18).

AIs work after tamoxifen and are more effective as initial treatment in pre-clinical models of tumor growth [13]. We know that the mechanism of the estrogen antagonism (namely inhibition of estrogen synthesis) is distinct from that of tamoxifen [14], and it is likely to be this feature that enables AIs to overcome tamoxifen "resistance." We know that AIs are well tolerated [15,16]. Finally, at least one of the AIs, letrozole, is considerably better than tamoxifen in first-line treatment, as shown in the P025 study [16].

IV. UNKNOWNS FROM TRIALS OF AIs IN METASTATIC DISEASE

Overall, the trials of AIs in the metastatic setting have been very successful. Letrozole has been found to be superior to tamoxifen as initial therapy for the key variables of time to progression and response rate [16]. Anastrozole is at least as good as tamoxifen, although it is not clear that it has any superiority [15,17]. As for the trials with exemestane, a randomized phase II trial shows a trend toward a higher response rate for the inhibitor, but it is still too early to draw any conclusions. However, these trials have left a number of unanswered questions.

We do not know, for example, what the long-term toxicity of AI treatment might be. Based on the mechanism of action, one might anticipate an increase in bone demineralization; if so, the question will be whether this can be compensated for with the application of supportive medications such as calcium and vitamin D or bisphosphonates. In principle there might be a risk of endometrial cancer comparable to that due to tamoxifen, although in theory, with such potent antiestrogens, this risk should not be increased and in fact might be reduced by the powerful antagonism of circulating estrogens. Similarly, the risk of venous thromboembolism seen with tamoxifen might, if anything, be reduced by the inhibitors, creating a relative anticoagulant effect in contrast to the increase seen with estrogen replacement therapy. It is imprudent to assume the long-term toxicities of these drugs; we should await the reports from the large ongoing clinical trials in this regard. There is a great deal of enthusiasm for the potential of AIs as adjuvant therapy, and large, well-designed trials are ongoing. The ATAC trial, which compares anastrozole with tamoxifen and with anastrozole plus tamoxifen (see below) is the largest adjuvant breast cancer trial ever undertaken. At the time of its initiation, there were no data on the efficacy of the combination or on any possible toxicity or pharmacokinetic interactions between the two drugs. The animal model of Brodie et al. [13] has predicted that a combination of an AI + SERM will be inferior to the AI or tamoxifen alone. It will, nonetheless, be interesting to compare the outcome of the clinical trial with the preclinical model.

V. THE ONGOING TRIALS OF AROMATASE INHIBITORS

A. BIG/FEMTA

The BIG/FEMTA trial of letrozole, conducted by the Breast International Group, has been designed for patients who have had complete resection. The study (started in March 1999) was planned for 5310 patients and had 3672 accrued at the time of this report. The treatment design, with four treatment arms, is shown in Fig. 1. The primary endpoint of the trial is disease-free survival at 5 years and

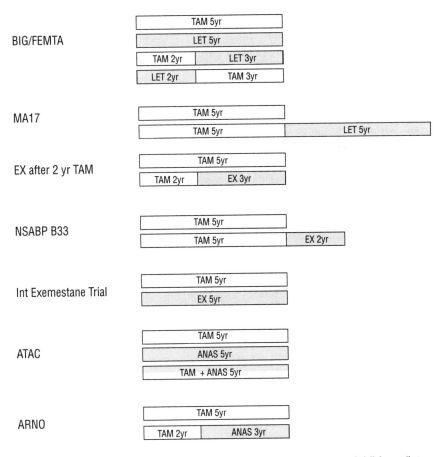

Figure 1 A summary of ongoing trials with adjuvant aromatase inhibitors (letrozole, LET; anastrozole, ANA; exemastane, EX) often versus a control arm of tamoxifen (TAM).

the secondary endpoints include distant and locoregional disease-free survival, overall survival, and safety. There were no substudies originally designed to be included in this trial, but some, at least for bone mineral density and lipid levels, are now being considered (Table 1).

B. MA17

The MA17 trial, organized by the National Cancer Institute of Canada—Clinical Trials Group, is an international intergroup trial activated in August 1998. Its objective is to determine disease-free survival and overall survival in breast cancer patients who are disease-free after 5 years of tamoxifen treatment and are then randomized to receive either letrozole or placebo for a further 5 years. The trial is designed to enroll 4800 patients; thus far 3017 have been accrued.

     Several substudies are ongoing in the context of the main trial. The current bone study is concerned with whether bone demineralization is exacerbated by the aromatase inhibitor. A second study being planned will examine whether bone density, in those patients whose bones are already at risk, can be improved with bisphosphonate therapy despite treatment with an aromatase inhibitor. A mammographic density substudy being planned will establish whether breast density is correlated with response, relapse, or any other factor, in intra- and intergroup comparisons [18]. A collection of tissue blocks, wherever possible, from all the trial participants is planned to allow the possibility of retrospective analyses and

Table 1 Summary of Planned Substudies of the Ongoing Clinical Trials for Aromatase Inhibitors in Early Breast Cancer

	BIG/ FEMTA	MA17	EX after 2-yr TAM	NSABP B33	Int. Exe Trial	ATAC	ARNO
Toxicity		✔					
Pharmacokinetics						✔	
Bone density	✔	✔	✔	✔		✔	
Serum lipids	✔	✔		✔		✔	
Mammographic density		✔					
Contralateral breast		✔					
Endometrial cancer			✔			✔	
End-organ effects		✔					
Quality of life		✔	✔	✔		✔	
Tissue-block archive		✔					

Key: BIG/FEMTA=Breast International Group/Femara versus Tamoxifen; MA17=Femara versus placebo after 5 years of adjuant Tamoxifen; EX after 2-yr TAM=Tamoxifen (5 yrs) versus Tamoxifen (2–3 yrs) followed by exemestane (2–3 yrs); NSABP B33=Exemestane versus placebo after 5 years of adjuvant Tamoxifen; Int.Exe Trial=International trial of Exemestane (5 yrs) versus Tamoxifen (5 yrs); ATAC=Arimidex, Tamoxifen, Alone or in Combination; ARNO=Arimidex Nolvadex.

correlation with patient outcome. Other substudies will examine the toxicity of the treatment, the incidence of contralateral breast cancer, end-organ effects (including serum lipids), and quality of life.

C. Exemestane After Tamoxifen

This trial, being chaired by Dr. Charles Coombes, will study the effect of exemestane following on from 2 years of tamoxifen and compare the result against 5 years of tamoxifen. The study (activated in March 1999) is just finishing accrual, with 4135 patients out of 4400 planned enrolled to date.

The trial has three subprotocols ongoing: one addressing bone metabolism (measuring bone mineral density), one on quality of life (using the FACT-ES psychometric test), and one on the incidence of endometrial cancer risk as assessed by transvaginal ultrasonography (TVUS).

D. NSABP B33

The B33 exemestane trial, organized by the National Surgical Adjuvant Breast and Bowel Project (NSABP), started accrual in May 2001. It has been planned for 3000 patients and the objectives are to see whether exemestane affects disease-free and overall survival. It is intended for postmenopausal women whose primary tumor was Er- and/or PgR-positive. The study is designed along the lines of the MA17 trial and addresses a similar question, but with a distinct agent and a shorter exposure of 2 years of inhibitor after tamoxifen.

The three subprotocols that go along with this trial are for bone metabolism, quality of life, and serum lipid levels.

E. International Exemestane Trial

A phase III randomized trial of exemestane versus tamoxifen for 5 years after surgery was activated in May 2001 for 3000 patients. It is not known whether any substudies are planned. The study outcomes are disease-free and overall survival.

F. ATAC

The ATAC trial was activated in 1996 and closed in 1999 with 9366 postmenopausal breast cancer patients. Initial data were presented for the first time at the 24th Annual San Antonio Breast Cancer Symposium (December 10–13, 2001).

There are five important substudies in the trial that concern bone metabolism (bone mineral density), lipid metabolism, the incidence of endometrial cancer (TVUS), the pharmacokinetics of the AI, and quality of life (assessed by FACT-ES).

G. ARNO

The ARNO trial (ARimidex NOlvadex) has been set up by German and Austrian Breast Cancer Groups to look at the effect of 3 years of anastrozole after 2 years of tamoxifen treatment and to compare this with 5 years of tamoxifen alone. The accrual has been slow for this study because, unlike the other posttamoxifen trials, the patients are randomized at the start of their tamoxifen treatment and not after they have received 2 years of tamoxifen outside of a clinical trial. This has made accrual very difficult. At the time of this manuscript, 1700 patients are enrolled. No substudies are planned for this trial.

VI. THE REPORTING ORDER OF THE TRIALS

The order in which the trials will report could have a big influence on clinical practice. It is very likely that because the results of the anastrozole versus tamoxifen trial will be known before the letrozole versus tamoxifen trial, clinical practice, at least initially, will swing in favor of anastrozole. There is also the influence of pharmaceutical company marketing, which is significant and influences clinical practice considerably.

The exemestane trial after 2 years of tamoxifen, because of the fast accrual to the trial, will probably be the first of the posttamoxifen trials to be reported. The date when some of the BIG/FEMTA results will be disclosed will depend on whether the organizers intend to report all the four arms together or if they will report data from the two nonsequenced arms first. When the sequenced data do come out, they will provide our first insight into the value of AI-tamoxifen as an adjuvant therapy sequence. The B33 is likely to be the last of the current trials to report.

VII. HOW WE WILL JUDGE THESE TRIALS

The data from these trials are probably going to be rather difficult to digest because of the sheer quantity of information. They should, however, provide answers to a number of key questions. In terms of efficacy, these trials will show whether AIs affect disease-free and overall survival after 5, 10, and 15 years from the start of treatment. The maximum time of treatment with an AI in any of these trials is 5 years, in keeping with the current practice with tamoxifen. In the next few years, however, we will begin to get results from the ATTOM and AT-LAS trials, which could influence our interpretation of the AI data.

These trials will also tell us if the AIs provoke any common toxicities, as on the vasomotor or urogenital systems, or any serious toxicities, as on the incidence of endometrial cancer, colon cancer, or other malignancies, or if they induce deep venous thrombosis or pulmonary embolism.

We will have data on the long-term effects of AI treatment on bone density, serum lipid levels, cognitive function, other organs, the incidence of contralateral breast tumors, and whether AIs have a potential application in chemoprevention of breast cancer in healthy women.

VIII. DEVELOPING PRECLINICAL MODELS

Although all of these clinical trials are still in their early phases, it remains important to continue our evaluation of novel endocrine therapies in preclinical models. Our group is using, for example, the model of the 10-month-old, ovariectomized, cycling Sprague-Dawley rat, as recommended by the U.S. Food and Drug Administration, for bone density assessments. We are in the process of determining the effects of AI treatment on bone density and lipid levels in serum to determine whether differences exist between nonsteroidal and steroidal inhibitors. These end-organ effects could have important implications for the application of these agents in long-term therapy in healthy women.

IX. CONCLUSIONS

The third-generation aromatase inhibitors exhibit great potential as therapeutic agents for the management of early breast cancer. It is anticipated that they may dislodge tamoxifen as the current "gold standard" of adjuvant therapy. Hopefully tamoxifen will also have added benefit with the inhibitors. We must, however, be cautious in assuming that it is all going to be good news. Well-designed trials and objective interpretation of the data still hold the key to success.

REFERENCES

1. EBCTCG. UK and USA breast cancer deaths down 25% in year 2000 at ages 20–69 years. http://www.ctsu.ox.ac.uk/pressreleases/Peto_releases_2000_UKUSA_FINAL. shtml; 2000.
2. Fuchs WS, Leary WP, van der Meer MJ, et al. Pharmacokinetics and bioavailability of tamoxifen in postmenopausal healthy women. Arzneimittelforschung 1996; 46:418–422.
3. Howell A, DeFriend DJ, Robertson JF, et al. Pharmacokinetics, pharmacological and anti-tumour effects of the specific anti-oestrogen ICI 182780 in women with advanced breast cancer. Br J Cancer 1996; 74:300–308.
4. Fuqua SA, Chamness GC, McGuire WL. Estrogen receptor mutations in breast cancer. J Cell Biochem 1993; 51:135–139.
5. Dowsett M, Daffada A, Chan CM, Johnston SR. Oestrogen receptor mutants and variants in breast cancer. Eur J Cancer 1997; 33:1177–1183.

6. Levenson AS, MacGregor Schafer JI, et al. Control of the estrogen-like actions of the tamoxifen-estrogen receptor complex by the surface amino acid at position 351. J Steroid Biochem Mol Biol 2001; 76:61–70.

7. Masamura S, Santner SJ, Heitjan DF, Santen RJ. Estrogen deprivation causes estradiol hypersensitivity in human breast cancer cells. J Clin Endocrinol Metab 1995; 80:2918–2925.

7a. Goddard P, Hill MJ. The in vivo metabolism of cholesterol by gut bacteria in the rat and guinea pig. J Steroid Biochem 1974; 5(6):569–572.

8. Simpson ER, Zhao Y, Agarwal VR, et al. Aromatase expression in health and disease. Recent Prog Horm Res 1997; 52:185–213.

9. Tekmal RR, Kirma N, Gill K, Fowler K. Aromatase overexpression and breast hyperplasia, an in vivo model—Continued overexpression of aromatase is sufficient to maintain hyperplasia without circulating estrogens, and aromatase inhibitors abrogate these preneoplastic changes in mammary glands. Endocr Rel Cancer 1999; 6:307–314.

10. Mor G, Yue W, Santen RJ, et al. Macrophages, estrogen and the microenvironment of breast cancer. J Steroid Biochem Mol Biol 1998; 67:403–411.

11. Saphner T, Tormey DC, Gray R. Annual hazard rates of recurrence for breast cancer after primary therapy. J Clin Oncol 1996; 14:2738–2746.

12. Fisher B, Dignam J, Bryant J, Wolmark N. Five versus more than five years of tamoxifen for lymph node-negative breast cancer: updated findings from the National Surgical Adjuvant Breast and Bowel Project B-14 randomized trial. J Natl Cancer Inst 2001; 93:684–690.

13. Brodie A, Lu Q, Liu Y, et al. Preclinical studies using the intratumoral aromatase model for postmenopausal breast cancer. Oncology (Huntingt) 1998; 12:36–40.

14. Bhatnagar AS, Hausler A, Schieweck K. Inhibition of aromatase in vitro and in vivo by aromatase inhibitors. J Enzyme Inhib 1990; 4:179–186.

15. Bonneterre J, Thurlimann B, Robertson JF, et al. Anastrozole versus tamoxifen as first-line therapy for advanced breast cancer in 668 postmenopausal women: Results of the Tamoxifen or Arimidex Randomized Group Efficacy and Tolerability study. J Clin Oncol 2000; 18:3748–3757.

16. Mouridsen H, Gershanovich M, Sun Y, et al. Superior efficacy of letrozole versus tamoxifen as first-line therapy for postmenopausal women with advanced breast cancer: Results of a phase III study of the International Letrozole Breast Cancer Group. J Clin Oncol 2001; 19:2596–2606.

17. Nabholtz JM, Buzdar A, Pollak M, et al. Anastrozole is superior to tamoxifen as first-line therapy for advanced breast cancer in postmenopausal women: results of a North American multicenter randomized trial. Arimidex Study Group. J Clin Oncol 2000; 18:3758–3767.

18. Boyd NF, Martin LJ, Stone J, et al. Mammographic densities as a marker of human breast cancer risk and their use in chemoprevention. Curr Oncol Rep 2001; 3:314–321.

8

SERMs: Overview in Early Breast Cancer

Ian E. Smith
Royal Marsden Hospital NHS Trust
London, England

I. ABSTRACT

This chapter reviews the effects of selective estrogen receptor modulators (SERMs) on their own, as well as in combination with other therapies, on breast cancer, osteoporosis, the cardiovascular system, and cognitive function. The advantages and disadvantages of SERMs compared with aromatase inhibitors in the treatment of breast cancer are also discussed.

II. INTRODUCTION

SERMs are a group of drugs, typified by tamoxifen, that can have both agonist and antagonist effects on estrogen receptors (ERs) at different sites throughout the body. In theory their spectrum is defined by estrogen as a pure agonist at one end and fulvestrant (ICI 182,780) as a pure antiestrogen at the other. In practice, clinical interest lies more with drugs situated more centrally within this spectrum, combining antagonist effects against breast cancer with agonist physiological effects.

Tamoxifen, the first and by far the most widely used SERM, has antagonist effects against breast cancer, with long-established activity in advanced disease, improving survival as adjuvant therapy [1], and reducing the incidence of breast cancer in healthy women at risk of developing the disease [2]. In addition, tamoxifen has agonist effects on bone, preventing bone loss in postmenopausal women [3], and it lowers blood cholesterol [4]. Tamoxifen does have disadvantages apart from a generic problem of acquired resistance common to all endocrine agents: it can precipitate bone loss in premenopausal women as well as vasomotor dysfunction and thromoembolic events. It also has agonist effects on uterine epithelium and is associated with an increased risk of uterine cancer [1,5]. Recently the supremacy of tamoxifen in the endocrine therapy of breast cancer has been challenged by a new generation of aromatase inhibitors, including letrozole, anastrozole, and exemestane. Letrozole has been shown to have superior efficacy to tamoxifen as first-line treatment of advanced breast cancer in terms of response rate and time to progression [6], as has anastrozole in one of two trials [7,8]. Letrozole has likewise been shown to achieve a significantly higher response rate than tamoxifen as neoadjuvant therapy before surgery [9] (see elsewhere in this publication for details). First results are imminent from an adjuvant trial comparing tamoxifen with anastrozole with both in combination (ATAC), and a large international adjuvant trial comparing letrozole with tamoxifen is under way. Even if their efficacy is no greater than that of tamoxifen, they are likely to be at least as good, and in these circumstances aromatase inhibitors could well be favored through absence of uterine cancer risk, and a lower risk of thromboembolic disease. Will these trials lead to the replacement of tamoxifen (and other SERMs) by aromatase inhibitors as the standard adjuvant endocrine therapy?

III. ADJUVANT SERMs VERSUS AROMATASE INHIBITORS: GENERAL PRINCIPLES

In clinical practice, the issues concerning the selection of aromatase inhibitors versus SERMs as adjuvant therapy will probably be complex. First, aromatase inhibitors are likely to be associated with all the disadvantages of estrogen deprivation, both short and long term. Second, newer SERMs, such as the benzothiophene raloxifene, have already been developed that do not appear to carry increased risk of uterine cancer, and there is the theoretical possibility that some of these newer SERMs may have an efficacy superior to that of tamoxifen.

IV. OSTEOPOROSIS

SERMs are already established as protective agents against bone loss in postmenopausal women. In the Royal Marsden tamoxifen prevention trial, postmenopausal patients randomized to tamoxifen had a mean annual increase in bone mineral density of 1.17% in the spine ($p<0.005$) and 1.71% in the hip ($p<0.001$) compared with placebo [3]. In contrast, premenopausal patients receiving tamoxifen experienced an annual bone loss of 1.44% compared with those on placebo ($p<0.001$). In early postmenopausal women, the SERM raloxifene was shown to prevent bone loss in the lumbar spine and proximal femur; in the large randomized controlled trial (MORE) in 7705 postmenopausal women with osteoporosis, 3 years of treatment with raloxifene 60 mg daily was associated with a significant reduction in the risk of vertebral fracture and bone mineral density compared with controls [10,11].

There is so far no large body of data concerning the effects on bone mineral density of long-term aromatase inhibitors, but—given their plasma estrogen–lowering mechanism of action—it seems likely that they will be associated with increased bone density loss. Preliminary data from our own research show that serum CTX (C-terminal crosslink of type 1 collagen) levels fell during a 3-month course of letrozole in normal volunteers; this marker is known to predict long-term loss of bone mineral density (M. Dowsett, personal communication, 2001). It is, of course, possible that bone loss with aromatase inhibitors could be prevented or modified with the concurrent use of bisphosphonates. Three bisphosphonates are currently licensed for use in the treatment of postmenopausal osteoporosis [cyclic etidronate (Didronel in the United Kingdom), alendronate (Fosamax in the United Kingdom), and risedronate (Actonel in the United Kingdom)]. Of these, alendronate has shown significant treatment benefits in bone mineral density when compared with placebo in the Fracture Intervention Trial (FIT) in postmenopausal women with osteoporosis [12]. In another randomized trial, 12 months of treatment with alendronate showed a significant reduction in nonvertebral fractures (relative risk 0.53, 95% CI 0.30 to 0.90) [13]. Likewise, two randomized controlled trials of risedronate on vertebral and nonvertebral fracture rates in postmenopausal women with established osteoporosis have recently been published. In a North American study, risedronate 5 mg orally daily was associated with a reduced relative risk of new vertebral fracture of 0.35 after 1 year and 0.59 after 3 years [14]. In a European/Australian trial, a significant reduction in vertebral and nonvertebral fractures was also seen, along with improvements in bone mineral density compared with placebo [15].

To date, the interaction between aromatase inhibitors and bisphosphonates on bone mineral density has not been investigated clinically. Long-term loss of bone mineral density remains an important theoretical disadvantage of aromatase inhibitors compared with SERMs until proven otherwise.

V. CARDIOVASCULAR EFFECTS

The effects of different SERMs on blood lipid and cholesterol levels appear to be similar and beneficial. Tamoxifen, toremifene, and raloxifene have all been shown to suppress total plasma cholesterol and low-density-lipoprotein (LDL) cholesterol as well as lipoproteins in postmenopausal women, but they have little or no effect on high-density-lipoprotein (HDL) cholesterol [4,10,16–19].

Some evidence has accumulated from adjuvant breast cancer trials indicating that tamoxifen may be associated with a reduction in the incidence of cardiovascular disease compared with placebo. The Scottish Cancer Trials Breast Group showed a reduction in the rate of myocardial infarction in patients treated with adjuvant therapy compared with controls (hazard ratio for the control group 1.92; 95% confidence interval 0.99 to 3.73) [20]. A Swedish trial showed that adjuvant tamoxifen resulted in a significantly reduced incidence of hospital admissions due to cardiac disease (hazard ratio 0.68; 95% confidence interval 0.48 to 0.97; $p=0.03$), and there was a further significant difference in favor of longer (5 years) versus shorter (2 years) treatment [21]. The NSABP B-14 trial showed a trend toward a lower average annual death rate from coronary artery disease for patients receiving adjuvant tamoxifen compared with placebo, but the difference was not statistically significant [22]. In contrast, the NSABP P-1 prevention trial so far has not shown a significant difference in the overall rates of cardiovascular events for tamoxifen versus placebo. However, follow-up is only at 4 years [23].

Long-term effects of aromatase inhibitors on cholesterol and lipoproteins have not been studied in detail. Estrogen replacement therapy is recognized to have a beneficial effect on blood lipids and cholesterol [24], and, by extrapolation, there is the risk that the estrogen-lowering properties of modern aromatase inhibitors may have an adverse effect.

VI. HORMONE REPLACEMENT THERAPY AFTER BREAST CANCER

Menopausal symptoms induced by adjuvant chemotherapy and/or tamoxifen are frequently a major problem in patients with breast cancer. Traditional wisdom has argued against the use of hormone replacement therapy (HRT) in patients with a history of breast cancer, but recently this dogma been challenged. This is a key issue for the future planning of adjuvant endocrine therapy. Theoretically SERMs could be given in combination with HRT: tamoxifen is effective in premenopausal patients with high circulating estrogen levels, and on this basis it is likely to provide protection against any putative risk of HRT with much lower levels of circulating estrogen. It is my view that the use of HRT in conjunction with aromatase inhibitors would be inappropriate on the basis of their estrogen-lowering mechanism of action.

In a recent report of great potential relevance to the management of women with early breast cancer, O'Meara and colleagues retrospectively assessed the effects of HRT in a population-based study involving 2755 women aged 35 to 74 years diagnosed with invasive breast cancer while enrolled in a large health maintenance organization (Group Health Cooperative of Puget Sound, Seattle) from 1977 to 1994 [25]. Pharmacy data identified 174 users of HRT after diagnosis, and each of these was matched to four randomly selected nonusers of HRT with similar age, disease stage, and year of diagnosis. A key feature in the analysis was that all women were recurrence-free at the start of HRT or at the equivalent time for controls. The recurrence rate per 1000 person-years was 17 for HRT users versus 30 for controls (relative risk 0.50; 95% Cl 0.30 to 0.85). Mortality rates from breast cancer were 5 (HRT) versus 15 (non-HRT) (relative risk 0.34 Cl 0.13 to 0.91) and total mortality rates were 16 (HRT) versus 30 (non-HRT) (relative risk 0.48 Cl 0.29 to 0.78). The lower rates of recurrence and death were seen in women who used any type of HRT, including oral, vaginal, or both. No dose effect was seen. Confounding factors are always a risk in such an analysis, but these appear to have been minimized by the use of matched control subjects. These findings are given further credence by having been observed before in a previous smaller study [26]. At the very least, these data encourage randomized trials of HRT in patients after breast cancer, and these are under way in Sweden and about to start in the United Kingdom following a successful pilot study [27]. It is my view that these data also support adjuvant trials using SERMs plus HRT, with quality of life (vasomotor effects, libido, etc.), long-term cardiovascular events, and long-term bone mineral density included as key endpoints in addition to freedom from breast cancer recurrence. Aromatase inhibitors might achieve greater efficacy than SERMs plus HRT, but this would be their only obvious potential advantage. If such a survival benefit were to emerge, it would have to be large enough to support a trade-off with quality of life by women with breast cancer, both in the short and the longer term.

VII. COGNITIVE FUNCTION WITH HRT AND SERMs

The brain is rich in ERs, particularly in regions such as the hippocampus and the amygdala, which are involved in learning and memory. Estrogen is known to regulate synapse formation and induces choline transferase and acetylcholinesterase, which are critical to memory function. The use of estrogen replacement therapy has been associated with a lower risk of Alzheimer's disease [28]. The results of randomized trials on the cognitive effects of estrogen in postmenopausal women are conflicting, but in one study estrogen replacement improved brain activation patterns during working memory tasks [29]. Two prospective trials are currently in progress examining the efficacy of estrogen replacement as a means of preventing cognitive deterioration or Alzheimer's disease in postmenopausal women. Data are slowly emerging on the relationship of SERMs to cognitive function. Tamoxifen has been shown to be antiestrogenic within the CNS in model systems, and one study suggested that cognitive function is worse in patients on long-term tamoxifen (at least 5 years) compared with those on shorter treatment [30]. In contrast, raloxifene is estrogenic in the CNS in model systems. Recently the effect of raloxifene on cognitive function was assessed in the MORE trial referred to above, evaluating the effect of 3 years of raloxifene versus placebo in 7705 postmenopausal women with osteoporosis [31]. Six tests of cognitive function were administered regularly over a 3-year period. No significant difference in the risk of decline in cognitive function was seen in four of the tests between raloxifene and placebo. In two tests, there was a trend toward less decline in cognitive function in patients receiving raloxifene: these involved verbal memory (relative risk 0.77) and attention (relative risk 0.87).

The relationship between postmenopausal estrogen levels and long-term cognitive function remains uncertain at present. These results suggest that some but not all SERMs may protect against declining cognitive function. The addition of HRT to SERMs may give additional protection. Demonstration of a benefit with HRT, SERMs, or both would be of considerable long-term importance. Furthermore, a cognitive protective effect with HRT would imply the risk of a detrimental effect with aromatase inhibitors. These issues remain to be resolved but could prove influential in the long term in deciding optimal adjuvant endocrine therapy.

VIII. NEWER SERMs

Tamoxifen, the original SERM, is a triphenylethylene nonsteroidal antiestrogen. Newer nonsteroidal SERMs fall into two categories: some are structurally similar to the triphenylethylene structure of tamoxifen (so-called first-generation SERMs) and others are structurally different, with a benzothiophene structure (so-called second- and third-generation SERMs). Theoretically, the steroidal pure antiestrogen fulvestrant (ICI 182,780) could be considered at the extreme end of the SERMs spectrum, but it is not discussed in this chapter because it lacks selective agonist effects in normal tissues.

Several first-generation triphenylethylene SERMs have been assessed clinically. Toremifene is structurally very similar to tamoxifen, differing only in a single chlorine atom at position 4. It was developed as having less genotoxic potential than tamoxifen. Droloxifene is 3-hydroxy tamoxifen and has a shorter half-life and a lower genotoxic potential than the parent compound. Idoxifene is more stable than tamoxifen because of a pyrrolidino side chain, with increased binding affinity for the estrogen receptor due to substitution of an iodine atom at position 4. It was developed in the hope that it would have reduced agonist activity on the uterus.

Within the second/third-generation benzothiophene derivatives, raloxifene has been the most extensively studied. Its main advantage is that it does not appear to have uterine agonist activity or to be associated with an increased incidence of clinical uterine abnormalities. Arzoxifene (LY 353381), often called SERM 3, is a benzothiophene analogue that is a more potent antiestrogen than raloxifene and with an improved agonist profile on bone and cholesterol metabolism [32]. EM-8000 is an orally active so-called pure nonsteroidal antiestrogen that is more effective than 4-hydroxytamoxifen and fulvestrant in inhibiting estradiol-induced cell proliferation in breast cancer cells in vitro [33].

IX. ARE THE NEWER SERMs LIKELY TO BE MORE EFFECTIVE THAN TAMOXIFEN AS ADJUVANT THERAPY?

Several of these newer SERMs have been directly compared with tamoxifen for metastatic breast cancer, as outlined in detail elsewhere in this volume. The bottom line is that, so far, none have been shown to have superior efficacy to tamoxifen.

However, one important issue remains unresolved. Long-term adjuvant therapy for more than 5 years may be associated with a slightly *increased* risk of cancer recurrence [34–35]. One possible explanation, supported by experimental data, is that tamoxifen may eventually become agonistic for breast cancer in some patients. Novel SERMs have differing agonist/antagonist activity on ER receptors in different tissues, and it is therefore possible that one or more of these might overcome any putative tamoxifen–agonist effects and achieve longer-term adjuvant control. So far no trials of novel SERMs against tamoxifen have shown improved time to progression to support this hypothesis, but in general patient numbers have been small.

Tamoxifen agonism may compromise the use of novel SERMs. In general, response rates to SERMs in such patients have proven low, including toremifene (5%, $n=102$); droloxifene (15%, $n=26$); idoxifene (9%, $n=56$); raloxifene ($n=14$); arzoxifene 50 mg (3%) and 20 mg (10%) ($n=63$); and EM-800 (14%, $n=43$) [36–41].

Novel SERMs will have to prove better long-term efficacy than tamoxifen or aromatase inhibitors in early breast cancer in the adjuvant trials. The current dilemma is whether such trials could be approved and funded in the absence of superior efficacy data in metastatic phase III trials.

X. CONCLUSIONS

Current results in metastatic disease and with neoadjuvant therapy suggest that adjuvant aromatase inhibitors may be at least as effective as tamoxifen and possibly more so. Even if this proves to be the case, dilemmas will still arise concerning optimum choice of adjuvant endocrine therapy.

Emerging data suggest that it may be possible to give HRT with adjuvant SERMs without prejudicing the risk of relapse. In such circumstances a combination of SERMs plus HRT has obvious advantages over aromatase inhibitors. These include improved quality of life (vasomotor, libido, etc.), bone loss protection, cardiovascular protection, reduced concerns about uterine function associated with tamoxifen, and possibly protection against deterioration in cognitive function. If aromatase inhibitors prove more effective than SERMs in preventing breast cancer recurrence, some women, but probably not all, will choose aromatase inhibitors for therapy, depending on the magnitude of the effect.

An attractive partial solution to this dilemma could be an adjuvant SERM and aromatase inhibitor combination. This option is currently being addressed in the ATAC trial with anastrozole. This could combine maximum efficacy with long term-bone and cardiovascular protection. It would not, however, provide the quality-of-life benefits of HRT, the use of which would be illogical with an aromatase inhibitor.

My personal view is that a pragmatic approach will emerge with an adjuvant "menu" for patients with differing priorities. For some patients, an aromatase inhibitor alone or in combination with a SERM may be the clear-cut choice because of maximum efficacy. For others, a SERM plus HRT may be a more attractive option, trading off improved quality of life, both short- and long-term, against the possibility of a small survival difference. The challenge for clinicians will be to guide patients through these complex decisions.

REFERENCES

1. Early Breast Cancer Trialists' Group. Tamoxifen for early breast cancer: An overview of the randomised trials. Lancet 1998; 351:1451–1467.
2. Fisher B, Costantini JP, Wickerham DL, et al. Tamoxifen for the prevention of breast cancer: Report of the National Surgical Adjuvant Breast and Bowel Project P-1 study. J Natl Cancer Inst 1998; 90:1371–1388.
3. Powles TJ, Hickish T, Kanis JA, et al. Effect of tamoxifen on bone mineral density measured by dual-energy x-ray absorptiometry in healthy premenopausal and postmenopausal women. J Clin Oncol 1996; 14:78–84.
4. Bruning PF, Bonfrer JMG, Hart AAM, et al. Tamoxifen, serum lipoproteins and cardiovascular risk. Br J Cancer 1988; 58:497–499.
5. Fisher B, Costantini JP, Redmond CK, et al. Endometrial cancer in tamoxifen-treated breast cancer patients: Findings from the National Surgical Adjuvant Breast and Bowel Project (NSABP) B-14. J Natl Cancer Inst 1994; 86:527–537.
6. Mouridsen H, Gershanovich M, Sun Y, et al. Superior efficacy of letrozole (Femara) versus tamoxifen as first-line therapy for postmenopausal women with advanced breast cancer: Results of a phase III study of the International Letrozole Breast Cancer Group. J Clin Oncol 2001; 19:2596–2606.
7. Nabholtz JM, Buzdar A, Pollack M, et al. Anastrozole is superior to tamoxifen as

first-line therapy for advanced breast cancer in post-menopausal women: Results of a North American multicenter randomised trial. J Clin Oncol 2000; 18:3758–3767.

8. Bonneterre J, Thurlimann B, Robertson JFR, et al. Anastrozole versus tamoxifen as first-line therapy for advanced breast cancer in 688 postmenopausal women: Results of the tamoxifen or arimidex randomised group efficacy and tolerability study. J Clin Oncol 2000; 18:3748–3757.

9. Ellis MJ, Jaenicke F, Llombart-Cussac A, et al. A randomized double-blind multi-center study of pre-operative tamoxifen versus Femara (letrozole) for post-menopausal women with ER and/or PgR positive breast cancer ineligible for breast-conserving surgery. Correlation of clinical response with tumor gene expression and proliferation (abstr). Breast Cancer Res Treat 2000; 64:A14.

10 Delmas PD, Bjarnason NH, Mitlak BH, et al. Effects of raloxifene on bone mineral density, serum cholesterol concentrations, and uterine endometrium in post-menopausal women. N Engl J Med 1997; 337:1641–1647.

11. Ettinger B, Black DM, Mitlak BH, et al. Reduction of vertebral fracture risk in post-menopausal women with osteoporosis treated with raloxifene: Results from a 3-year randomized clinical trial. JAMA 1999; 282:637–645.

12. Cummings SR, Black DM, Thompson DE, et al. Effect of alendronate on risk of fracture in women with low bone density but without vertebral fractures: Results from the Fracture Intervention Trial. JAMA 1998; 24:2077–2082.

13. Pols HA, Felsenberg D, Hanley DA, et al. Multinational, placebo-controlled, ran-domized trial of the effects of alendronate on bone density and fracture risk in post-menopausal women with low bone mass: Results of the FOSIT study. Fozamax International Trial Study Group. Osteoporos Int 1999; 9:461–468.

14. Harris ST, Watts NB, Genant HK, et al. Effects of risedronate treatment on vertebral and nonvertebral fractures in women with postmenopausal osteoporosis: a random-ized controlled trial. Vertebral Efficacy with Risedronate Therapy (VERT) Study Group. JAMA 1999; 282:1344–1352.

15. Reginster J, Minne HW, Sorensen OH, et al. Randomized trial of the effects of rise-dronate on vertebral fractures in women with established postmenopausal osteo-porosis. Vertebral Efficacy with Risedronate Therapy (VERT) Study Group. Osteoporos Int 2000; 11:83–91.

16. Walsh BW, Kuller LH, Wild RA, et al. Effects of raloxifene on serum lipids and co-agulation factors in healthy postmenopausal women. JAMA 1998; 279:1445–1451.

17. Love RR, Wiebe DA, Feyzi JM, Newcomb PA, Chappell RJ. Effects of tamoxifen on cardiovascular risk factors in post-menopausal women after 5 years of treatment. J Natl Cancer Inst 1994; 86:1534–1539.

18. Chang J, Powles TJ, Ashley SE, et al. The effect of tamoxifen and hormone replace-ment therapy on serum cholesterol, bone mineral density and coagulation factors in healthy postmenopausal women participating in a randomised, controlled tamoxifen prevention study. Ann Oncol 1996; 7:671–675.

19. Saarto T, Blomqvist C, Ehnholm C, et al. Antiatherogenic effects of adjuvant antie-strogens: A randomized trial comparing the effects of tamoxifen and toremifene on plasma lipid levels in postmenopausal women with node-positive breast cancer. J Clin Oncol 1996; 14:429–433.

20. McDonald CC, Alexander FE, Whyte BW, et al. Cardiac and vascular morbidity in women receiving adjuvant tamoxifen for breast cancer in a randomised trial. Br Med J 1995; 311:977–980.

21. Rutqvist LE, Mattsson A. Cardiac and thromboembolic morbidity among postmenopausal women with early-stage breast cancer in a randomized trial of adjuvant tamoxifen. J Natl Cancer Inst 1993; 85:1398–1406.

22. Costantino JP, Kuller LH, Ives DG, et al. Coronary heart disease mortality and adjuvant tamoxifen therapy. J Natl Cancer Inst 1997; 89:776–782.

23. Reis SE, Costantino JP, Wickerman DL, et al. Cardiovascular effects of tamoxifen in women with and without disease: Breast cancer prevention trial. National Surgical Adjuvant Breast and Bowel Project Breast Cancer Prevention Trial Investigators. J Natl Cancer Inst 2001; 93:16–21.

24. Walsh BW, Schiff I, Rosner B, et al. Effects of postmenopausal estrogen replacement on the concentrations and metabolism of plasma lipoproteins. N Engl J Med 1991; 325:1196–1204.

25. O'Meara ES, Rossing MA, Daling JR, et al. Hormone replacement therapy after a diagnosis of breast cancer in relation to recurrence and mortality. J Natl Cancer Inst 2001; 93:754–762.

26. Eden JA, Bush T, Nand S, Wren BG. A case control study of combined continuous estrogen-progestin replacement therapy among women with a personal history of breast cancer. Menopause 1995; 2:67–72.

27. Marsden J and Sacks NP. Hormone replacement therapy and breast cancer. Endocr Rel Cancer 1997; 4:269–279.

28. Tang MX, Jacobs D, Stern Y, et al. Effect of oestrogen during menopause on risk and age of onset of Alzheimer's disease. Lancet 1996; 348:429–432.

29. Shaywitz SE, Shaywitz BA, Pugh KR, et al. Effect of estrogen on brain activation patterns in postmenopausal women during working memory tasks. JAMA 1999; 281:1197–1202.

30. Paganini-Hill A, Clark LJ. Preliminary assessment of cognitive function in breast cancer patients treated with tamoxifen. Breast Cancer Res Treat 2000; 64:165–176.

31. Yaffe K, Krueger K, Sarkar S, et al. Multiple Outcomes of Raloxifene Evaluation Investigators. Cognitive function in postmenopausal women treated with raloxifene. N Engl J Med 2001; 344:1207–1213.

32. Sato M, Turner CH, Wang TY, et al. A novel raloxifene analogue with improved SERM potency and efficacy in vivo. J Pharmacol Exp Ther 1998; 287:1–7.

33. Simard J, Labrie CL, Belanger A, et al. Characterisation of the effects of the novel non-steroidal antiestrogen EM-800 on basal and estrogen-induced proliferation of T47-D, ZR-75-1 and MCF-7 human breast cancer cells in vitro. Int J Cancer 1997; 73:104–112.

34. Stewart HJ, Prescott RJ, Forrest APM. Scottish Adjuvant Tamoxifen Trial: A randomized study updated to 15 years. J Natl Cancer Inst 2001; 93:456–462.

35. Fisher B, Dignam J, Bryant J, Wolmark N. Five versus more than five years of tamoxifen for lymph node-negative breast cancer: Updated findings from the National Surgical Adjuvant Breast and Bowel Project B-14 Randomized Trial. J Natl Cancer Inst 2001; 93:684–690.

36. Vogel CL, Shemano I, Schoenfelder J, et al. Multicenter phase II efficacy trial of toremiphene in tamoxifen-refractory patients with advanced breast cancer. J Clin Oncol 1993; 11:345–350.
37. Haarstad H, Gundersen S, Wist E, et al. Droloxifene—A new antiestrogen. Acta Oncol 1992; 31:425–428.
38. Johnston SRD, Gumbrell L, Evans TRJ, et al. A phase II randomised double-bline study of idoxifene (40 mg/d) vs tamoxifen (40 mg/d) in patients with locally advanced/metastatic breast cancer resistant to tamoxifen (20 mg/d). Proc Am Soc Clin Oncol 1999; 18:109 (A413).
39. Buzdar A, Marcus C, Holmes F, et al. Phase II evaluation of LY156758 in metastatic breast cancer. Oncology 1988; 45:344–345
40 Buzdar A, O'Shaughnessy J, Hudis C, et al. Preliminary results of a randomised double-blind phase II study of the selective estrogen receptor modifier (SERM) arzoxifene in patients with locally advanced or metastatic breast cancer (abstr). Proc Am Soc Clin Oncol 2001; 20:45a.
41. Labrie F, Champagne P, Labrie C, et al. Response to the orally active specific antiestrogen EM-800 (SCH-57070) in tamoxifen-resistant breast cancer (abstr). Breast Cancer Res Treat 1997; 46:53.

9

Surrogate and Intermediate Markers in Early Breast Cancer

Mitch Dowsett
Royal Marsden Hospital NHS Trust
London, England

I. ABSTRACT

Surrogate markers are biochemical measures that provide information on the biological response to therapy. Of greater value, however, are intermediate markers, which can predict clinical response early during treatment. For the management of breast cancer, where neoadjuvant (preoperative) therapy precedes tumor excision and the adjuvant therapy after excision provides such an important step in controlling the disease, the need for intermediate markers is especially high. Thus the goal is to make biochemical assessments of blood and the excised tissue, which helps us to predict the optimal treatment in the adjuvant setting.

Markers are being investigated that reflect the likelihood of either a positive response of the tumor to treatment (tumor cell death or growth arrest) or of negative effects (endometrial cancer, thromboembolism, and osteoporosis). At present these markers are still in the process of validation but are providing valuable information for drug development and for our understanding of the disease process.

II. INTRODUCTION

This chapter seeks to provide a short review of recent and ongoing work on surrogate and intermediate markers as they are applied to early breast cancer and particularly as this pertains to hormonal treatment of the disease. The word surrogate means "substitute" and implies that one measurement can essentially replace the other, normally "gold standard" measurement. One example of this from prostate cancer is the measurement of prostate-specific antigen (PSA), which has largely been accepted as a surrogate marker of response and, as such, for the ongoing management of individual patients as well as for the purposes of licensing new drugs by drug regulatory authorities. However, in breast cancer there are very few, if any, markers for which the evidence is so substantial. Surrogate markers generally but not necessarily have a direct temporal relationship with the gold standard measurement; for example, change in PSA is seen to be a marker of change in the bulk of disease at that particular time point. Intermediate, on the other hand, indicates that one measurement is made between two other measurements in time; necessarily the intermediate marker precedes and predicts the second outcome. Thus, for example, the change in a particular marker between point A and point B would predict the clinical outcome between point A and a later point C. Valid intermediate markers have particular value because they can allow early intervention, which may change the the clinical outcome.

Surrogate/intermediate markers have value in a series of circumstances. Hard data relating the intermediate marker to the clinical outcome with excellent confidence are required for the use of most markers in individual patient treatment and for acceptance by regulatory authorities in the registration of new drugs. While rigorously validated markers are always preferable, less developed markers may nonetheless be useful indices during the clinical development of new drugs. This is particularly relevant for many of the new biologically based agents, since, with these, clinical regression of solid tumors may be unexpected due to their mechanism of action (e.g., angiogenesis inhibitors). For example, the anticipated cessation of progression of disease may be measurable by the assessment of parameters such as growth determinants or markers of angiogenesis itself. Although such data may not be used currently as a surrogate endpoint for clinical effectiveness (so far as regulatory authorities are concerned), they may be of considerable value in assessing the prospects for a new drug and for the understanding of molecular relationships in human tissues in vivo. The application of the markers is best conducted with a prior knowledge of the variability of the particular marker within and between patients and over time. This allows the application of marker measurements to an individual with a known confidence in its predictability. It also allows the powering of clinical trials in which the intermediate marker forms an important endpoint for the study.

Surrogate/intermediate markers can logically be divided into two groups: first, those in which the marker is predictive of clinical outcome, particularly in response or resistance to a particular therapeutic maneuver, and second, those in which the measurement reflects one of a multitude of possible treatment complications. In both circumstances there is a special need for such markers in early breast cancer, since (a) the benefit for an individual from a particular adjuvant treatment for breast cancer is exceptionally difficult to judge, given that there is no clinically detectable disease for assessment once the initial excision has occurred, and (b) treatment complications have much greater relevance in early breast cancer than in advanced disease, where side effects of a drug are normally initially characterized.

III. MARKERS OF BENEFIT FROM TREATMENT

The key drugs in the hormonal therapy of early breast cancer (either in routine use or in current development) are those that act as antiestrogens or estrogen deprivation agents. So far as estrogen deprivation is concerned, plasma estrogen concentrations provide relatively straightforward pharmacological measures of effectiveness [1]. This can be extended to the measurement of intratumoral estrogen levels and, for aromatase inhibitors, the measurement of aromatase activity itself [2,3]. Although these measurements are of value in selecting dosages of greatest pharmacological effect or in comparisons between drugs, the eventual clinical effectiveness of the drugs depends on the heterogeneous, molecular makeup of breast cancer. Thus a strong relationship between pharmacological effectiveness and clinical outcome is rarely seen, although in a large enough population of patients this might be demonstrable [4].

With selective estrogen-receptor modulators (SERMs), or antiestrogens, the situation is yet more difficult, since the major effects of these agents are on the tumor itself. It has been suggested that insulin-like growth factor 1 (IGF1) levels might be a valuable marker of effectiveness, but since IGF1 is generally considered to be only a minor mediator of the tumor's response to therapy, this is likely to be of limited value [5]. With such drugs, the measurement of parameters within the tumor itself is necessary. This is likely to be the case with most new agents in which the manipulation of the host environment is an infrequent target.

Although the primary lesion in early breast cancer is nearly always removed by surgical excision, there have been many attempts recently to assess the value of presurgical medical treatment. This has the established advantage of permitting more conservative surgery and the potential advantage of assessing the sensitivity of individual lesions to particular treatment. For this latter neoadjuvant (preoperative) test of efficacy to have clinical utility and for it to be used itself as a marker of treatment effectiveness for the validation of biomarkers as surrogate endpoints, a significant relationship between neoadjuvant response and long-term outcome needs to have been established in clinical trials. The NSABP B-18 study [6] has been particularly helpful in this regard in that it established that the complete clinical response (CR) of the primary lesion to chemotherapy of the 743 patients in the neoadjuvant arm was associated with increased relapse-free survival (p=0.0014). The only independent pathological predictor of outcome in this trial, in a model including lymph node status, was pathological CR (pCR), but this does not negate the validity of using response categories as markers of treatment benefit. In the Royal Marsden Hospital trial of neoadjuvant mitoxantrone plus methotrexate plus tamoxifen, the relationship between response and long-term clinical outcome was confirmed: patients achieving pCR or good clinical response (CR or minimal residual disease) had a significantly improved disease-free and overall survival compared with those who achieved a partial response or had no response [7].

There appears to be only one study relating neoadjuvant response to endocrine therapy with long-term outcome (see Chapter 13), and this shows a significant positive association. However, this is a relatively small study bringing together results from a variety of endocrine agents.

Our work on intermediate markers of response has focused largely on the changes that occur in the two major determinants of the growth of the lesion—i.e., cell proliferation and cell death. This focus has been due to our presumption that for any lesion to regress or progress there must be a change in proliferation and/or apoptosis. This should be the case whether we are considering cytotoxic treatment, hormonal therapy, antiangiogenic agents, or any of the newer treatments under development. It has become clear that changes in both proliferation and apoptosis occur in a measurable fashion within 24 h of starting cytotoxic chemotherapy (Fig. 1)[8,9]. We have not made such early measurements with hormonal therapy to date, since it might be expected that such treatments, in which the agents or their downstream targets need several days or weeks to get to steady state, are unlikely to show the same rapid biological response. We are continuing to evaluate the degree to which these 24-h changes can predict response to therapy in the chemotherapeutic scenario, but our strongest data for such a relationship relate to measurements of changes in proliferation 2 to 3 weeks after starting therapy. In these circumstances we have shown statistically significant relationships between clinical response of the primary lesion and the change in proliferation as measured by Ki67, not only for chemotherapy but also for endocrine therapy and combined chemoendocrine therapy (Fig. 2)[9]. These data have allowed us to apply these measurements with confidence to the early clinical evaluation of new hormonal agents including raloxifene, idoxifene, and the pure antiestrogen Faslodex [10–12]. In these cases, a change in proliferation during a period of drug exposure between diagnosis and surgery of between 1 and 3 weeks was the primary endpoint of the study. During that time, medical therapy is not generally applied. This opportunistic approach to deriving clinical

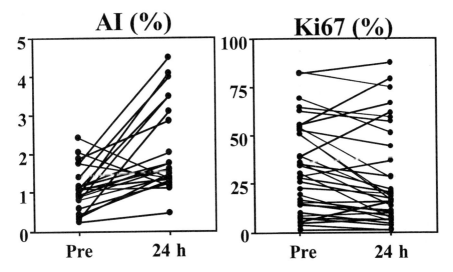

Figure 1 Changes in apoptotic index (AI) and proliferation (Ki67) after 24 h of chemotherapy. Data are shown for more patients on Ki67 than on AI. There were statistically significant increases in AI and decreases in Ki67 ($p< 0.01$ for both).

data on new agents is one that has great potential for the investigation of other compounds that have nonhormonal mechanisms. However, such patients are in many cases cured by surgery, and their exposure to potentially toxic compounds is unethical. Similarly, agents that might affect the surgical process negatively or might lead to a detrimental interaction between surgery and clinical outcome from the disease are not suitable for testing in this circumstance.

Although change in proliferation or apoptosis is likely to be reflective of a change in growth of a tumor, the relationship between these measurements and *clinical response* is unlikely to be close for two reasons, as discussed below: (a) because of the variability in the analyses and (b) because of two issues which relate these changes to eventual clinical outcome in the adjuvant setting.

We have estimated the error in the assessment of proliferation and apoptosis: for an apparent change in either of these measurements in an individual tumor to be considered statistically significant, they need to differ by at least 50% [13]. These variability estimates apply to studies as conducted by us using 14-gauge core cuts and counts of 1000–3000 cells for Ki67 and apoptosis, respectively. In an attempt to take into consideration the influence of these errors and to reduce their impact as well as to try to derive a single marker for these growth changes, we have described a function that we call the growth index. This is calculated by the following formula:

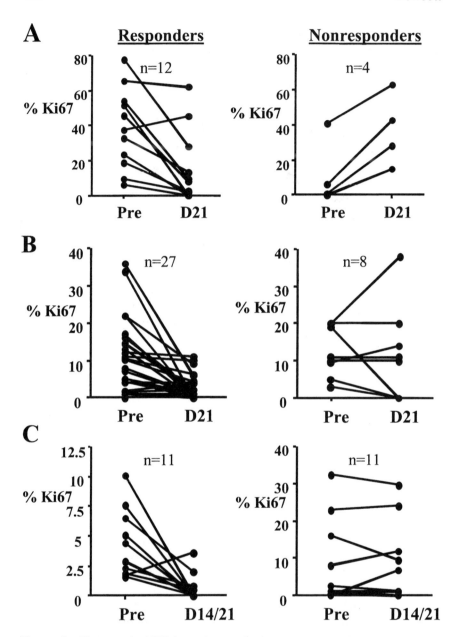

Figure 2 Changes in Ki67 in patients after 21 days of chemotherapy (A) or chemoendocrine therapy (B) or after 14/21 days of tamoxifen therapy (C). In each case there were statistically significant reductions in Ki67 in responders but not nonresponders.

$$\text{Growth index} = \frac{(\text{Ki67}_{post}/\text{apoptotic index}_{post})}{(\text{Ki67}_{pre}/\text{apoptotic index}_{pre})}$$

This relationship approximates to an expectation that values >1 indicate increased tumor growth as opposed to values <1, indicating decreased tumor growth.

This relationship is illustrated in Figure 3, in which a line of equivalence is drawn where apoptosis and proliferation change to an equal proportional extent. For some tumors the change in proliferation is positive and/or in apoptosis is negative, but in most of these patients the changes are in the segment above the line of equivalence in the diagram, in which increased proliferation is balanced out by a greater increase in apoptosis. Thus the overall change would be toward reducing the growth of the tumor. Values fall below this line in only three cases. This application of a growth index has recently been described for Faslodex [14], revealing a statistically significant greater reduction in the index after treatment with a single injection of Faslodex (250 mg) than with tamoxifen while significant changes in the individual parameters were not seen. It is important to note that the growth index is not completely mathematically valid in reflecting the true changes in the dynamics of growth. It should also be noted that the measurements and development of a growth index relate to a single time point and that varying chronology for the changes in proliferation and apoptosis may markedly affect the growth index if measured at different time points. Despite these issues, it is possible that the index may have clinical utility, but establishment of this would require substantial further research.

It is also important to note that these changes in proliferation and apoptosis, even when incorporated into a growth index, indicate only changes in the growth rate of the tumor and do not necessarily predict clinical regression. This point is clear from consideration of the changes in proliferation and apoptosis that occur after estrogen deprivation (i.e., the removal of the estradiol pellet), from groups of mice carrying MCF7 estrogen-dependent xenografts [9,15]. In these cases, the tumors have Ki67 levels of about 50% and apoptopic indices of about 0.8% during estrogen treatment. Rapid regression occurs on withdrawal of the estrogen pellet and is associated with an approximately fivefold increase in apoptosis and fivefold decrease in proliferation (a 25-fold decrease in the growth index). For tamoxifen, the change in growth of tumors is what would be described as stable disease in clinical breast cancer. However, this is associated with marked reductions in Ki67 and increases in apoptopic index. Smaller changes in proliferation or apoptosis would be associated with what would be described in clinical circumstances as progressive disease. It is clear that in these circumstances the patient (in this case the mouse) would derive benefit from treatment in the slowing of the growth of the tumor. However, in clinical circumstances this would not be observable, because the growth of the tumor in the absence of treatment cannot

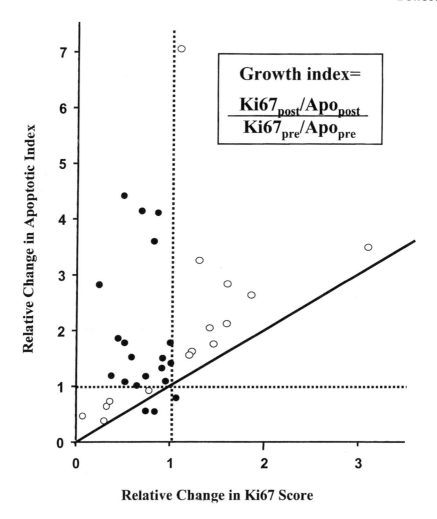

Figure 3 Relationship between relative change in apoptotic index and in proliferation (Ki67) after 24 h chemotherapy. The dotted lines at unity indicates no change in the indices and the solid inclined line represent a line of equivalence, where the changes in the two indices are equal and the growth index = 1. For the majority of patients, the tumors responded to treatment with a drop in proliferation (Ki67 index <1) and an increase in apoptosis (apoptotic index >1). The open circles indicate tumors in which there was either an increase in Ki67 accompanied by an even greater increase in apoptotic index or a decrease in apoptotic index accompanied by an even greater decrease in Ki67.

be established. It is also notable that although, in clinically assessable lesions, such slowing of growth would be called progressive disease, in patients on adjuvant therapy such a change in growth could lead to enhanced relapse-free survival. Thus, in these circumstances, our main indices of benefit from treatment may become dissociated.

Measuring single parameters in this fashion, albeit parameters directly related to the growth of the tumor, may soon be superseded by the simultaneous measurement of many thousands of markers, as are available on cDNA microarrays. The conventional approach with these arrays is to assess whether the expression of individual genes or sets of genes can predict outcome of treatment in a single pretreatment sample. Clearly the arrays can also be applied to sequential samples, and in these circumstances a different approach may be possible. In general, tumors that are nonresponsive to endocrine therapy are considered refractory to the treatment; thus changes in gene expression might be minimal. In contrast, in a responding tumor, one might expect to see a multitude of genes, related to downstream effects of the agent. We have gathered preliminary evidence for this from a set of 10 patients on chemotherapy. In biopsies taken pretreatment and shortly after starting treatment, five times as many genes showed changes of greater than 1.5-fold in tumors that eventually showed a good clinical response compared with those showing a poor response. Thus simply the number of genes perturbed may be sufficient to predict outcome [16].

In some ways this consideration of changes in a multitude of unknown genes is paralleled by the changes that may be seen in some imaging approaches, such as positron emission tomography (PET). An extreme example of this is available in another disease setting—i.e., the application of STI571, or Glivec, in which the PET images become markedly reduced in intensity over a 24-h period in those patients with GIST tumors that eventually respond, in some cases many months later [17].

IV. MARKERS OF COMPLICATIONS DUE TO TREATMENT

The complications that may frequently occur as a result of hormonal therapy are generally those which have at least some dependence on estrogen. In some cases the complications are well established as a result of their monitoring during tamoxifen therapy and/or evidence from the use of hormone replacement therapy in postmenopausal women. However, for many drugs, the exact expectation from the hormonal manipulation is ill defined because early breast cancer patients have currently been exposed to them for only limited periods. Tamoxifen has well-established detrimental effects on the increased incidence of thromboembolic disease and endometrial cancer. So far as markers are concerned, alterations in clotting factors have been evaluated for their relationship with the increase in thromboembolism, but no clear pattern has emerged [18]. The issue of early detection of endometrial hyperplasia as a precursor of cancer has been particularly controversial. For several years the tamoxifen-induced thickening of the endometrium has been detected by ultrasound. However, it has recently become clear that this thickening in most cases is not a true reflection of the thickness of endometrial tissue, with over 70% of patients showing apparent thickening having an atrophic endometrium [19].

On the beneficial side, tamoxifen-decreased cardiac events have been expected due to the well-established cholesterol-lowering effects of the drug [18]. However, the relationship between plasma lipids and cardiac events has become muddied. Although there still seems to be clear evidence that patients with high cholesterol levels have an increased risk of cardiac events, the alteration of such levels with hormonal agents has not revealed a parallel effect in changing cardiac events [20]. Although there is evidence from clinical trials in the adjuvant setting (Stockholm/Scottish/NSABP trials) that tamoxifen can reduce mortality from ischemic heart disease, these observations can be complicated by the late effects of radiation therapy. In the NSABP-P1 study, there was no reduction in cardiac events with tamoxifen [21]. Thus there is no confirmed relationship between changes in lipid levels and clinical outcome.

Tamoxifen has significant beneficial effects on the maintenance of bone density in postmenopausal women. In the NSABP-P1 study, there was a 19% reduction in bone fractures in women who received tamoxifen (CI – 37% to + 5%). This important positive component of tamoxifen's pharmacology has led to the development of several new specific SERMs that are now being targeted principally to prevent or treat osteoporosis (e.g., raloxifene). We have recently shown that, in patients on neoadjuvant tamoxifen therapy, plasma levels of the bone resorption marker CTX are significantly decreased, as would be expected with an agent that increases bone mineral density [22]. Increasing attention is being paid to the possible dependence of maintained cognition in women on estrogen and the way in which loss of estrogen might be associated with increased Alzheimer's disease, although the evidence relating to this remains conflicting. There is little evidence to date on whether the use of tamoxifen or other SERMs is detrimental, beneficial, or neutral in these circumstances, and intermediate tests predicting or measuring changes are in the early stages of development. However, this will become an increasingly important issue in the application of these agents to patients with early breast cancer.

At present there are a number of large trials of aromatase inhibitors in postmenopausal women [23], and each of these has subprotocols to examine potentially important metabolic complications. Intermediate markers for evaluating, predicting, and managing any complications that might occur would be of great value. The evidence to date suggests that aromatase inhibitors are unlikely to be associated with the agonist effects of tamoxifen on thromboembolic disease and endometrial hyperplasia. Thus concern has focused more on the detrimental effects that they might have on processes known to be disadvantageously affected by estrogen deprivation during menopause.

There is good evidence that estrogen replacement therapy can reduce bone fractures in postmenopausal women but—as noted above—somewhat less evidence that this reduces cardiac disease. There are, however, very few data indicating that the small residual amount of estrogen in postmenopausal women continues to have a protective effect on these functions. The effects of aromatase inhibitors on lipids appear relatively neutral [22]. Thus no serious deleterious effects on cardiac function should be anticipated insofar as lipid levels predict these. However, for bone, the few data that are available on changes in serum and urine markers indicate that bone resorption is enhanced by third-generation aromatase inhibitors. Heshmati et al. [24] reported that letrozole increased the urinary levels of deoxypyrodinoline and pyrodinoline significantly in a group of 22 women over a 6-month period of treatment with the drug. Our data with vorozole, an aromatase inhibitor of relatively similar pharmacological effectiveness as letrozole, showed a statistically nonsignificant increase in serum CTX [22]. However, in 30 healthy women treated with letrozole over a 3-month period, a significant increase of approximately 20% in serum CTX was measured [25]. Relationships have been established on the interaction between change in serum CTX over 1- and 6-month periods and eventual decrease in bone density over a 3-year period [27]. However, these have been in relation to additional estrogen rather than deprivation of estrogen. What seems clear is that these changes in bone markers are statistically significant and likely to be detrimental to some degree, at least in some patients in the long term. One of the issues to consider is that although fractures might not measurably increase during the 5-year period of a clinical trial on an aromatase inhibitor, the lifetime risk of having an osteoporotic fracture might still be increased, since the lowered bone density during the 5 years of treatment may not be reversed by cessation.

V. SUMMARY

The potential value of surrogate and intermediate markers of treatment benefit and complications is unquestionable. However, at the present time, few have been sufficiently well characterized to allow us to use them with enough confidence for clinical utility. In part, this is because there has been limited exposure of patients with early breast cancer to the new hormonal agents, such that it has not been possible to develop with confidence the relationship with clinical outcome. It is clear, however, that the detailed study of these markers during the ongoing trials of these agents is exceptionally important not just for early breast cancer patients but also for those that might receive the same agents for prophylaxis.

REFERENCES

1. Dowsett M, Goss PE, Powles TJ, et al. Use of the aromatase inhibitor 4-hydroxyan-drostenedione in postmenopausal breast cancer: Optimization of therapeutic dose and route. Cancer Res 1987; 47:1957–1961.

2. Geisler J, Detre S, Berntsen H, et al. Influence of neo-adjuvant anastrozole (Arimidex) on intratumoral estrogen levels and proliferation markers in patients with locally advanced breast cancer. Clin Cancer Res 2001; 7:1230–1236.

3. Dowsett M, Pfister C, Johnston SRD, et al. Impact of tamoxifen on the pharmacokinetics and endocrine effects of the aromatase inhibitor letrozole in postmenopausal women with breast cancer. Clin Cancer Res 1999; 5:2338–2343.

4. Bajetta E, Zilembo N, Bichisao E, et al. Tumour response and estrogen suppression in breast cancer patients treated with aromatase inhibitors. Ann Oncol 2000; 8:1017–1022.

5. Decensi A, Bonanni B, Guerrieri-Gonzaga A, et al. Biologic activity of tamoxifen at low doses in healthy women. J Natl Cancer Inst 1998; 7:1461–1467.

6. Fisher B, Bryant J, Wolmark N, et al. Effect of preoperative chemotherapy on the outcome of women with operable breast cancer. J Clin Oncol 1998; 16:2672–2685.

7. Powles TJ, Hickish TF, Makris A, et al. Randomized trial of chemoendocrine therapy started before or after surgery for treatment of primary breast cancer. J Clin Oncol 1995; 13:547–552.

8. Ellis PA, Smith IE, McCarthy K, et al. Preoperative chemotherapy induces apoptosis in early breast. Lancet 1997; 349:849.

9. Dowsett M, Smith IE, Powles TJ, et al. Biological studies in primary medical therapy of breast cancer: The Royal Marsden Hospital experience. In: Howell A, Dowsett M, eds. European School of Oncology Updates 4: Primary Medical Therapy for Breast Cancer. Amsterdam: Elsevier, 1999:127–130.

10. DeFriend DJ, Howell A, Nicolson RI, et al. Investigation of a new pure antiestrogen (ICI 182780) in women with primary breast cancer. Cancer Res 1994; 54:408–414.

11. Dowsett M, Donaldson K, Tsuboi M, et al. Effects of the aromatase inhibitor anastrozole on serum estrogens in Japanese and Caucasian women. Cancer Chemother Pharmacol 2000; 46:35–39.

12. Dowsett M, Bundred N, Decensi A, et al. Effect of raloxifene on breast cancer cell Ki67 and apoptosis: A doubled-blind, placebo-controlled, randomized clinical trial in postmenopausal patients. Cancer Epidemiol Biomarkers Prev 2001; 10:961–966.

13. Ellis PA, Smith IE, Detre S, Dowsett M. Reduced apoptosis and proliferation and increased bcl-2 in residual breast cancer following preoperative chemotherapy. Breast Cancer Res Treat 1998; 48:107–116.

14. Bundred N, Anderson E, Nicholson R I, et al. ICI 182,780 (Faslodex) an estrogen receptor downregulator reduces cell turnover index more effectively than tamoxifen. Proc Am Soc Clin Oncol 2001; 20:1660.

15. Johnston SRD, Boeddinghaus IM, Riddler S, et al. Idoxifene antagonises estradiol-dependent MCF-7 breast cancer xenograft growth through sustained induction of apoptosis. Cancer Res 1999; 59:3646–3651.

16. Sotiriou C, Powles TJ, Dowsett M, et al. cDNA Microarray profiles as predictors of clinical outcome from systemic therapy for breast cancer. Submitted.

17. Joensuu H, Roberts PJ, Sadomo-Rikala M, et al. Effect of the tyrosine kinase inhibitor ST1571 in a patient with a metastatic gastrointestinal stromal tumor. N Engl J Med 2001; 344:1052–1056.

18. Powles TJ, Hardy JR, Ashley SE, et al. A pilot trial to evaluate the acute toxicity and feasibility of tamoxifen for prevention of breast cancer. Br J Cancer 1989; 60:126–131.

19. Gerber B, Krause A, Muller H, et al. Effects of adjuvant tamoxifen on the endometrium in postmenopausal women with breast cancer: A prospective long-term study using transvaginal ultrasound. J Clin Oncol 2000; 18:3464–3470.

20. Hulley S, Grady D, Bush T, et al. Randomized trial of estrogen plus progestin for secondary prevention of coronary heart disease in postmenopausal women. Heart and Estrogen/progestin Replacement Study (HERS) Research Group. JAMA 1998: 280:605–613.

21. Fisher B, Costantino JP, Wickerham DL, et al. Tamoxifen for prevention of breast cancer: report of the National Surgical Adjuvant Breast and Bowel Project P-1 Study. J Natl Cancer Inst 1998; 90:1371–1388.

22. Harper-Wynne C, Sacks NP, Shenton K, et al. Comparison of the systemic and intratumoural effects of tamoxifen and the aromatase inhibitor vorozole in postmenopausal patients with breast cancer. J Clin Oncol. In press, 2002.

23. Harper-Wynne C, Dowsett M. Recent advances in the clinical application of aromatase inhibitors. J Steroid Biochem Mol Biol 2001; 76:179–186.

24. Heshmati HM, Khosla A, Robins SP, et al. Role of low levels of residual estrogen in regulation of bone resorption in late postmenopausal women. Submitted.

25. Harper-Wynne C, Ross G, Sacks N, et al. Effects of the aromatase inhibitor letrozole in healthy postmenopausal women: rationale for prevention. Proc Am Soc Clin Oncol 2001; 3091:335b.

26. Bjarnason NH, Christiansen C. Early response in biochemical markers predicts long-term response in bone mass during hormone replacement therapy in early postmenopausal women. Bone 2000; 6:561–569.

Panel Discussion 2

Early Breast Cancer

Hans-Jorg Senn and William R. Miller, *Chairmen*
Monday, June 25, 2001

H-J. Senn: Contrary to this morning's session, when there was a long discussion about "consensus" in the treatment of metastatic breast cancer, in early breast cancer (or primary breast cancer), consensus meetings have a long tradition. We just had one in St. Gallen in February 2001 and there was a national one several months ago at the National Cancer Institute (at the end of 2000). It would probably be interesting to discuss these treatment recommendations, but we unfortunately have no time to do so. You will be able to discuss, or criticize, the St. Gallen conference when it is published in the *Journal of Clinical Oncology* (hopefully in August or September 2001).

I think we heard four contributions about possible future integration of new antihormonal compounds in the adjuvant treatment setup of early breast cancer and we probably should use this time to discuss them, one after the other. Are there still, after such a long time of living with and using tamoxifen, any questions about tamoxifen?

J. Forbes: There are more events in the ATLAS/ATOM duration trial than in the other three trials combined and there remains substantial uncertainty, when all events are looked at, as to whether it is beneficial, harmful, or not different to continue tamoxifen treatment beyond the 5-year time point. In addition, in the context of how patients might be treated in countries other than developed western countries, the potential for even a small treatment effect having a very wide benefit remains for such a simple drug as tamoxifen. That is still an important question.

H-J. Senn: Many of the problems with tamoxifen have been discussed by the speakers. Can we come up with questions about the aromatase inhibitors and their current integration in adjuvant trials? Unfortunately we do not have these data yet, just projections. Does anybody want to speak about this? There are certainly good reasons for wide-scale inclusion of aromatase inhibitors in adjuvant trials right now.

M. Dixon: Are there not certain situations currently where people probably do use aromatase inhibitors as adjuvant? That is, in patients who may have contraindications to tamoxifen. So perhaps we could start and say there are currently a group of patients who we would not want to give adjuvant tamoxifen to on the basis they have had previous thrombotic events, which we think would predispose them to further problems with tamoxifen. These patients would be appropriate candidates for aromatase inhibitors. Can we not start with a fairly select group like that?

C. Benz: Yes, I echo that. In our weekly tumor boards we argue this point all the time, given low-risk tumors in women over the age of 65, where the thromboembolic risk of tamoxifen becomes high enough that risk begins to exceed therapeutic benefit.

H-J. Senn: Now this would be a target population to study. Are there such studies at the moment in the target population of women at higher risk on tamoxifen?

C. Benz: I know that elderly women are being evaluated on tamoxifen therapy alone. It seems very reasonable to preferentially consider aromatase inhibitors in this clinical setting.

J. Forbes: Does anyone have information on Leiden Factor V (an inhibitory clotting factor; certain individuals have mutations in the gene that encodes for Leiden Factor V and possibly are at higher risk for spontaneous deep venous thrombosis) as a predictor for thromboembolic events with tamoxifen?

D. Hayes: Yes and no. I was just going to say that I'm not sure we know who is at high risk for thromboembolic phenomena. Certainly it is not every woman over the age of 65. One might argue that if the aromatase inhibitors enhance osteoporosis, then that risk might outweigh the thrombosis risk. The CALGB is trying to run a cohort matched study for Leiden factors (and anything else for that matter, because we are going to have the DNA). Subjects who have deep venous thrombosis (DVT) and are on tamoxifen are matched with two other patients on tamoxifen (by age) who have not had DVT. (DVT is the event and not strokes.) That study is about halfway accrued, but it is going to take about 300–400 cases—overall about 1000 patients. So stay tuned, but there are no data yet.

H-J. Senn: Are there any more problems with the inclusion of aromatase inhibitors in the adjuvant therapy setting in early (primary) breast cancer?

A. Howell: Just to say that the ATAC trial should give us some feel for this DVT problem.

M. Dixon: Just to point out the problem for a country like the United Kingdom. If we were to switch all our patients from tamoxifen to aromatase inhibitors, that would increase our total oncology drug budget 2.5 times. One of the things that is not in any of these studies is cost-effectiveness. There may be certain groups who benefit and certain groups who might not. It's fine for most countries with unlimited budgets. John Forbes was speaking about this relation to countries in the world that perhaps couldn't afford to give everybody certain drugs. It would be useful at some point to find out which groups of patients benefit most. Although the United Kingdom is not a third world country, our drug budget would be in major trouble if we were to switch everyone to aromatase inhibitors.

H-J. Senn: Thank you Mike Dixon; I think you are the first participant during this conference to mention comparative economics in prospective drug research. Yours is no third world country, but it is the country (as far as I know) with the lowest health expenditure in Europe. Anyone to comment on this issue?

M. Ellis: There have been some health economic outcomes done in the metastatic setting that suggest aromatase inhibitors have an impact by delaying the use of expensive palliative chemotherapy. Even a modest delay of a few months translates into significant cost savings. So the relative difference in the price of tamoxifen and an aromatase inhibitor is almost irrelevant when looking at the problem from this angle.

J. Forbes: Matthew (Ellis), do they end up having a shorter overall time on this expensive palliative care, or is it just delayed and they have it for the same total time?

M. Ellis: I am not sure; it's not my data. It was presented at a Canadian investigators meeting at ASCO. This was a Novartis-sponsored meeting and I am sure we could get the data and examine the finer details of it.

P. Lønning: That was addressed in a paper by Bruce Hillier in *Cancer,* which related to exemestane and showed it was cost-effective to use it in metastatic patients.

H-J. Senn: I would like to add a word of caution for these economical considerations, because the calculations vary from country to country depending on the medical and the insurance systems and are very badly comparable to one another. Data about "cost-effectiveness" of drugs from the United States (due to very high hospital costs) are not easily applicable in most European countries. Let's move on to discuss the selective estrogen-receptor modulators (SERMs) and the intermediate or surrogate markers during the remaining time.

C. Benz: I would like to ask Mitch Dowsett about tumor sampling after initiating treatment with SERMs or other agents. He talked about measuring surrogate markers after 24 h versus 21 days, and I know that a lot of groups are grappling with this issue. Do you have any data that you could share with us about how you arrived at those time points or which ones are optimal?

M. Dowsett: In clinical studies you can do only limited sampling, and in these circumstances we picked those for pragmatic reasons. For the 24-h study, the patients were staying overnight for their chemotherapy, so we took the second sample 24 h later. In the second study with Trevor (Powles), the patients were coming back for their next course of chemotherapy 21 days later. That's quite an interesting issue (the 21 days) for, of course, by that time any immediate effects of chemotherapy might have worn off. So the sort of things that we see in those microarray experiments are the persistent effects. We don't know whether these are changes in the phenotype within the same cells or whether in fact there is already some sort of cell selection through cytotoxicity. I think it is likely there are going to be waves and these genes are going to go up and down differentially over time. One other issue very briefly, I showed that 300 or so genes could be selected that are associated with a good or poor response. I think it is likely that we are going to be able to reduce that down markedly because many of those are probably correlated closely with one another and they are not contributing very much to what might eventually come out as a discriminatory function. It may be possible to reduce that number from hundreds down to perhaps only a few handfuls.

H-J. Senn: Thank you. Mitch Dowsett had a very provocative statement in one of his slides: that adjuvant studies are too long, probably too expensive, too cumbersome, and need too many patients. Yet we are working in always larger groups, international BIG groups and this allows us to get studies done faster and get results earlier. Maybe that is also one way to solve the problem. You were proposing (according to the title of your talk) "Surrogate and Intermediate Markers." As a clinician, I have a hard time believing that any drug regulatory agency or we as clinicians would ever substitute survival (be it overall survival or disease-free survival) with surrogate markers as a basis to evaluate the clearance of new treatments. Would anybody like to comment on that?

I. Smith: Can I make a comment on that? Mitch Dowsett and I have discussed this for many years (and I've got to say that I'm strongly on his side here). It's not just the number of patients that is the problem, it's the natural history of breast cancer. There is no way you can speed that up, which is fortunate, of course, for the patients. I think that unless we get these surrogate markers, if you look at all the new drugs that are becoming available—and even in this small area that we are discussing today, there are several—I don't begin to see how we are going make the best use of these new agents, if we have a traditional adjuvant trial with survival as an endpoint each time. If the surrogate markers can be shown to predict the survival, then of course we would be happy to use them. The trick is designing trials proving that the surrogate marker does predict the survival. That's the difficult bit.

M. Ellis: Yes, I think the idea is not that we're going to replace large adjuvant trials—of course we'll continue to do those—but what are the baseline requirements for activating these trials. Currently we don't have a requirement where there has been biomarker analysis in say, the preoperative setting. But it might be reasonable to set such a requirement. For example, for a new endocrine therapy, we might require more apoptosis or more evidence of an antiproliferative effect when treating with the new agent when comparing against the standard therapy. In the preoperative setting, one is looking at early disease, which might be most relevant to the adjuvant situation, rather than metastatic disease, in which characteristics of tumors may have changed as a result of prior treatment.

H-J. Senn: Thank you, Dr. Ellis. I think we have to come to the last contribution of the discussion period.

D. Hayes: I was actually going to echo what Matthew Ellis said. Rather than as an endpoint for approval, surrogate endpoints might be used to design larger trials. We design large trials based on response rates or stability. Those are currently used surrogates in the metastatic setting for activity. The newer drugs seem not to induce those as quickly or as well. One thing I think Mitch Dowsett glossed over quickly was circulating tumor markers. There are three circulating markers out now: Muc1 assays, CEA assays, and the extracellular HER2. In the metastatic setting, all of these have had not major but at least minor specificity issues and each of them has had sensitivity issues, so they don't cover 100% of the patients and they bounce around a little bit. Unlike prostate-specific antigen in prostate cancer, which the urologists have been willing to accept as an endpoint (sometime too quickly and too often), the breast cancer markers have not been terribly good. We talked about circulating epithelial cancer cells and, as I said, I think that's a real avenue of research in the future. I agree wholeheartedly that this technique needs a lot of validation, but I think it's on its way. Finally, the whole field of proteonomics may give us the opportunity to take serum or plasma and look at patterns of circulating markers that are much too small in quantity to detect with the currently available immunoassays but which we might be able to detect using proteomics. One of the problems there is that albumin and the commonly expressed proteins swamp out everything right now, but people are working very hard on excluding those. One can begin to look at small changes in a variety of proteins that are related to the tumor and that could be related to the predictive biological effect of a given drug. The whole field of aptimer research, I think some of you may have seen, I think offers enormous promise and could really offer a way to make early trials less expensive and more efficient.

H-J. Senn: Thank you very much ladies and gentlemen. This session must come to a close. There certainly remain important questions about trial concepts and strategies in relation to preclinical data and options to be answered in the near future. Maybe they can be discussed more extensively in tomorrow's session on neoadjuvant therapy of breast cancer.

Part IV

NEOADJUVANT THERAPY

10

Neoadjuvant Endocrine Therapy for Breast Cancer: A Medical Oncologist's Perspective

Matthew J. Ellis
Duke University Medical Center
Durham, North Carolina

I. ABSTRACT

It took many years for the effectiveness of adjuvant endocrine therapy to become apparent because of the indolent nature of estrogen-dependent breast cancer. This fact is the most important obstacle to the development of new adjuvant endocrine treatments. Clinical trials require thousands of participants and at least a decade of clinical investigation. How can we be sure that a new endocrine strategy really warrants this extraordinary level of investment? The success of a recent neoadjuvant trial that compared the selective aromatase inhibitor letrozole with tamoxifen suggests that this treatment approach may provide an answer. The Letrozole 024 trial established that 4 months of neoadjuvant letrozole, in postmenopausal women with confirmed hormone receptor–positive breast cancer, ineligible for breast conserving surgery, was associated with a 60% clinical response rate and a 48% rate of conversion to breast-conserving surgery. For tamoxifen, on the other hand, the corresponding figures were 41 and 36% respectively. The superior efficacy of letrozole was particularly marked for tumors that coexpress estrogen receptors (ER) and ErbB1 and/or ErbB2, supporting the notion that tumors with this immunophenotype are relatively tamoxifen-resistant yet estrogen-dependent. Future neoadjuvant endocrine therapy designs could focus on a number of objectives, for example: (a) nonrandomized trials to focus on gene microarray studies and other genetic technologies to investigate the molecular basis of estrogen-dependent growth; (b) randomized trials to address critical drug development questions in early-stage disease as a prelude to adjuvant studies; and (c) randomized trials that compare neoadjuvant chemotherapy with neoadjuvant aromatase inhibitor therapy to establish a place for neoadjuvant endocrine therapy in routine clinical practice.

II. HISTORICAL PERSPECTIVES

The first experience with preoperative systemic therapy for breast cancer was published in 1957, with several case reports indicating that diethylstilbestrol (DES) was effective in locally advanced breast cancer [1]. After DES was replaced by tamoxifen in the 1970s, tamoxifen alone without initial surgery (primary tamoxifen therapy) was investigated as an alternative to immediate surgery for older patients with breast cancer. These investigations established that primary breast cancer frequently regresses when treated with tamoxifen. However, randomized studies that compared primary tamoxifen with immediate surgery followed by tamoxifen (the CRC trial and the GRETA trial) found that about one-quarter of the patients who received primary tamoxifen developed tumor progression in the breast by 34 to 36 months [2,3]. Despite poor local control, all these studies showed that overall survival was not affected by the surgical delay associated with primary tamoxifen treatment. However, a meta-analysis subsequently suggested that breast cancer–specific mortality, though not overall mortality, may be compromised by primary tamoxifen therapy [4]. These data indicate that primary tamoxifen therapy without initial surgery should be reserved for truly frail elderly or medically infirm patients. However, short courses of neoadjuvant (preoperative) tamoxifen for 3 to 6 months before surgery continued to be investigated as a safe, effective, and nontoxic means to downstage tumors before surgery [5]. For example, the M.D. Anderson Cancer Center reported a series of patients who received neoadjuvant tamoxifen with favorable outcomes in terms of response and increased opportunities for breast-conserving surgery [6]. Importantly, tumor responsiveness to tamoxifen in the neoadjuvant setting is associated with prolonged survival as compared with nonresponsive tumors [7,8]. Thus a potentially critical advantage for neoadjuvant endocrine therapy concerns information on the likelihood that adjuvant endocrine treatment will prevent disease recurrence and death. Trials that explore the utility of this information are under discussion.

III. NEOADJUVANT ENDOCRINE THERAPY TRIALS WITH AROMATASE INHIBITORS

By the mid-1990s the development of selective aromatase inhibitors had reached a stage where direct comparisons with tamoxifen were warranted. In addition to adjuvant and metastatic trials, several neoadjuvant investigations were initiated. These trials were driven by the opportunity afforded by the neoadjuvant context to obtain tumor tissue before and after endocrine treatment, so that both baseline predictive markers and surrogate markers of drug effect could be investigated. These neoadjuvant trials should be distinguished from "perioperative" treatment studies, where exposure to an endocrine agent or other experimental treatment lasts no more than a few weeks. For example, early clinical development of ICI 182,780 used a perioperative design to demonstrate the antiproliferative activity of this pure antiestrogen [9]. Since perioperative studies focus purely on surrogate markers (changes in proliferation, apoptosis, and gene expression), not true clinical outcomes, they are not further considered here. Information on the activity of neoadjuvant anastrozole and exemestane are limited at this point to the pioneering phase II experiences of the Edinburgh group headed by Miller and Dixon [10]. This group conducted a randomized double-blind study in 24 patients with "ER-rich" tumors that examined 1 mg and 10 mg of anastrozole per day for 3 months before surgery. The average reduction in tumor volume was 89.3% (caliper measurements). In this study, 15 patients who would have been expected to require a mastectomy at the outset of the study were suitable for breast conservation after 3 months treatment [11]. These data encouraged an ongoing 300-patient randomized study in which tamoxifen is being compared with anastrozole as well as with the combination of the two drugs [12].

A. The Letrozole 024 Neoadjuvant Study

A phase II study with letrozole was also encouraging [13] and led to a randomized comparison with tamoxifen (Fig. 1). The clinical details of this investigation are now in press in the *Annals of Oncology* [14]. Briefly, in a research program involving 55 centers in 16 countries, 337 postmenopausal women with a diagnosis of ER- and/or progesterone receptor (PgR)–positive breast cancer, ineligible for breast-conserving surgery, were entered into a protocol that evaluated the efficacy of 4 months neoadjuvant endocrine therapy with either tamoxifen or letrozole. To be eligible, patients were required to have ER- and/or PgR- positive, T2, T3, or T4a-c, NO-2, MO breast cancer; no history of other malignancies; and no serious concurrent illnesses or inflammatory breast cancer. Treatment was randomly assigned between letrozole 2.5 mg/day and tamoxifen 20 mg/day in a double-blind manner. Response was assessed by clinical measurement, breast ultrasound, and mammography. A total of 55% of the patients treated with letrozole responded by clinical measurements versus 36% with tamoxifen ($p<0.001$).

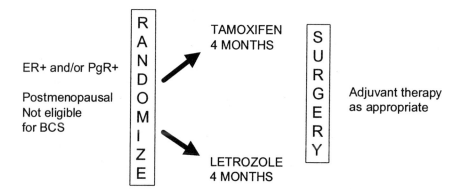

Figure 1 Schema for the Letrozole 024 study.

Letrozole was also superior to tamoxifen for ultrasound response, 35 versus 25% (*p*=0.042) and mammographic response, 34 versus 17% (*p*= <0.001). Logistic regression demonstrated that the odds of achieving a clinical response (CR+PR) were more than twice as high with letrozole than with tamoxifen (odds ratio 2.23, 95% confidence interval (CI) of 1.43–3.50, *p*=0.0005). Finally, more patients underwent breast-conserving surgery when treated with letrozole than with tamoxifen (45 versus 35%, *p*=0.022). These results demonstrate that 4 months of letrozole treatment is a viable and nontoxic neoadjuvant regimen (compared with chemotherapy) that facilitates breast-conserving surgery more effectively than neoadjuvant tamoxifen.

B.   Biomaker Studies in the Letrozole 024 Study

The principal objective of predictive biomarker studies is to define relationships between tumor characteristics and therapeutic outcomes. In the context of neoadjuvant endocrine studies, a major objective has been to prospectively identify tumors likely to respond to this therapeutic approach. Until the execution of the Letrozole 024 study, predictive biomarker research on aromatase inhibitors was limited. Nonetheless, data from the Edinburgh group strongly suggested that ER should be measured at baseline and neoadjuvant endocrine therapy offered only to patients with unquestionably positive, or "ER-rich" tumors. In addition, studies by Soubeyran et al. [15] suggested that PS2 (trefoil factor 1) is an additional and valuable predictor of response to neoadjuvant tamoxifen.

1.   Confirmation of Study Eligibility

An obvious use for a tumor bank developed during an endocrine therapy study is to recheck hormone receptor status so that patients with hormone receptor–negative tumors, who entered the trial because of a false-positive result, can be excluded from the analysis. Baseline biopsies for a central analysis of ER and PgR status were received from 278 patients in the Letrozole 024 study. Full details of the methodological approaches for this study have been reported in the *Journal of Clinical Oncology* [16]. This material allowed an adjusted analysis to be performed for study-biopsy–confirmed ER- and/or PgR-positive cases using a conventional cutoff of 10% or more positive-staining nuclei. This analysis suggests that the original analysis modestly underestimated the benefit of neoadjuvant endocrine therapy because of the presence of a small number of ER- and PgR-negative cases. For cases that were confirmed to be ER- and/or PgR-positive, the clinical response rate with letrozole was documented to be 60%, with 48% of patients experiencing breast-conserving surgery. Only 8% of patients on the letrozole arm experienced disease progression during neoadjuvant treatment. Results for this subset analysis are summarized in Table 1.

2. Estrogen Receptor

To examine the relationship between ER expression levels and response in more detail, the Allred score was utilized. This is a semiquantitative immuno-histochemical analysis that combines an intensity score (1 to 3) with a frequency score (0 to 5) [17]. The relationship between ER expression level and log (odds of response) fitted a linear model that was significant by logistic regression within treatment groups (letrozole $p=0.0013$ and tamoxifen $p=0.0061$, Wald's test) (Fig. 2). There were no responses to either drug in the Allred categories of 0 and 2. These tumors should therefore be considered "ER-negative" and, in retrospect, were not suitable for neoadjuvant endocrine therapy. Interestingly, for every Allred category from 3 to 8, letrozole was more effective than tamoxifen. This information demonstrates that the superiority of letrozole over tamoxifen is not dependent on the level of ER expression. Furthermore, within Allred categories of 3 to 5, or "ER-intermediate" range, responses to letrozole

Table 1 Results of the Letrozole 024 Study for on Study Biopsy Confirmed ER- and/or PgR-Positive Tumors

	Letrozole	Tamoxifen	*p* Value[a]
Confirmed (ER/PgR)	124 (100%)	126 (100%)	
Overall tumor response (CR+PR)			
Clinical	74 (60%)	52 (41%)	0.004
Ultrasound	48 (39%)	37 (29%)	0.119
Mammography	47 (37%)	25 (20%)	0.002
Breast-conserving surgery	60 (48%)	45 (36%)	0.036
Clinical disease progression	10 (8%)	15 (12%)	0.303

Source: Reproduced with permission from Ref. 16.

% of cases in each category

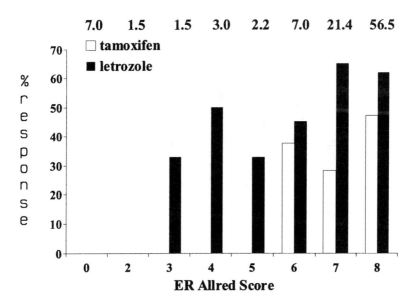

Figure 2 Relationship between ER expression according to Allred score and clinical response rates to tamoxifen and letrozole. Logistic regression analysis of linear model: letrozole, p=0.0013; tamoxifen, p=0.0061. (Reproduced with permission from Ref. 16.)

were observed but not to tamoxifen. This suggests that lower ER cutoff values may be acceptable for therapy with letrozole than with tamoxifen, although the small number of cases in the range of 3 to 5 was too low to allow a robust conclusion. In the author's view, neoadjuvant letrozole treatment should still be restricted to patients with tumors that contain 10% or more cells unequivocally expressing ER and/or PgR or whose tumors express ER with an Allred score of 6, 7, or 8 in order to ensure the highest response rates when using neoadjuvant letrozole therapy.

3. Progesterone Receptor

The relationship between PgR Allred score and response to letrozole and tamoxifen was complex because maximal response rates for both drugs occurred at intermediate levels of expression, not at the highest levels of expression (Fig. 3). When the absolute difference in log odds from the peak letrozole response rate associated with an Allred score of 5, was assessed by logistic regression, an inverse V-shaped model was the best model that fit the data (p=0.0015, Wald's test). This

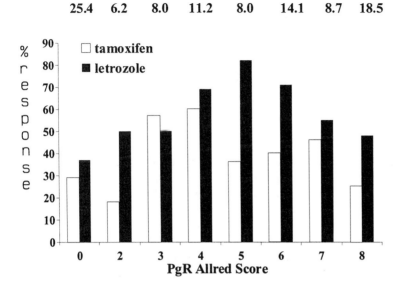

% of cases in each Allred category

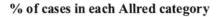

Figure 3 Relationship between PgR expression according to Allred score and clinical response rates to tamoxifen and letrozole. Logistic regression analysis of "inverse V" model: letrozole, p=0.0015; tamoxifen, p=0.0165. (Reproduced with permission from Ref. 16.)

indicated that high as well as low PgR expression scores were associated with a lower chance of responding than intermediate scores. A similar model fit the tamoxifen data if the peak response rate was taken to be an Allred score of 4, although with a lower level of statistical confidence (p=0.0165). An inverse V-shaped relationship was not anticipated from prior information on the predictive properties of PgR in breast cancer [18]. It was generally accepted that expression of PgR was a marker for estrogen-dependent cancers with "functional ERs," because PgR requires activated ER for expression [19]. It was also assumed that like ER, the relationship between PgR level and response was linear, with the most responsive tumors expressing the highest levels of expression. While this classical hypothesis explains the initial increase in response rates associated with Allred scores of 0 to 5—i.e., the rise in response rates associated with the appearance of PgR expression—it does not predict the subsequent decline in response rates associated with PgR Allred scores of 6, 7, and 8. A number of explanations for the inverse V-shaped relationship can be entertained. For example, it is possible that PgR expression is a surrogate for tumor estrogen content and aromatase activity. PgR-rich tumors may, therefore, be associated with high levels of estrogen production inducing relative resistance to aromatase inhibitor therapy. An alternative hypothesis is that high levels of PgR are a marker for tumors that become estrogen "hypersensitive." Shim et al. as well as others have described a marked upregulation of estrogen sensitivity after estrogen deprivation that allows breast cancer cells to proliferate in response to ultra low levels of estrogen [20]. Tumors with this phenotype would also be expected to exhibit resistance to estrogen deprivation. Finally, certain mutants of ER have been described that exhibit estrogen hypersensitivity that could also be associated with high levels of PgR expression [21].

4. Responses to Letrozole and Tamoxifen According to ErbB1 and ErbB2 Status

Samples from the Letrozole 024 trial were also used to address a long-standing controversy concerning the relationship between ErbB1 (the EGF receptor) and ErbB2 (HER-2/*neu*) expression and resistance to endocrine therapies [22–25]. The number of cases overexpressing ErbB2 (defined as ++ or +++ on immunohistochemical scoring) was 14%, with 7% overexpressing ErbB1 (by the same definition). A proportion of these ErbB1+ and/or ErbB2+ cases were ER-, so that the true frequency of tumors overexpressing ErbB1 and/or ErbB2, as well as expressing ER (10% expression or greater) in the entire analysis (ErbB1+ and/or ErbB2+ *and* ER+) was 15.2%. Logistic regression was used to assess the level of significance associated with the difference in efficacy between letrozole and tamoxifen within the subset of tumors that were ErbB1+ and/or ErbB2+ *and* ER+ (Table 2). Letrozole was considerably more active than tamoxifen in this subset of tumors (RR 88% versus 21%, odds ratio for response 28, $p=0.0004$). When ErbB1+ and/or ErbB2+ tumors were removed from the analysis of tumor response, letrozole still showed a numerically higher response rate than tamoxifen in ER+ tumors (54% versus 42%, $p=0.078$). These data suggest that while ErbB1 and ErbB2 status might not be the only explanation for the superiority of letrozole over tamoxifen, overcoming resistance pathways associated with ErbB1

Table 2 Clinical Response Rates of Letrozole Versus Tamoxifen for Subsets Defined by ErbB1, ErbB2, and ER

Category	Letrozole	Tamoxifen	Odds Ratio Let vs. Tam	p Value[a]
ErbB 1/2+[b] ER+	15/17 (88%)	4/19 (21%)	28 (4.5–177)	0.0004
ErbB 1/2-[c] ER+	55/101 (54%)	42/100 (42%)	1.7 (0.9–2.9)	0.0780

[a]Stratified Mantel–Haenszel chi-squared test.
[b]ErbB1 and/or ErbB2 positive.
[c]ErbB1 and/or ErbB2 negative.
Source: Reproduced with permission from Ref. 16.

and ErbB2 expression is a significant component of the improvement in outcomes associated with letrozole treatment observed in this clinical trial. These results illustrate the effective way neoadjuvant endocrine therapy can be used to investigate the impact of biomarkers on tumor response.

IV. CONFIRMING THE ACTIVITY OF LETROZOLE IN ER+ AND ERBB1+ AND/OR ERBB2+ BREAST CANCER IN THE ADJUVANT SETTING

Since large tumor banks from patients treated with aromatase inhibitors in the adjuvant or metastatic disease setting are currently not available, it will not be possible to replicate the biomarker findings of the Letrozole 024 study in more conventional settings in the immediate future. It is certainly disappointing that the ATAC and BIG/FEMTA studies did not have companion tissue-block protocols. Retrospective biomarker analyses of these large adjuvant studies, if they are ultimately possible, may be biased by incomplete block collection, which tends to underrepresent patients who have died or who entered the trial early on in the accrual phase. These conclusions suggest that a prospective study should be considered.

A. An Adjuvant Study for ER+ and/or PgR+, ErbB1+ and/or ErbB2+ Breast Cancer

Tumors with the ER+, ErbB1, and/or ErbB2+ phenotype represent 15–20% of all hormone receptor–positive breast cancers [16,26] and are an important challenge for drug development because of the coexpression of two classes of therapeutic target—steroid receptors and tyrosine kinase–linked growth-factor receptors. Establishing the most appropriate endocrine therapy for ER+ and/or PgR+, ErbB1+, and/or ErbB2+ disease is a logical prerequisite for future adjuvant trials that will examine the activity of novel ErbB1 and/or ErbB2 inhibitors in the adjuvant setting. Current trastuzumab adjuvant studies employ tamoxifen for adjuvant endocrine therapy. If aromatase inhibitors are more active than tamoxifen for ER+, ErbB2+ disease, the additive benefit of trastuzumab could be questioned if a future switch to the use of aromatase inhibitors takes place. Future studies of ErbB1/2-targeted therapies would greatly benefit from an understanding of the optimal endocrine therapy for the ER+ and/or PgR+, ErbB1+, and/or ErbB2+ tumor subtype. A study design under consideration is presented in Figure 4. For this investigation, the adjuvant endocrine treatment of postmenopausal women with stage 1 T1c, stage 2 and stage 3 ER+ and/or PgR+, ErbB1+, and/or ErbB2+ breast cancer will be randomized between letrozole and tamoxifen. Outcomes will be stratified according to the administration of chemotherapy. The relative value of ErbB2 analysis by immunohistochemistry

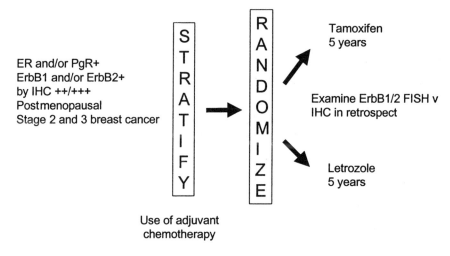

ER and/or PgR+
ErbB1 and/or ErbB2+
by IHC ++/+++
Postmenopausal
Stage 2 and 3 breast cancer

S T R A T I F Y

R A N D O M I Z E

Tamoxifen
5 years

Examine ErbB1/2 FISH v
IHC in retrospect

Letrozole
5 years

Use of adjuvant
chemotherapy

Figure 4 A clinical trial schema that compares the efficacy of tamoxifen and letrozole as adjuvant therapy for postmenopausal women with ER-and/or PgR-positive, ErbB1- and/or ErbB2-positive breast cancer.

and fluorescence in situ hybridization (FISH) in predicting the outcome of endocrine therapy will be examined as a planned retrospective subset analysis.

V. STUDIES IN THE METASTATIC DISEASE SETTING

Immunophenotyping of metastatic breast cancer is difficult to achieve on a routine basis. Studies that probe the relationship between ErbB2 expression and endocrine therapy on the basis of the serum assay for the extracellular domain of ErbB2 are not strictly comparable to direct examination of tumor tissue, because (a) the ER status is not reconfirmed and (b) shed extracellular domain (ECD) is not the functional equivalent of membrane-bound receptor and so may have different properties as a predictive biomarker. Several trials are currently under way to examine the combination of an aromatase inhibitor and the ErbB2 targeting antibody trastuzumab. These studies should shed further light on the management of ER+, ErbB2+ disease.

A. Preoperative Chemotherapy Versus Neoadjuvant Endocrine Therapy

For older patients, particularly those with comorbid illnesses, the improvement in surgical outcomes associated with neoadjuvant letrozole treatment is a significant advance in treatment. For younger postmenopausal patients with ER-positive breast cancer requiring preoperative systemic therapy, chemotherapy remains the standard of care. The response rate is high, conversion to breast-conserving surgery is reasonably frequent, and safety and efficacy have been validated by a large randomized controlled clinical trial [27]. However neoadjuvant chemotherapy has significant shortcomings for postmenopausal women with ER-positive breast cancer: (a) older patients are more prone to chemotherapy-induced myelodysplasia and doxorubicin-induced cardiomyopathy [28]; (b) the benefits of chemotherapy for older patients with ER-positive disease are considerably less than for younger patients or patients with ER-negative breast cancer, in part because these patients experience the majority of their adjuvant benefits from endocrine therapy [29,30]; and (c) there is evidence that the activity of neoadjuvant chemotherapy is blunted in ER-positive disease. For example, a complete pathological response to preoperative cyclophosphamide, Adriamycin (doxorubicin), and 5-fluorouracil (CAF) is considerably more common for ER-negative than for ER-positive tumors [31]. These data replicated earlier results from other preoperative chemotherapy studies [32] and together do suggest that ER-positive disease is relatively resistant to chemotherapy [33]. Given these factors, could neoadjuvant letrozole be as effective as chemotherapy? In the NSABP B18 trial, the clinical response rate was 80%, approximately 20% higher than the response to letrozole (55–60%). However, 27% of patients enrolled in the NSABP B20 trial had tumors that were less than 2 cm in size, and many other study subjects had T2 tumors that were small enough to be amenable to breast-conserving surgery. Given these data, the response rate to neoadjuvant letrozole of 55 to 0% and a conversion to breast-conserving surgery of 45 to 48% is a result well within the realm of what might have been achieved with chemotherapy in the same study population and is an impressive result for an agent with such low toxicity. A randomized trial comparing neoadjuvant chemotherapy versus neoadjuvant letrozole is therefore warranted.

B. A Potential Design for a Randomized Neoadjuvant Trial Comparing Chemotherapy with Letrozole

1. Preoperative Phase

A major change in clinical practice in breast cancer requires a trial in which standard therapy is compared with a new approach. In the study outlined in Fig. 5, neoadjuvant chemotherapy will be directly compared with letrozole treatment. Since the best data concerning the value of chemotherapy in postmenopausal women with ER+ disease is from the use of CAF chemotherapy [28], each study site would choose a CAF-like regimen that would be used in a consistent fashion. The duration of preoperative chemotherapy would range from 18 to 24 weeks, depending on whether a 3- or 4-week CAF regimen were chosen. The duration of letrozole treatment would also be flexible, so that partial responders at

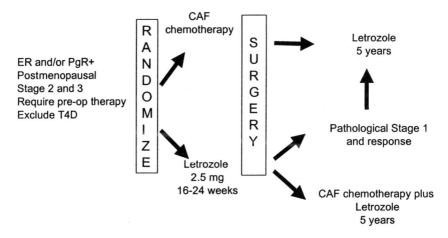

Figure 5 A clinical trial schema that compares the efficacy of neoadjuvant cyclophosphamide/Adriamycin/5-fluorouracil chemotherapy (CAF) with neoadjuvant letrozole.

4 months would be allowed to continue therapy up to a maximum period of 24 months before surgery. Patients who experienced a poor response to either approach could choose either immediate surgery or cross over to CAF before surgery. The endpoint of the preoperative phase would be response rate, and rates of breast-conserving surgery.

2. Postoperative Phase

All patients will receive letrozole for 5 years after surgery. For the patients who received neoadjuvant letrozole, consideration must be given to the prognostic information provided by the responses observed. Clearly patients whose tumors do not respond to letrozole should receive CAF chemotherapy. CAF would also be administered if, after surgery, a substantial amount of tumor were found in the breast or the lymph nodes. However, if a patient's tumor had undergone a clinical or radiological CR or PR to letrozole, the nodes were negative, and the residual disease was 2 cm or less, the patient would escape chemotherapy and simply continue with 5 years of postoperative letrozole therapy. All appropriate patients would receive radiotherapy. From a statistical point of view, the trial would be powered for equivalent outcomes on the two treatment arms: i.e., despite the use of neoadjuvant letrozole and a reduction in the administration of chemotherapy administration on the experimental arm, the two arms would have similar relapse-free and overall survival statistics. If this were the case, a clear improvement in clinical management will have been made, with an improvement in quality of life and cost due to the reduced administration of chemotherapy, without compromising long-term outcomes. If this study were a success, new clinical designs could follow in which neoadjuvant endocrine therapy becomes the new standard and the value of chemotherapy in more finely defined subsets, or a strategy of switching to alternative endocrine therapy, could be evaluated. However, in the author's view, we should resist the temptation to build in secondary randomizations into the initial, practice-setting trial (i.e., treatments depending on postneoadjuvant status), as we currently do not know enough about the relationships between molecular and clinical parameters and long-term clinical outcomes.

VI. SUMMARY

The clinical significance of neoadjuvant endocrine therapy lies in the opportunity to "unlock" the patient-to-patient variability associated with adjuvant endocrine therapy in order to better target our therapeutic approaches. Currently neoadjuvant studies focus on clinical, radiological, and pathological response, but future studies will increasingly rely on molecular biomarkers. For example, one can easily imagine that proliferation rates after 4 months of endocrine therapy could be a powerful predictor of subsequent relapse, because proliferation despite estrogen deprivation is a sign of estrogen-independent growth. The opportunity afforded by neoadjuvant endocrine therapy to scan the transcriptosome (the state of gene expression levels at a given time) of tumor cells during treatment is also highly significant. Gene expression patterns detected by microarray analysis may detect resistance early or define tumors in which ER function has been inadequately suppressed [34].

ACKNOWLEDGMENT

Grant support from Novartis Pharmaceuticals.

REFERENCES

1. Kennedy BJ, Kelly RM, White G, Nathanson IT. Surgery as an adjunct to hormone therapy of breast cancer. Cancer 1957; 10:1055–1075.
2. Bates T, Riley DL, Houghton J, et al. Breast cancer in elderly women: A Cancer Research Campaign trial comparing treatment with tamoxifen and optimal surgery with tamoxifen alone. The Elderly Breast Cancer Working Party. Br J Surg 1991; 78:591–594.
3. Mustacchi G, Milani S, Pluchinotta A, et al. Tamoxifen or surgery plus tamoxifen as primary treatment for elderly patients with operable breast cancer: The GRETA Trial. Group for Research on Endocrine Therapy in the Elderly. Anticancer Res 1994; 14:2197–2000.

4. Mustacchi G, Latteier J, Baum M. Tamoxifen alone versus surgery plus tamoxifen for breast cancer of the elderly: Meta-analysis of long-term results of the GRETA and CRC trials. 21st Annual San Antonio Breast Cancer Symposium, San Antonio, TX, Dec 12–15, 1998.

5. Ellis MJ. Preoperative endocrine therapy for older women with breast cancer: renewed interest in an old idea. Cancer Control 2000; 7:557–562.

6. Hoff PM, Valero V, Buzdar AU, et al. Combined modality treatment of locally advanced breast carcinoma in elderly patients or patients with severe comorbid conditions using tamoxifen as the primary therapy. Cancer 2000; 88:2054–2060.

7. Horobin JM, Preece PE, Dewar JA, et al. Long-term follow-up of elderly patients with locoregional breast cancer treated with tamoxifen only. Br J Surg 1991; 78:213–217.

8. Kenny FS, Robertson JFR, Ellis IO. Long-term follow-up of elderly patients randomized to primary tamoxifen or wedge mastectomy as initial therapy for operable breast carcinoma. Breast 1998; 7:335–339.

9. Ellis PA, Saccani-Jotti G, Clarke R, et al. A'Hern R, Salter J, Detre S, Nicholson R, Robertson J, Smith IE, Dowsett M. Induction of apoptosis by tamoxifen and ICI 182780 in primary breast cancer. Int J Cancer 1997; 72:608–613.

10. Dixon JM, Love CD, Renshaw L, et al. Leonard RC. Lessons from the use of aromatase inhibitors in the neoadjuvant setting. Endocr Rel Cancer 1999; 6:227–230.

11. Dixon JM, Renshaw L, Bellamy C, et al. The effects of neo-adjuvant anastrozole (Arimidex) on tumor volume in postmenopausal women with breast cancer: A randomized, double-blind, single-center study. Clin Cancer Res 2000; 6:2229–2235.

12. Boeddinghaus IE, Dowsett M, Smith IE, et al. Allum W. Neoadjuvant Arimidex ot Tamoxifen Alone or in Combined, for breast cancer (IMPACT): PgR-related reductions in Proliferation Marker Ki67. 36th Annual Meeting of ASCO, New Orleans, LA, May 20–23, 2000.

13. Dixon J, Love C, Tucker S, et al. Letrozole as primary medical therapy for locally advanced and large operable breast cancer (abstr). Breast Cancer Res Treat 1997; 46:213.

14. Eiermann W, Paepke S, Appffelstaedt J, et al. Vinholes J, Mauriac L, Ellis M, Lassus M, Chaudrai HA, Dugan M, Borgs M, Semiglazov V. Preoperative treatment of postmenopausal breast cancer patients with letrozole: A randomized double-blind multicenter study. Ann Oncol 2001; 12:1–6.

15. Soubeyran I, Quenel N, Coindre JM, et al. pS2 protein: A marker improving prediction of response to neoadjuvant tamoxifen in post-menopausal breast cancer patients. Br J Cancer 1996; 74:1120–1125.

16. Ellis M, Coop A, Singh B, et al. Letrozole is more effective neo-adjuvant endocrine therapy than tamoxifen for ErbB1 and/or ErbB2 positive, estrogen receptor positive primary breast cancer: Evidence from a phase 3 randomized trial. J Clin Oncol. In press.

17. Allred DC, Harvey JM, Berardo M, Clark GM. Prognostic and predictive factors in breast cancer by immunohistochemical analysis. Mod Pathol 1998; 11:155–168.

18. Clark GM, McGuire WL, Hubay CA, et al. Progesterone receptors as a prognostic factor in stage II breast cancer. N Engl J Med 1983; 309:1343–1347.

19. Kastner P, Krust A, Turcotte B, et al. Two distinct estrogen-regulated promoters generate transcripts encoding the two functionally different human progesterone receptor forms A and B. EMBO J 1990; 9:1603–1614.

20. Shim WS, Conaway M, Masamura S, et al. Estradiol hypersensitivity and mitogen-activated protein kinase expression in long-term estrogen deprived human breast cancer cells in vivo. Endocrinology 2000; 141:396–405.

21. Fuqua SA, Wiltschke C, Zhang QX, et al. Hilsenbeck S, Mohsin S, O'Connell P, Allred DC. A hypersensitive estrogen receptor-alpha mutation in premalignant breast lesions. Cancer Res 2000; 60:4026–4029.

22. Wright C, Nicholson S, Angus B, et al. AL, Horne CH. Relationship between c-erbB-2 protein product expression and response to endocrine therapy in advanced breast cancer. Br J Cancer 1992; 65:118–121.

23. Berns EM, Foekens JA, van Staveren IL, et al. Oncogene amplification and prognosis in breast cancer: Relationship with systemic treatment. Gene 1995; 159:11–18.

24. Yamauchi H, O'Neill A, Gelman R, et al. Prediction of response to antiestrogen therapy in advanced breast cancer patients by pretreatment circulating levels of extracellular domain of the HER-2/c-neu protein. J Clin Oncol 1997; 15:2518–2525.

25. Carlomagno C, Perrone F, Gallo C, et al. c-erb B2 overexpression decreases the benefit of adjuvant tamoxifen in early-stage breast cancer without axillary lymph node metastases. J Clin Oncol 1996; 14:2702–2708.

26. Berry DA, Muss HB, Thor AD, et al. HER-2/neu and p53 expression versus tamoxifen resistance in estrogen receptor-positive, node-positive breast cancer. J Clin Oncol 2000; 18:3471–3479.

27. Fisher B, Bryant J, Wolmark N, et al. Effect of preoperative chemotherapy on the outcome of women with operable breast cancer. J Clin Oncol 1998; 16:2672–2685.

28. Albain KS, Green S, Ravdin P, et al. Overall survival after cyclophosphamide, Adriamycin, 5FU and tamoxifen (CAFT) is superior to T alone in postmenopausal, receptor (+), Node (+) Breast cancer: New findings from Phase III Southwest Oncology Group Intergroup Trial S8814 (INT-0100). 37th Annual Meeting of ASCO, San Francisco, CA, May 12–15, 2001.

29. Polychemotherapy for early breast cancer: An overview of the randomised trials. Early Breast Cancer Trialists' Collaborative Group. Lancet 1998; 352:930–942.

30. Tamoxifen for early breast cancer: an overview of the randomised trials. Early Breast Cancer Trialists' Collaborative Group. Lancet 1998; 351:1451–1467.

31. Kuerer HM, Newman LA, Smith TL, et al. Clinical course of breast cancer patients with complete pathologic primary tumor and axillary lymph node response to doxorubicin-based neo-adjuvant chemotherapy. J Clin Oncol 1999; 17:460–469.

32. Bonadonna G, Veronesi U, Brambilla C, et al. Primary chemotherapy to avoid mastectomy in tumors with diameters of three centimeters or more. J Natl Cancer Inst 1990; 82:1539–1545.

33. Lippman ME, Allegra JC, Thompson EB, et al. The relation between estrogen receptors and response rate to cytotoxic chemotherapy in metastatic breast cancer. N Engl J Med 1978; 298:1223–1228.

34. Dressman MA, Walz TM, Barnes L, et al. Genes that co-cluster with estrogen receptor alpha in microarray analysis of breast biopsies. Pharmacogenomics J 2001; 1:135–141.

11

Neoadjuvant Therapy: Surgical Perspectives

J. Michael Dixon
Edinburgh Breast Unit
Western General Hospital
Edinburgh, Scotland

I. INTRODUCTION

There are several potential advantages and disadvantages of administering systemic therapy before definitive locoregional treatment in early and locally advanced breast cancer. The presence of a measurable mass within the breast permits assessment of response and provides direct in vivo measurements of the sensitivity of the tumor to the particular drug or drugs used. Theoretically the early detection of a resistant tumor should enable both the discontinuation of an ineffective treatment, thereby avoiding unnecessary toxicity, and a change to a potentially more effective therapy. In addition, the earlier the disease is treated the lower the likelihood that resistant tumor clones will emerge spontaneously. Even a short delay in administration of systemic therapy could adversely affect outcome [1]. Another major advantage of early drug treatment is the possibility of making a locally advanced breast cancer operable or making a large operable breast cancer shrink to a sufficient degree to allow breast-conserving surgery rather than mastectomy. The major disadvantage of primary systemic therapy is that the commonly used prognostic factors, in particular axillary node status, are not available before a decision is taken on the use of systemic therapy. However, it is now possible to determine preoperatively the grade of the cancer and hormone receptor status with the histological diagnosis of the cancer obtained with core biopsy.

Preoperative chemotherapy has been used extensively for the treatment of initially inoperable locally advanced breast cancers to achieve a reduction in tumor volume and allow later tumor excision. More recently, this strategy has also been introduced for operable breast cancer. Few studies have evaluated neoadjuvant endocrine therapy for this strategy, although there are a number of published studies that have analyzed the results of treating patients with agents such as tamoxifen alone. In the early 1980s uncontrolled studies suggested that tamoxifen as sole treatment was effective for elderly patients with breast cancer [2–5]. Thereafter, increasing numbers of patients have been treated similarly. The problem was that follow-up was short in the early published studies and patients were not selected on the basis of whether the tumor expressed estrogen receptors (ERs) and was therefore likely to respond. In one series of 113 women aged 70 or more and treated with tamoxifen as primary treatment, a complete response rate was reported for 38, a partial response for 17, and no change for 34; 24 had progressive disease [6]. A total of 70 patients (61.9%) did not maintain local cancer control with tamoxifen either at death or most recent follow-up. The study concluded that tamoxifen provided an alternative treatment for operable breast cancer in the short term and that tamoxifen alone was suitable only for patients with concurrent disease who were unwilling to undergo surgery [6].

Subsequently there have been four randomized trials of primary endocrine therapy [7–70]. In these trials the major question asked was whether neoadjuvant endocrine therapy could obviate the need for breast surgery and whether the avoidance of surgery would affect survival in relatively infirm and aged women. In two of the trials, tamoxifen therapy alone was compared with surgery alone, while in the other two tamoxifen was compared with surgery combined with tamoxifen [7–10]. Not surprisingly, the time to relapse was significantly shorter in the tamoxifen alone arm in all trials. It was surprising to note, however, that in three of the four trials the number of patients with distant relapse was lower in the groups that had no immediate surgery. This result was contradicted by a more recent analysis of a series of studies that found a significant reduction in deaths from breast cancer in patients undergoing immediate surgery combined with tamoxifen [11]. As these trials were designed to address the question of whether delayed surgery was detrimental, it is not possible to use them to evaluate neoadjuvant hormonal therapy followed a few months later by definitive locoregional treatment.

Substantial reductions in tumor volume over a 3-month period have been reported for hormone-sensitive tumors treated with agents such as luteinizing hormone–releasing hormone (LH-RH) analogues, tamoxifen, aminoglutethimide, and 4-hydroxyandrostenedione [12,13]. Two of the agents, aminoglutethimide and 4-hydroxyandrostenedione, have now been replaced by the third-generation aromatase inhibitors letrozole, anastrozole, and exemestane.

II. SELECTION OF PATIENTS FOR PRIMARY SYSTEMIC THERAPY

The studies that have been published to date have failed to show any survival advantage for patients treated with chemotherapy in the neoadjuvant setting over those treated (with the same drugs) adjuvantly [14]. However, neoadjuvant systemic therapy should provide some additional benefit to patients through the conversion of locally inoperable cancers to an operable disease or through the reduction in size of a large operable breast cancer, so that breast-conserving surgery can be performed. Patients with multiple tumors in one breast, on the other hand, are less likely to benefit unless they have locally advanced breast cancer, because they will require mastectomy even if the neoadjuvant therapy produces a significant response. In selecting patients for neoadjuvant endocrine therapy, ER status and to a lesser degree progesterone receptor status are important determinants of response. This requirement has been underlined by the observation that ER-positive tumors treated with primary tamoxifen show complete and partial response rates ranging from 72–92% [12,13,15,16]. There is also evidence that a direct correlation exists between the level of ER expression and both the likelihood of response and the degree of response [13]. For this reason only patients with ER-rich tumors are selected for neoadjuvant endocrine therapy at the Edinburgh Breast Unit. Although this recommendation applies primarily to postmenopausal women, for whose condition we have the most clinical experience, neoadjuvant endocrine therapy has been used for the treatment of premenopausal women, and the requirement is essentially the same [2,12]. There are certain types of tumor for which the response to treatment can be difficult to assess. These include invasive lobular carcinomas and mucinous carcinomas. Invasive lobular carcinomas have pathologically poorly defined margins, and this makes clinical response and response by ultrasonography or mammography harder to judge. The patient whose mammograms are shown in Figure 1 was diagnosed as having an invasive lobular cancer that was strongly ER-positive (80% of cells were strongly stained). The extent of disease using the original mammogram was difficult to estimate. The patient was given neoadjuvant tamoxifen, and the mammogram taken 3 months later (Fig. 1B) showed little change in the extent of disease. Although ultrasound measurements also indicated only a minor response, clinically the tumor appeared much smaller. An attempt was made to excise the cancer widely by breast-conserving surgery, and a specimen x-ray (Fig. 1C) indicated that the area of abnormality had been removed. Pathology, however, demonstrated that the 8-cm invasive lobular carcinoma reached all margins, and the patient was treated subsequently by mastectomy. Invasive mu-

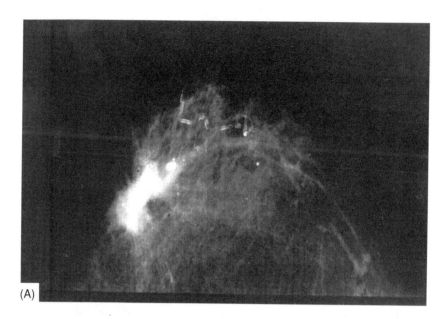

(A)

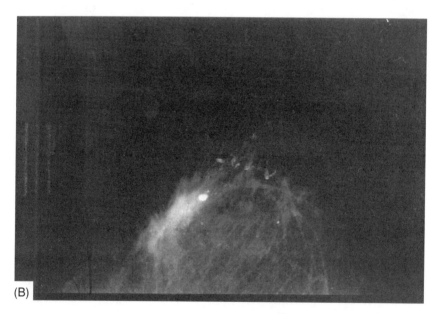

(B)

Figure 1 Patient with invasive lobular carcinoma at diagnosis (A), after 3 months of hormonal therapy (B), and the specimen x-ray of the wide excision (C).

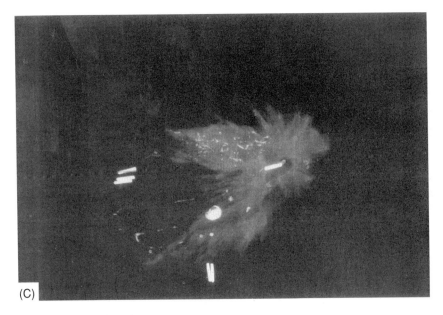

(C)

Figure 1   Continued

cinous cancers do respond to endocrine therapy, but their response is slower. The reason for this seems to be that a large part of the cancer consists not of cell mass but of lakes of mucin. Figure 2 shows an example from a patient with an advanced invasive mucinous cancer that was well circumscribed mammographically. The cancer shrank over an 18-month period and became operable by wide excision (Fig. 2B). The problem was that there was no apparent change in size of this cancer over the first 3 to 4 months, which has become the standard period for treatment by neoadjuvant endocrine therapy.

III.   ASSESSMENT OF RESPONSE

Response can be measured clinically and by imaging. Clinical measurements of tumor size are observer-dependent, whereas ultrasonography and mammography estimate tumor diameter and volume objectively and with greater accuracy [17,18]. Various studies have compared these two imaging techniques, and while some have found the two equally accurate, others have demonstrated that ultrasonography is more accurate in measuring tumor size [18,19]. These two imaging techniques have also been evaluated as methods for measuring response. The two appear to be equally effective for use in mammographically discrete tumors,

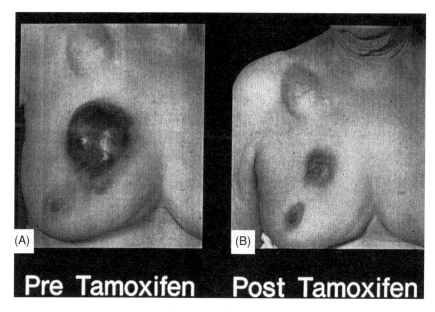

Figure 2 Patient with a mucinous carcinoma before (A) and after (B) 18 months of endocrine therapy. The abnormality just under the clavicle is a lipoma.

but ultrasonography is more useful, since it can assess response even in mammographically diffuse lesions [18]. Correlating the final pathological size with the size assessed by clinical, mammographic, and ultrasound measurements demonstrates that the best correlation is for ultrasound assessment of tumor size and volume [18,20]. Thus, rather than relying on clinical assessment alone, patients treated with primary systemic therapy should also have their cancer monitored by both mammography and ultrasound.

Recent work has centered on the use of magnetic resonance imaging (MRI) and positron emission tomography (PET) to image cancers and to demonstrate changes during treatment. Tumor blood flow can be assessed during treatment either using dynamic MRI or color Doppler ultrasound. Reductions in blood flow are evident within a few weeks of starting treatment and studies are evaluating whether these early changes correlate with long-term response.

Although partial responses are common, pathologically complete responses are uncommon. Preoperative chemotherapy produces complete responses in only 10–20% of patients and complete pathological responses are rarely seen with neoadjuvant endocrine therapy [21–23]. The standard criteria for assessing response have been issued by the International Union against Cancer (UICC), but the problem with these is that they demand reduction in tumor volume to be maintained for 1 month. Less stringent criteria are those of the World Health Organization (WHO), which specify that a 50% or greater reduction in bidimensional measurements is required for a partial response but for which there is no 1-month maintenance period [24]. An alternative is to use reduction in tumor volume, which can be estimated from two-dimensional measurements taken 45 degrees apart by clinical or mammographic measurement using the following formula:

$$V = D^3 \times \pi/6.$$

Ultrasound volumes are calculated using two diameters and a depth according to the formula

$$V = D^2 \times d \times \pi/6$$

where D = mean diameter d = mean thickness.

IV. DURATION OF TREATMENT

It has been standard practice to treat patients with neoadjuvant chemotherapy for between three and six cycles prior to surgery. This time period appears long enough to differentiate responders from nonresponders. In patients who do respond, it permits most locally advanced breast cancers to become operable, and a significant number of patients who would otherwise have required mastectomy at least a chance of being of being considered for breast-conserving surgery. There have, however, been few studies of the optimal duration of neoadjuvant endocrine therapy. In early studies, patients remained on tamoxifen until their tumor became nonresponsive and regrew [4–6]. An unpublished study from Edinburgh identified that 3 months was the most appropriate initial period of neoadjuvant endocrine treatment. This consecutive series of 100 patients over the age of 70 years and with ER-positive breast cancer (>20 fmol/mg cytosolic protein) was treated with neoadjuvant tamoxifen. After 3 months, 72 patients had a reduction in tumor volume of over 25% and were classified as responders. One patient had progressive disease with an increase in tumor volume of more than 25%, and the remaining 27 patients were classified as having static disease and continued on tamoxifen for a further 3 months. Of the patients continuing on tamoxifen, 4 had a reduction in tumor volume (≥25%), 5 progressed, and the remaining 18 showed no change. From these data it is evident that if a patient has not responded by 3 months, the chance of getting a significant response thereafter is small, and this is balanced by the risk of the tumor progressing. For this reason it has been standard in Edinburgh to treat patients for a 3-month period at least initially.

V. RESPONSE AND DOWNSTAGING OF TUMORS

Response rates to preoperative chemotherapy are in the region of 80%, and there do not appear to be major differences between different chemotherapy regimens [25]. Neoadjuvant endocrine therapy in appropriately selected patients also produces significant responses. Tumors from consecutive groups of patients treated at our unit with tamoxifen, letrozole, anastrozole, or exemestane showed both positive and negative changes in volume assessed by ultrasound in response to treatment. The results are shown in Table 1 and the median reductions in tumor volume with the four drugs are shown in Figure 3. The results of the P024 randomized trial comparing tamoxifen and letrozole showed that there was a significantly higher clinical (55 versus 35%), mammographic (34 versus 16%) and ultrasound (35 versus 25%) response rate with letrozole than with tamoxifen [26]. In correlating clinical response with different levels of ER, no patient with an Allred score below 6 responded to tamoxifen. This justifies our own ER-positivity cutoff of 20 fmol/mg cytosolic protein, a histoscore of 80, or an Allred score of 6 or greater [27].

In the Milan study of patients who were treated with preoperative chemotherapy, breast-conserving surgery was possible in 91% of patients. More than 73% of patients who had tumors larger than 5 cm became candidates for breast-conserving surgery [25]. The large NSABP study of preoperative chemotherapy included 1523 patients, who were randomized to receive either surgery followed by four cycles of Adriamycin chemotherapy (AC), or four cycles of AC followed by surgery [14]. After preoperative chemotherapy, 36% of patients obtained a clinical complete response and 43% had a clinical partial response. Thus an overall response rate of 79% was recorded. Of those who achieved a complete clinical response, 25% were found to have no tumor present on pathological examination. Patients receiving preoperative chemotherapy were significantly more likely to have a lumpectomy, 68 versus 60%, $p<0.01$. Although this difference is significant, it is not as dramatic as the conversion rate reported by the Italian or other series [28,29].

Table 1 Median Percentage Reduction in Tumor Volume as Assessed by Ultrasound

Drug	Number of patients	Number with >50% reduction	Number with <50% reduction or increase <25%	Number with >25% increase
Tamoxifen	65	30 (46%)	34 (52%)	1 (2%)
Letrozole	36	32 (89%)	3 (8%)	1 (3%)
Anastrozole	23	18 (78%)	5 (13%)	0
Exemestane	12	10 (83%)	2 (17%)	0

Responses to Aromatase Inhibitors

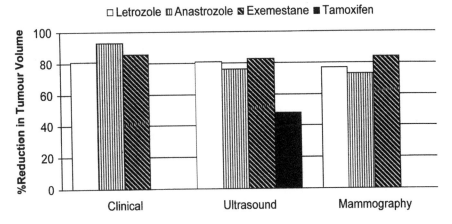

Figure 3 Median reductions in clinical, mammographic, and ultrasound volume for patients treated by letrozole (*n*=24), anastrozole (*n*=23), and exemestane (*n*=12). For comparison, ultrasound response is shown for a series of patients with tamoxifen (*n*=64).

There are few data on conversion rates from mastectomy to breast-conserving surgery with neoadjuvant endocrine therapy. Results from the Edinburgh unit with patients treated with 3 months of neoadjuvant tamoxifen or 3 months neoadjuvant letrozole, anastrozole, or exemestane are presented in Table 2. This shows a high rate of conversion from mastectomy to breast conservation varying between 63 and 93% with different endocrine treatments. The apparent superiority of aromatase inhibitors over tamoxifen in downstaging breast cancers was confirmed in the randomized trial P024. All patients entered into that study either had locally advanced disease or required mastectomy. A total of 45% of the patients treated with letrozole compared 35% of patients treated with tamoxifen were eligible for breast-conserving surgery after 4 months (*p*<0.02).

VI. COMPLETENESS OF EXCISION

There are few studies that have looked at the histology of wide excision specimens after downstaging of breast cancers by primary chemotherapy or hormonal therapy. In the study by Veronesi, 37 of 227 patients (16.3%) had histological evidence of multifocality at the time of wide excision [30]. He noted that multifocality was

Table 2 Patients Requiring Mastectomy Before and After 3 Months of Neoadjuvant Treatment

Drug	Number of patients	Number requiring Mx[a] at outset of study	Number requiring Mx after treatment	Conversion rate
Tamoxifen	65	41	15	63%
Letrozole	36	24	2	93%
Anastrozole	23	19	2	89%
Exemestane	12	10	2	80%

[a]Mastectomy.

observed more frequently in larger tumors, probably because these had not been destroyed uniformly by chemotherapy. This concurs with our own experience in Edinburgh of wide excision performed after neoadjuvant chemotherapy in patients with large operable or locally advanced breast cancer. In a series of 25 patients in whom breast-conserving surgery was attempted, 6 had diffuse "multifocal" disease despite there being no palpable tumor in 5 of these patients. In another study performed at the Royal Marsden Hospital, 309 patients were randomized to receive either adjuvant or neoadjuvant chemotherapy. In the adjuvant group, 31 of 144 (22%) of patients had a mastectomy, but only 16 of 149 (11%) of patients in the neoadjuvant arm required mastectomy [31]. The remaining patients had wide excision followed by postoperative radiotherapy, but in the neoadjuvant arm there was a higher rate of margin involvement at the time of wide excision despite the apparent clinical responses in these patients [32]. In our experience, most patients treated by primary neoadjuvant endocrine therapy who then become eligible for breast-conserving surgery have a complete excision. In the series of 65 patients treated with tamoxifen, 50 had breast-conserving surgery, while in the subsequent series of patients treated with aromatase inhibitors, 53 were suitable for breast conservation and only 4 of these patients had an incomplete excision. One was the patient with invasive lobular carcinoma pictured in Figure 1. An extensive in situ component is significantly less common in older patients. Also, the nature of the response appears different after neoadjuvant endocrine therapy compared with that seen in patents with chemotherapy. In comparing the type of disease remaining in the breast following neoadjuvant hormone therapy with that of the results reported by other authors using neoadjuvant chemotherapy, our impression is that after neoadjuvant hormone therapy the whole of the tumor seems to shrink concentrically, whereas in some patients treated with primary chemotherapy the extent of disease often remains the same but the cellularity of the tumor is markedly reduced by this treatment.

VII. LOCAL RECURRENCE AFTER BREAST-CONSERVING SURGERY FOLLOWING NEOADJUVANT SYSTEMIC THERAPY

At a mean follow-up of 36 months, Veronesi reported 12 cases of local recurrence in the 203 patients treated by quadrantectomy and radiotherapy after neoadjuvant chemotherapy, a rate of 5% at 3 years [30]. This was less than the local recurrence rate seen after mastectomy (5 out of 23, or 22%). In the randomized trial from the Royal Marsden Hospital, the relapse rate was 5 of 144 patients (3.5%) in the adjuvant arm and 4 of 149 (2.7%) in the neoadjuvant arm at a median follow-up of 48 months [31]. There were, however, only 19 patients in the neoadjuvant arm who avoided mastectomy and one of these subsequently had a local relapse. There were more concerning data from the French-American randomized trial [33]. At a median follow-up of 124 months, there was local recurrence in 9 of 40 (22.5%) patients treated by tumorectomy, axillary dissection, and breast irradiation, and in 15 of 44 (34%) patients who had no surgery but just had radiation to the breast and nodal areas. In another report of 185 patients treated at the Royal Marsden Hospital by neoadjuvant chemotherapy, 29 patients who had a clinical complete response were treated by radiotherapy without surgery [33]. These patients had a significantly higher rate of local recurrence compared with partial responders who had surgery ($p < 0.02$). Results from these two studies suggests that local surgery should be performed following neoadjuvant chemotherapy even in patients with an apparent complete response. There are no published data on local recurrence after breast conservation in patients after neoadjuvant endocrine therapy. Table 3 shows the local recurrence rates in patients treated in Edinburgh. These are the first published data on local recurrence of a large series of patients treated with neoadjuvant endocrine therapy and suggest that breast-conserving surgery optimally followed by radiotherapy produces satisfactory local control rates.

Table 3 Local Recurrence (LR) Following Breast Conservation

Drug	Number	No XRT	LR	XRT[a]	LR	Median follow-up in months
Tamoxifen	43	13	2	30	0	78
Letrozole	33	12	2	21	0	61
Anastrozole	22	1	0	21	1	37
Exemestane	10	3	0	7	0	24
Total	108	29	4	79	1	48

[a]X-ray therapy.

VIII. COSMETIC OUTCOMES

There have been no studies of cosmetic outcomes in patients whose cancers have been downstaged by neoadjuvant endocrine therapy. Examples of two patients treated in Edinburgh are shown in Figure 4A and B.

IX. PROGNOSIS

Response to neoadjuvant chemotherapy and endocrine therapy predicts subsequent survival. Data from patients treated in Edinburgh are presented in Figure 5A and B. Patients are subdivided by whether the time to halve tumor volume was less or greater than the median.

X. SUMMARY

Neoadjuvant chemotherapy and endocrine therapy are being used increasingly to downstage locally advanced and large operable breast cancers. This treatment can result in inoperable breast cancer becoming operable, allowing patients who would otherwise have required mastectomy to become candidates for breast-conserving surgery. Patients treated with neoadjuvant endocrine therapy need careful selection, and only those with ER-rich tumors are candidates for this treatment. These patients have a high response rate and a significant reduction in tumor volume over a 3-month period. Response should be monitored carefully during treatment with a combination of clinical and imaging measurements. MRI and PET are currently being evaluated as more accurate methods of assessing response to treatment. High rates of conversion from mastectomy to breast-conserving surgery are possible with a 3- to 4-month course of neoadjuvant endocrine therapy [20]. In a randomized trial in the neoadjuvant setting, letrozole appeared to produce higher response rates than tamoxifen in postmenopausal women. This translates into a higher rate of conversion to breast-conserving surgery: 45% versus 35% in the randomized trial of letrozole versus tamoxifen [26]. There is some evidence to suggest that the pattern of response may be different in some patients treated by neoadjuvant chemotherapy compared with neoadjuvant hormonal therapy. In up to one-quarter of patients following neoadjuvant chemotherapy, the treatment reduces cellularity but there is no significant reduction in the extent of disease [30]. In the majority of patients treated with neoadjuvant chemo- or endocrine therapy, the tumor mass shrinks, making these patients eligible for breast-conserving surgery. Rates of complete excision appear higher in patients treated by neoadjuvant endocrine therapy than in those treated with neoadjuvant chemotherapy. Breast-conserving surgery after neoadjuvant chemotherapy or endocrine therapy is associated with a satisfactory rate of complete excison and a low rate of local recurrence.

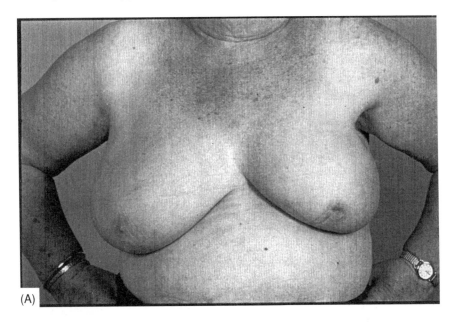

(A)

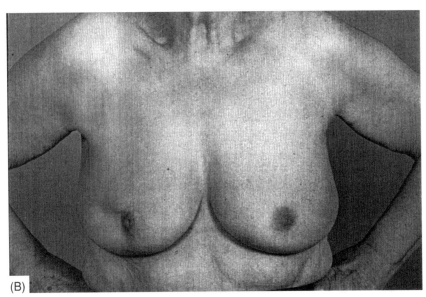

(B)

Figure 4 Cosmetic outcomes of patients treated by neoadjuvant endocrine therapy followed by surgery. This patient (A) had a locally advanced cancer of the left breast in the inframammary fold at diagnosis, and the patient in (B) would have required a mastectomy prior to neoadjuvant endocrine therapy.

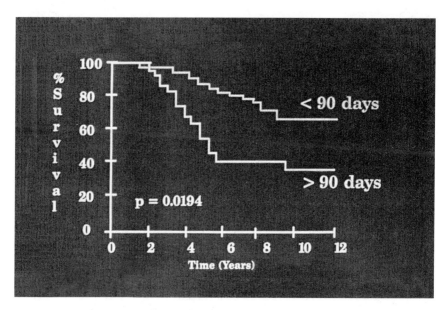

Figure 5 Survival of patients treated by primary medical therapy either endocrine subdivided on the basis of the median time taken for the tumor to halve in volume for each series of patients.

REFERENCES

1. Goldie JH. Scientific basis for adjuvant and primary (neoadjuvant) chemotherapy. Semin Oncol 1987; 14:1.
2. Preece PE, Wood RAB, Mackie CR, Cuschieri A. Tamoxifen as initial sole treatment of localised breast cancer in elderly patients. Br Med J 1982; 284:869–870.
3. Helleberg A, Lundgren B, Norin T, Sander S. Treatment of early localised breast cancer in elderly patients by tamoxifen. Br J Radiol 1982; 15:511–515.
4. Bradbeer J, Kyngdon J. Primary treatment of breast cancer in elderly women with tamoxifen. Clin Oncol 1983; 9:31–34.
5. Allan SG, Rodger A, Smyth JF, et al. Tamoxifen as primary treatment of breast cancer in elderly or frail patients: a practical management. BMJ 1985; 290:358.
6. Horobin JM, Preece PM, Dewar JA, et al. Long-term follow-up of elderly patients with locoregional breast cancer treated with tamoxifen only. Br J Surg 1991; 78:213–217.
7. Mustacchi G, Milani S, Pluchinotta A, et al. Tamoxifen or surgery plus tamoxifen as primary treatment for elderly patients with operable breast cancer. The GRETA trial. Anticancer Res 1994; 14:2197–2200.
8. Van Dalsen AD, De Cries J. Treatment of breast cancer in elderly patients. J Surg Oncol 1995; 60:80–82.

9. Bates T, Riley DL, Houghton J, et al. Breast cancer in elderly women: a Cancer Research Campaign trial comparing treatment with tamoxifen and optimal surgery with tamoxifen alone. Br J Surg 1991; 78:591–594.

10. Gazet JC, Ford HT, Coombes RC, et al. Prospective randomised trial of tamoxifen vs surgery in elderly patients with breast cancer. Eur J Surg Oncol 1994; 20:207–214.

11. Kenny FS, Robertson JFR, Ellis IO, et al. Primary tamoxifen versus mastectomy and adjuvant tamoxifen in fit elderly patients with operable breast cancer of high ER content. Breast 1999; 8:216.

12. Anderson EDC, Forrest APM, Levack PA, et al. Response to endocrine manipulation and oestrogen receptor concentration in large operable primary breast cancer. Br J Cancer 1989; 60:223–226.

13. Keen JC, Dixon JM, Miller EP, et al. The expression of Ki-S1 and BCL-2 and the response to primary tamoxifen therapy in elderly patients with breast cancer. Breast Cancer Res Treat 1997; 44:123–233.

14. Mamounas EP. Overview of National Surgical Adjuvant Breast Project neoadjuvant chemotherapy studies. Semin Oncol 1998; 25:31–35.

15. Dixon JM, Love CDB, Tucker S, et al. Letrozole as primary medical therapy for locally advanced and large operable breast cancer. Breast Cancer Res Treat 1997; 46(suppl):54.

16. Low SC, Dixon AR, Bell J, et al. Tumor oestrogen receptor content allows selection of elderly patients with breast cancer for conservative tamoxifen treatment. Br J Surg 1992; 79:1314–1316.

17. Cheung CWD, Johnson AE. Carcinoma of the breast: Measurement and the management of treatment: The value of the data. Br J Radiol 1991; 64:29–36.

18. Forouhi P, Walsh JS, Anderson TJ, Chetty U. Ultrasonography as a method of measuring breast tumor size and monitoring response to primary systemic treatment. Br J Surg 1994; 81:223–225.

19. Pain JA, Ebbs SR, Hem RPA, et al. Assessment of breast cancer size: A comparison of methods. Eur J Surg Oncol 1992; 18:44–48.

20. Dixon JM, Renshaw L, Bellamy C, et al. The effects of neoadjuvant anastrozole (Arimidex) on tumor volume in postmenopausal women with breast cancer: A randomized, double-blind, single-center study. Clin Cancer Res 2000; 6:2229–2235.

21. Kuerer HM, Newman LA, Buzdar AU, et al. Pathologic tumor response in the breast following neoadjuvant chemotherapy predicts axillary lymph node status. Cancer J Sci Am 1998; 4:230.

22. Machiavelli MR, Romero AO, Perez JE, et al. Prognostic significance of pathological response of primary tumor and metastatic axillary lymph nodes after neoadjuvant chemotherapy for locally advanced breast carcinoma. Cancer J Sci Am 1998; 4:125.

23. Brain E, Garrino C, Misset JL, et al. Long-term prognostic and predictive factors in 107 stage II/III breast cancer patients treated with anthracycline-based neoadjuvant chemotherapy. Br J Cancer 1997; 75:1360.

24. WHO Handbook for Reporting Results of Cancer Treatment (Response Criteria) Geneva: Publication number 48. World Health Organization, 1979.

25. Bonadonna G, Valagussa P, Brambilla C, et al. Adjuvant and neoadjuvant treatment of breast cancer with chemotherapy and/or endocrine therapy. Semin Oncol 1991; 15:515.

26. Paepke W, Appffelstaedt J, Eremin O, et al. Neoadjuvant treatment of post-menopausal breast cancer patients with letrozole (Femara): A randomised multicenter study versus tamoxifen. Eur J Cancer 2000; 36:S76A.

27. Allred DC, Harvey JM, Berardo M, Clark GM. Prognostic and predictive factors in breast cancer by immunohistochemical analysis. Mod Pathol 1998; 11:155–168.

28. Powles TJ, Hickish TG, Makris A, et al. Randomised trial of chemoendocrine therapy started before and after surgery for treatment of primary breast cancer. J Clin Oncol 1995; 13:547.

29. Mauriac L, Durand M, Avril A, et al. Effects of primary chemotherapy in conservative treatment of breast cancer patients with operable tumors larger than 3 cm: Results of a randomised trial in a single center. Ann Oncol 1991; 2:347.

30. Veronesi U, Bonadonna G, Zurrida S, et al. Andreola S, Rilke F, Raselli R, Merson M, Sacchini V, Agresti R. Conservation surgery after primary chemotherapy in large carcinomas of the breast. Ann Surg 1995; 222:612–618.

31. Makris A, Powles TJ, Ashley SE, et al. A reduction in the requirements for mastectomy in a randomised trial of neoadjuvant chemoendocrine therapy in primary breast cancer. Ann Oncol 1998; 9:1179–1184.

32. Mauriac L, MacGrogan G, Avril A, et al. on behalf of Institut Bergonie Bordeaux Groupe Sein (IBBGS). Neoadjuvant chemotherapy for operable breast carcinoma larger than 3 cm: A unicentre randomised trial with a 124 month follow up. Ann Oncol 1999; 10:47–52.

33. Ellis PA, Ashley S, Walsh G, et al. Identification of clinical factors predicting outcome following primary chemotherapy for operable breast cancer. Breast 1999; 8:235.

12

Pathology of Breast Cancer Following Neoadjuvant Endocrine Therapy

Hironobu Sasano, Takashi Suzuki, and Takuya Moriya
Tohoku University School of Medicine
Sendai, Japan

I. ABSTRACT

The clinical benefits of neoadjuvant endocrine therapy for patients with breast carcinoma have been supported by many recent clinical studies. The comparison of pretreatment biopsies with resected pathological specimens following this therapy could provide important information on the effectiveness of treatment and allow a predictive assessment of the response to further systemic therapy to be made. However, the pathological and/or pathobiological features of breast carcinoma tissues after endocrine treatment in the neoadjuvant setting have not been characterized and have not been compared with those following neoadjuvant chemotherapy. Neoadjuvant endocrine therapy may result in more degenerative changes than chemotherapy, such as hyalinosis associated with inflammatory cell infiltration. Treatment with tamoxifen or aromatase inhibitors in the neoadjuvant setting achieves its biological effectiveness via a reduction in estrogenic activity—for example, by reducing pS2 and progesterone receptor (PgR) expression. (Editors' note: tamoxifen treatment is often associated with an increase in PgP and pS2. See references in Chap. 12.) This results in more apoptotic and fewer proliferative carcinoma cells. However, new-generation aromatase inhibitors may

provide much more effective suppression of in situ estrogenic action and cell proliferation and a greater stimulation of carcinoma cell apoptosis than tamoxifen. It
will become increasingly important for surgical pathologists to evaluate tumor
specimens (following therapy) using cell markers related to apoptosis and/or cell
proliferation to assist in the management of the breast cancer patients undergoing
neoadjuvant endocrine therapy.

II. INTRODUCTION

Results of various clinical trials have demonstrated the advantages of administering medical therapy, including chemotherapy and/or endocrine treatment, to patients with operable breast cancer—i.e., neoadjuvant therapy [1,2]. Possible
advantages of neoadjuvant therapy include improved survival for patients following an early introduction of systemic therapy [2] and the downstaging of the primary tumor, which allows breast-conserving surgery rather than mastectomy,
without any increment in local recurrence rates [3,4]. The examination of resected
breast carcinomas can provide an indication of the possible response to further
systemic adjuvant treatment, identifying possible subgroups of patients who may
benefit from more intense chemotherapy or endocrine treatment [1,5–7].

Assessment of the response to neoadjuvant therapy has been largely been
performed using imaging techniques, typically comparing mammograms and/or
ultrasound images before and after treatment. These examinations provide very
important information on alterations in the tumor size but can also be associated
with false-positive and/or false-negative findings compared with histological
analysis. The assessment of resected tissue specimens following neoadjuvant
therapy and surgical resection can, therefore, be useful in the evaluation of the
response of breast cancer patients (identifying biologically or clinically inert tissue). It has therefore become very important for surgical pathologists to examine
specimens of breast cancer following neoadjuvant therapy to determine whether
patients responded to treatment and, if so, the degree of responsiveness (complete or partial). It is also important to employ appropriate biological and/or molecular markers relevant to the response, in the preparation of resected specimens
(for example, Ki67, PgR, Bcl-2, etc.). In this chapter, we review the pathological
changes following neoadjuvant chemotherapy and discuss the changes following
neoadjuvant endocrine therapy, focusing on the effect of estrogen deprivation
through receptor blockade and/or aromatase inhibition.

III. PATHOLOGICAL CHANGES FOLLOWING
NEOADJUVANT CHEMOTHERAPY

Chemotherapy is the most frequently administered form of neoadjuvant therapy
[8]. Experimentally, administration of chemotherapeutic agents can prevent the

increased growth rate of residual micrometastasis following surgery and can prolong overall survival in various animal models [9,10], although this benefit is disputed clinically [11]. The characteristics of the treated breast cancer in surgical pathology specimens may have major implications for the type of additional therapy given to patients.

Morphological changes in neoplastic breast cancer tissues following neo-adjuvant chemotherapy have been reported by several investigators. The most important indicators of response to therapy are the volume of the residual carcinoma and viability of cells in pathology specimens. Kennedy et al. [12] examined the histopathological changes of breast cancer by comparing initial biopsy specimens with posttherapy tissues in 57 patients treated with chemotherapy. Their most striking finding was the histiocyte-like appearance of tumor cells following chemotherapy (Fig. 1 shows a similar example), where only scattered microscopic foci of tumor remained in a sea of bland fibrous tissue. This was especially common when an almost complete clinical response occurred [12]. In some cases, the carcinoma cells undergoing degenerative changes may not be identified by routine light microscopic studies but

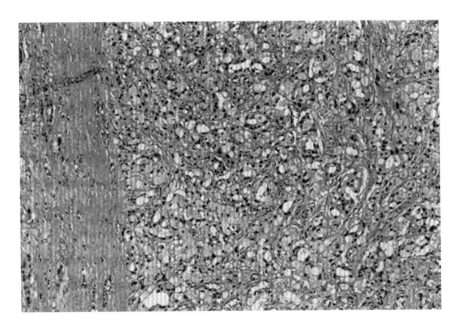

Figure 1   Light microscopic features of breast carcinoma following neoadjuvant chemotherapy. Marked degenerative changes were detected, including the histiocyte appearance of tumor cells.

require immunohistochemical examination; for example, the use of epithelial membrane antigen (EMA) and/or cytokeratin antibodies can be of great value in the assessment of residual carcinoma cells.

When tumors exhibit little overall clinical response in terms of size reduction evaluated by imaging methods, their morphology closely resembles that of the pretreatment biopsy. Frierson and Fechner reported that the histological grade of residual breast carcinoma after neoadjuvant chemotherapy reflected the grade of pretreatment biopsy [13]. These results indicate that the biological properties of residual carcinoma cells following neoadjuvant chemotherapy are not different from those prior to the therapy. However, it is also very important to note that a considerable amount of viable tumor may persist despite a complete clinical response or, vice versa, a patient with a partial clinical response may have little or no microscopically and/or immunohistochemically detectable tumor. The latter case (partial clinical response and no detectable tumor) is usually associated with fibrosis and/or chronic granulomatous changes with destruction of carcinoma cells in the stroma. This may mimic residual carcinoma under imaging analysis (mammography or ultrasonography) but can be correctly identified by microscopic or immunohistochemical examination. Cytologically, carcinoma cells following neoadjuvant chemotherapy exhibit an irregularity and smudging of the nuclear outlines, hyperchromasia, and coarse chromatin clumping (Fig. 2). However, it is very important to recognize that these cytological changes also occur in nonneoplastic ductal epithelial cells adjacent to the carcinoma, which makes the distinction between these cells and residual carcinoma problematic, especially in the cases of intraductal carcinoma [12]. In addition, not all breast carcinoma cells are equally affected by neoadjuvant chemotherapy [12], and the intratumoral heterogeneity associated with neoadjuvant chemotherapy is a very frequent feature.

Many chemotherapeutic agents achieve cytotoxic effects by inducing apoptosis [8]. Rasbridge et al. reported that apoptosis and other morphological changes varied among breast cancer specimens of both responsive and nonresponsive patients [14]. Ellis et al. reported a significant increase in apoptosis in breast biopsies following neoadjuvant chemotherapy, but no changes in Ki67 and Bcl-2 levels [15]. Shao et al. recently obtained an apoptotic index using the TUNEL (terminal deoxynucleotidyl transferase–mediated dUTP-biotin nick endlabeling) method in breast cancer specimens before and after neoadjuvant chemotherapy and reported that the postchemotherapy apoptotic index correlated well with clinical response [8]. Their data, moreover, indicated that this index correlated well with patient survival, both disease-free survival and overall survival [8]. All of these results suggest that an assessment of apoptotic index can be of great value in evaluating the response of breast cancinomas to neoadjuvant chemotherapy.

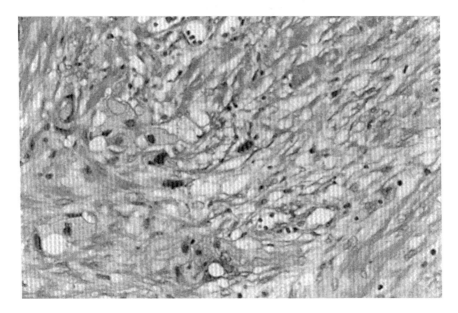

Figure 2 Light microscopic features of breast carcinoma following neoadjuvant chemotherapy. Hyperchromatic degenerated nuclei with dense collagen fibers were present.

IV. PATHOLOGICAL CHANGES FOLLOWING ENDOCRINE THERAPY

A. Tamoxifen

The great majority of patients who respond to tamoxifen treatment have estrogen receptor (ER)–positive carcinoma cells, but not all ER-expressing carcinomas respond well to tamoxifen in the long term [16]. It is possible that the comparison of clinical and/or pathological features of the before and after neoadjuvant treatment with tamoxifen may help predict the potential benefits of long-term tamoxifen treatment [16]. In particular, a detailed examination of the surgical pathology specimens following tamoxifen treatment in the neoadjuvant setting could identify markers in addition to that of ER expression that would help to predict response and select appropriate patients for adjuvant therapies [17].

In terms of morphology, Kennedy et al. suggested that the vacuolization of the cytoplasm, or teardrop appearance, may reflect an effect of tamoxifen treatment [12]. However, histopathological changes following tamoxifen monotherapy have not been well documented in breast cancer tissues. Soubeyran et al. reported that, in a trial of 208 postmenopausal patients receiving neoadjuvant tamoxifen therapy for nonmetastatic invasive ductal carcinoma, the expression of ER and pS2 (an estrogen-inducible cytoplasmic protein) were significantly correlated with tumor regression (defined as ≥50% regression) [18]. This suggests that an immunohistochemical evaluation of pS2 and ER status in resected surgical pathology specimens following neoadjuvant tamoxifen therapy can be predictive of tumor progression. Keen et al. demonstrated that the response of breast carcinomas to tamoxifen treatment for 3 months correlated both with the pretreatment level of Bcl-2 expression, one of the estrogen-regulated inhibitory proteins of apoptosis, and with the posttreatment level of KiS1 protein, a sensitive marker of cell-cycle activity [19]. Cameron et al. extended this by reporting that neoadjuvant tamoxifen treatment both increased apoptosis as a consequence of reduced Bcl-2 expression and decreased cell proliferation [16].

B. Aromatase Inhibitors

The increasing use of aromatase inhibitors is making it increasingly important to study pathological changes in breast carcinoma associated with neoadjuvant therapy by aromatase inhibition. Following neoadjuvant therapy using aromatase inhibitors, there is not only increased coagulative necrosis as detected in neoadjuvant chemotherapy but also extensive hyalinosis (Fig. 3). Hyalinosis is one of the degenerative processes of carcinoma tissues that can occur with or without foreign-body reaction [20]. These degenerative changes associated with aromatase inhibition may well correlate with alterations of microvascular density and/or local immune reaction, such as intratumoral lymphocytes and/or macrophage infiltration. Interestingly, Markis et al. also reported a reduction of microvascular density in primary breast carcinoma following neoadjuvant chemoendocrine therapy, but further investigations are required to confirm these findings [21].

Several investigators have reported changes in biological markers following neoadjuvant aromatase inhibitor therapy. Reed et al. reported a decrease in DNA polymerase alpha activity, and Nakamura et al. reported a decrease in ^{3}H-incorporation into breast cancer tissue as a result of aromatase inhibition [22,23]. We have also reported decreased cell proliferation following neoadjuvant aromatase inhibition, as demonstrated by Ki67 labeling index and increased apoptosis evaluated by the TUNEL method (Fig. 4) [20].

It will then be of great interest to compare the pathobiological changes caused by aromatase inhibitors with those of tamoxifen, given that the new aromatase inhibitors are possibly more effective agents in the neoadjuvant setting [24]. Anderson et al. recently reported a study comparing pathobiological changes between neoadjuvant aromatase inhibition and estrogen-receptor blockage by tamoxifen in 71 postmenopausal patients [25]. In that study, aro-

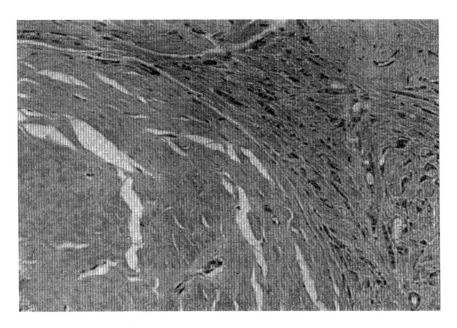

Figure 3 Light microscopic features of breast carcinoma following neoadjuvant endocrine therapy using aromatase inhibitors. Marked hyalinization was detected.

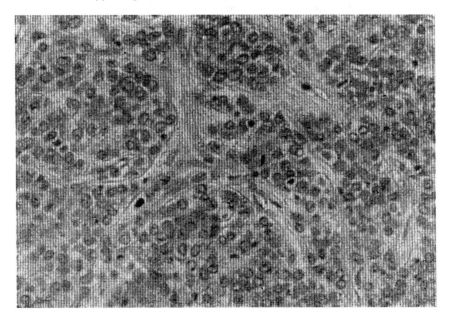

Figure 4 TUNEL stain of breast carcinoma following neoadjuvant endocrine therapy using aromatase inhibitors. DAB deposition (a brown pigment) was detected in carcinoma cell nuclei.

matase inhibitors significantly decreased PgR levels, which suggests a more complete suppression of estrogenic reaction, increased apoptotic index, and decreased Ki67 labeling index compared to tamoxifen. The histopathological changes observed in resected tumors of these patients was, however, similar [25]. Ellis et al. recently reported that in patients having undergone neoadjuvant endocrine treatment, approximately one-third of tamoxifen-treated tumors showed evidence of agonistic effects on PgR and pS2 status, whereas this was rarely seen with letrozole [26]. This is indicative of a more effective suppression of estrogen-related biological phenomena by aromatase inhibitors than by tamoxifen [26].

Results of these studies all indicate that new-generation aromatase inhibitors could yield much more effective suppression of both cell proliferation and estrogenic activity and stimulation of apoptosis in carcinoma cells than tamoxifen. Further investigations that include randomized trials are required for clarification.

V. CONCLUSION

Analysis of surgical pathology specimens following neoadjuvant endocrine therapy in breast cancer is important not only for assessing the effectiveness of the therapy but also for predicting the response to (possible) further systemic adjuvant endocrine therapy. Neoadjuvant endocrine therapy using one of the new-generation of aromatase inhibitors may yield much more effective suppression of cell proliferation and local estrogenic actions as well as stimulation of apoptosis compared with that employing tamoxifen. It will therefore be important for surgical pathologists to compare not only routine histopathological features but also various cell biological markers related to effects of endocrine treatment such as Ki67 apoptotic index, PgR, Bcl-2, pS2, and others.

REFERENCES

1. Vinnicombe SJ, MacVicar AD, Guy RL, et al. Primary breast cancer: Mammographic changes after neoadjuvant chemotherapy, with pathologic correlation. Radiology 1996; 198:333–340.
2. Ragaz J, Baird R, Rebbeck P, et al. Neoadjuvant (preoperative) chemotherapy for breast cancer. Cancer 1985; 56:719–729.
3. Mansi JL, Smith IE, Walsh G. Primary medical therapy for operable breast cancer. Eur J Cancer Clin Oncol 1989; 25:1623–1627.
4. Anderson EDC, Forrest APM, Hawkins RA, et al. Primary systemic therapy for operable breast cancer. Br J Cancer 1991; 63:561–566.
5. Powles TJ, Ashley SE, Makris A. A randomised trial of chemo-endocrine therapy started before (neoadjuvant) or after (adjuvant) surgery for treatment of primary breast cancer. J Clin Oncol 1995; 13:547–552.

6. Feldman LD, Hortobagyi GN, Buzdar AU, et al. Pathological assessment of response to induction chemotherapy in breast cancer. Cancer Res 1986; 46:2578–2581.

7. Hortobagyi GN, Ames FC, Buzdar AU. Management of stage 3 primary breast cancer with primary chemotherapy, surgery and radiation therapy. Cancer 1988; 62:2507–2516.

8. Shao Z-M, Li J, Wu J, et al. Neo-adjuvant chemotherapy for operable breast cancer induces apoptosis. Breast Cancer Res Treat 1999; 53:263–269.

9. Fisher B, Gunduz N, Coyle J, et al. Presence of a growth-stimulating factor in serum following primary tumor removal in mice. Cancer Res 1989; 49:1996–2001.

10. Fisher B, Saffer E, Rudock C, et al. Effect of local or systemic treatment prior to primary tumor removal on the production and response to a serum growth stimulating factor in mice. Cancer Res 1989; 49:2002–2004.

11. Fisher B, Brown A, Mamounas E, et al. Effect of pre-operative chemotherapy on local-regional disease in women with operable breast cancer: Findings from National Surgical Adjuvant Breast and Bowel Project B-18. J Clin Oncol 1997; 15:2483–12493.

12. Kennedy S, Merino MJ, Swain SM, Lippman ME. The effects of hormonal and chemotherapy on tumoral and non-neoplastic breast tissue. Hum Pathol 1990; 21:192–198.

13. Frierson HF Jr, Fechner RE. Histologic grade of locally advanced infiltrating ductal carcinoma after treatment with induction chemotherapy. Am J Clin Pathol 1994; 102:154–157.

14. Rasbridge SA, Gillet CE, Seymour AM, et al. The effects of chemotherapy on morphology, cellular proliferation, apoptosis and oncoprotein expression in primary breast carcinoma. Br J Cancer 1994; 70:335–341.

15. Ellis PA, Smith IE, McCarthy K, et al. Pre-operative chemotherapy induces apoptosis in early breast cancer. Lancet 1997; 349:849.

16. Cameron DA, Keen JC, Dixon JM, et al. Effective tamoxifen therapy of breast cancer involves both antiproliferative and pro-apoptotic changes. Eur J Cancer 2000; 36:845–851.

17. Cheung KL, Howell A, Robertson JF. Preoperative endocrine therapy for breast cancer. Endoc Rel Cancer 2000; 7:131–141.

18. Soubeyran I, Quenel N, Coindre JM, et al. L. pS2 protein: A marker improving prediction of response to neoadjuvant tamoxifen in post-menopausal breast cancer patients. Br J Cancer 1996; 74:1120–1125.

19. Keen JC, Dixon JM, Miller EP. The expression of KiS-1 and Bcl-2 and the response to primary tamoxifen therapy in elderly patients with primary breast cancer. Breast Cancer Res Treat 1997; 44:123–133.

20. Sasano H, Sato S, Ito K, et al. Anderson TJ, Miller WR. Effects of aromatase inhibitors on the pathobiology of human breast, endometrial and ovarian carcinoma. Endoc Rel Cancer 1999; 6:197–204.

21. Makris A, Powles TJ, Kakolyris S, et al. Reduction in angiogenesis after neoadjuvant chemoendocrine therapy in patients with operable breast carcinoma. Cancer 1999; 85:1996–2000.

22. Reed MJ, Owen AM, Lai LC, et al. In situ oestrone synthesis in normal breast and breast tumour tissues: Effect of treatment with 4-hydroxyandrostenedione. Int J Cancer 1989; 44:233–237.

23. Nakamura J, Imai E, Yoshihama M, et al. Histoculture drug response assay, a possible examination system for predicting the antitumor effect of aromatase inhibitors in patients with breast cancer. Anticancer Res 1998; 18:125–128.

24. Dixon JM, Love CD, Renshaw L, et al. Lessons from the use of aromatase inhibitors in the neoadjuvant setting. Endocrine-Related Cancer 1999; 6:227–230.

25. Anderson TJ, Cameron DA, Dixon JM, Miller WR. Important differences between neoadjuvant aromatase inhibition and oestrogen receptor blockade in breast cancer. Aromatase 2000: The 3rd Generation Meeting, Port Douglas, Australia, November 3–7, 2000.

26. Ellis MJ, Singh B, Miller WR, et al. Letrozole (Femara) is a more effective inhibitor of estrogen activity than tamoxifen: Evidence from a randomized phase III trial of 4 months preoperative endocrine therapy for postmenopausal women with primary invasive breast cancer. Abstract of American Society of Clinical Oncology, San Francisco, CA, May 12–15, 2001.

13

Neoadjuvant Therapy: Prediction of Response

William R. Miller, T. J. Anderson, S. Iqbal, and J. Michael Dixon
Edinburgh Breast Unit
Western General Hospital
Edinburgh, Scotland

I. ABSTRACT

Neoadjuvant protocols allow identification of predictive markers of response to therapy. Indices measured in tumor biopsies taken before and during treatment may be related to response as determined by sequential clinical measurements of tumor size. Studies in which patients have been given a variety of endocrine therapies (surgical/medical castration in premenopausal women and tamoxifen or aromatase inhibitors in postmenopausal women) have confirmed that estrogen-receptor (ER) status is the single best predictor of subsequent benefit, as cancers with poor ER levels rarely respond. Other markers such as progesterone receptors (PgRs) increase discrimination in ER-rich cancers, but not absolutely. It can be shown that changes in cell-cycle parameters precede clinical response and are less likely to occur in nonresponsive cancers. Paradoxical phenotypic changes that occur in "responding" cancers may indicate progression to hormone resistance, being associated with the same increased incidence of early recurrence as nonresponding cancers. Micro- and tissue assays are novel technologies that will be increasingly used to produce RNA and protein profiles of tumor biopsies taken before and during therapy, but their potential has yet to be fully exploited.

II. INTRODUCTION

Neoadjuvant therapy, in which treatment is administered with the primary tumor in situ, offers major opportunities for determining predictive markers of response and resistance to individual therapies. The accessibility of the primary tumor enables (a) accurate measurement of the size of the tumor—using calipers, mammography, and ultrasound methods—providing an accurate assessment of clinical response, and (b) removal of sequential samples from the tumor by biopsy or fine needle aspirate before, during, and after treatment [1]. Therefore, it is possible to relate biological and molecular characteristics of the tumor to its clinical response as well as to monitor changes that occur during treatment/response.

III. ER AND RESPONSE TO ENDOCRINE THERAPY

In our early studies on endocrine therapy, patients were recruited if they had large primary cancers or wished to avoid breast surgery [2]. In these studies, tumor ER status was not taken into account. However, retrospective analysis of the first 81 women studied (premenopausal patients oophorectomized or receiving luteinizing hormone–releasing hormone (LH-RH) agonists and postmenopausal patients receiving tamoxifen or an aromatase inhibitor, aminoglutethimide, or 4-hydroxyandrostenedione) showed that only a single ER-poor tumor (<20 fmol mg cytosol protein) responded to therapy (Table 1) [3]. Analysis of the subgroup of patients treated with aromatase inhibitors showed that none of the eight patients with ER-poor cancers responded to aromatase inhibitor therapy (Table 1). Because of these results, ER-poor cancers were excluded from following studies with endocrine therapy and only patients with ER-rich cancers were subsequently recruited. However, only about 50% of women with ER-rich cancers respond to endocrine treatment (Table 1); for optimal management, it is essential to identify further markers by which to subdivide the ER-rich cancers into responders and nonresponders.

Table 1 ER Status and Response to Endocrine Therapy

ER Status	Endocrine therapy[a]		Aromatase inhibitors[b]	
	Responsive	Nonresponsive	Responsive	Nonresponsive
ER-rich	27	26	6	8
ER-poor	1	27	0	8

[a]$p=0.001$.
[b]$p=0.051$.

IV. OTHER PUTATIVE PREDICTIVE MARKERS OF RESPONSE

Other markers that have been suggested to predict hormone responsiveness have been assessed in the neoadjuvant setting. These include PgR, pS2, epidermal growth factor receptor (EGFR), c-erbB$_2$, cell survival protein bcl-2, p53, transforming growth factor (TGF) β and angiogenesis [3–7]. While some of these markers increase discrimination, none do so absolutely. For example, Ellis (see Chap. 12) reported a study in which predictive markers such as PgR and pS2 were measured in patients with ER-positive cancers treated with either tamoxifen or letrozole and correlated the markers with response to treatment [4]. The data indicated that PgR-positive or pS2-positive cancers were more likely to respond to either drug than PgR-negative, pS2-negative cancers. However, a substantial number of the latter did respond to treatment, and the presence of both markers did not guarantee response. Our own data from patients treated with either letrozole, anastrozole, or exemestane are summarized in Table 2. Although the incidence of PgR-positive cancers was high (presumably on account of the selection of ER-rich cancers), cases of response and nonresponse were evident in both PgR-positive and PgR-negative cancers. This was apparent whether responses were assessed clinically (by ultrasound measurements) or pathologically (by changes in tumor cellularity).

It is likely that predictive indices vary depending on treatment. An interesting example may be derived from the PEO24 study in which the expression of EGFR and ErbB$_2$ was associated with a decreased likelihood of response to tamoxifen but an increase in response to letrozole [4].

V. CHANGES IN CELL CYCLE/SURVIVAL PARAMETERS WITH THERAPY

We have previously reported a study in which the expression of the proliferation marker KiS1 and the cell survival protein bcl-2 was assessed by immunohistochemistry in ER-rich cancers taken from elderly patients prior to and 3 months after treatment with tamoxifen [3,5]. The majority of responding cancers showed

Table 2 Progesterone Receptors and Response to Neoadjuvant Therapy with Aromatase Inhibitors

PgR Status	Clinical response		Pathological response	
	Responsive	Nonresponsive	Responsive	Nonresponsive
PgR +ve	49	3	32	20
PgR −ve	5	2	5	2

a decrease in the expression of either KiS1, bcl-2, or both, whereas nonresponding cancers did not. However, there were small cohorts of cancers in which phenotypic changes were not consistent with clinical response. Thus, certain cancers were categorized as clinically nonresponsive although they displayed a reduction in KiS1 and bcl-2 staining following treatment. Delayed clinical responses have been reported with tamoxifen, and it may be that these cancers would have regressed had treatment been extended [3] (see Chap. 13). Conversely, cancers that responded clinically but without the phenotype of either reduced KiS1 or bcl-2 expression may have shown an early response in which hormone-sensitive clones of cells were deleted from the tumor mass, leaving highly proliferating cells, which are programmed for survival. If this were the case, it might be expected that this cohort of cancers would be associated with a resistance to tamoxifen and an aggressive behavior. The patients in this study now have at least 5 years' follow-up, and the response rate at this time is summarized in Table 3. Consistent with the benefits from therapy, patients in the responding group had a significantly lower relapse rate than those not responding. However, within the responding group, the subgroup that did not display reduced expression of either KiS1 or bcl-2 had a poorer prognosis, with a relapse rate of 50%, which is similar to the nonresponder rate. Despite the reduction in tumor size observed over the treatment period, this might reflect "early" resistance to tamoxifen.

Measurements of changes that occur after 3 months of treatment are unhelpful in predicting tumor response to therapy, since by this time clinical response is usually already evident. Consequently, we have introduced an additional tumor biopsy into our study protocol at 10–14 days after initiation of therapy (Fig. 1), which precedes any clinical or morphological evidence of response. Results on the measurement of the cell cycle marker, Mib1 are shown in Table 4. These indicate that a decrease in Mib1 staining can be detected in the majority of cancers that subsequently respond to tamoxifen, whereas this change was not apparent in most nonresponding cancers. This difference between groups of nonresponding and responding cancers was statistically significant, but it should be noted that the changes were not always apparent in individual

Table 3 Recurrence Rates Following Neoadjuvant Tamoxifen[a]

	Response phenotype (KiS1, bcl-2)		
	Decrease	No change/increase	Total
Responsive	17% (5/29)	50% (4/8)	24%
Nonresponsive	67% (2/3)	45% (5/11)	50%

[a]The recurrence rate correlated with change in expression of KiS1 and bcl-2 from biopsy to excision and the clinical response at surgery.

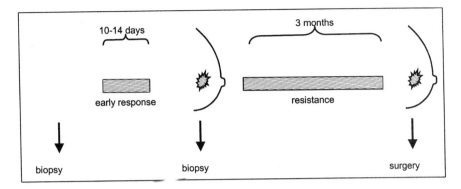

Figure 1 Timing of biopsies during neoadjuvant therapy.

Table 4 Early Change in Mib1 and Clinical Response to Neoadjuvant Tamoxifen

	Response phenotype (Mib1)	
	Decrease	No change/increase
Responsive	28	10
Nonresponsive	3	8

cancers; clearly, additional markers will be required so that patients are selected on an individual basis for endocrine therapy.

VI. FUTURE PERSPECTIVES

Available powerful technologies will allow the identification of predictive indices for novel markers, and rapid screening of archival material will confirm their utility. For example, gene microarrays such as those used to screen for chemosensitivity [8] have yet to be applied in a systematic manner, but preliminary data are beginning to appear [9]. Similarly, tissue arrays based on sequential biopsies from neoadjuvant endocrine protocols will provide rapid screens by which to validate putative markers emerging from gene microarrays. The size of the task should not be underestimated, as it is likely that no single pathway leads to response/resistance to endocrine therapy. If multiple pathways and genes are involved, sophisticated discrimination involving neural networks may be needed to unravel the complexities. Furthermore, different sets of markers may be needed to predict for individual forms of endocrine treatment, such as antiestrogens and aromatase inhibitors, especially if one requires markers for second-line therapy after a previous endocrine treatment. For example, it is already known that whereas aromatase inhibitors consistently decrease the expression of PgR, tamoxifen is frequently associated with enhanced expression [9]. Thus the phenotype of cancers relapsing on tamoxifen is likely to be different from that of cancers failing on aromatase inhibitors.

Problems with the recognized heterogeneity of breast cancers will also have to be overcome, especially if small sample biopsies are to be used in analysis. It is possible that more accurate sampling, using devices such as a mammotome in combination with ultrasound or stereotactic guidance, will be required. Additionally, microdissection can identify relevant areas of pathological specimens and molecular typing of tissue compartments can allow for compensatory corrections to be made (see Chap. 14).

There are also likely to be difficulties resulting from intertumor variability. Not all cancers respond to treatment at the same time or to the same degree. Given that multiple sampling of cancers is currently impractical, it will be necessary to gamble on the timing of biopsy, and crucial windows of response may be missed, particularly if they differ widely in individual cancers. Present practice is usually determined by patient management and practical considerations, such as the need to identify predictive markers that precede clinical response and reduce the time period of "experimental" exposure to treatment; the requirement to allow the tumor to "settle" after surgery or biopsy required to provide diagnosis and ER status prior to treatment; and the time for pharmacological/clinically effective levels of drugs or hormone suppression to be reached. Hopefully, noninvasive methods to allow the continuous monitoring of cancers will emerge.

Given that the ultimate aim of predicting outcome is to define endocrine responsiveness of individual cancers that may be unique, there is the potential problem that the first step in individualization will require the laborious procedure of group comparisons.

Finally, the merits of studying the primary cancers in neoadjuvant protocols to identify markers of endocrine response are largely predicated on the assumption that response in the primary tumor will predict for micrometastatic disease (unless the sole aim is to avoid or reduce the extent of breast surgery). In the absence of definitive comparisons of primary and micrometastatic disease, one has to look elsewhere for answers. Thus, though it is true that tumor phenotype changes with advancing disease and that endocrine response may be different in metastatic sites within individual patients [10], there is reason to believe that there is a consistency with regard to major predictors of response. Thus, current clinical practice of selecting endocrine therapy for patients with advanced breast tumors is often based on ER status of the primary cancers. This has produced acceptable predictive accuracy even where there has been intervening therapy. Furthermore, ER status in recurrent disease arising after endocrine therapy is usually similar to that of the primary tumor [11]. For these reasons, it seems pragmatic to proceed with neoadjuvant studies, especially as the potential gain is extremely high.

REFERENCES

1. Forouhi P, Walsh JS, Anderson TJ, Chetty U. Ultrasound as a method of measuring breast tumour size and monitoring response to primary systemic therapy. Br J Surg 1994; 81:223–225.

2. Forrest APM, Levack P, Chetty U, et al. Anderson TJ A human tumour model. Lancet 1986; 2:840 842.

3. Miller WR, Anderson TJ, Hawkins RA, et al. Neoadjuvant endocrine treatment: the Edinburgh experience. In Howell A, Dowsett M, eds. Primary Medical Therapy for Breast Cancer. London: Elsevier Science, 1999:89–99.

4. Ellis MJ, Coop A, Singh B, et al. Letrozole is more effective neoadjuvant endocrine therapy than tamoxifen for ErbBB1 and/or ErbB2 positive, estrogen receptor positive primary breast cancer. J Clin Oncol 2001; 19:3808–3810.

5. Keen JC, Dixon JM, Miller E, et al. Expression of Ki-S1 and BCL-2 and the responses to primary tamoxifen therapy in elderly patients with breast cancer. Breast Cancer Res Treat 1997; 44:123–134.

6. MacCallum J, Keen JC, Bartlett JMS, et al. Changes in expression of transforming growth factor beta mRNA isoforms in patients undergoing tamoxifen therapy. Br J Cancer 1996; 74:474–478.

7. Marson LP, Kurian KK, Harmey JH, et al. Microvessel counts and vascular endothelial growth factor expression in primary breast cancer treated with tamoxifen. Breast Cancer Res Treat 1999; 57:A29.

8. Perou CM, Serile T, Elsen MB, et al. Molecular portraits of human breast tumours. Nature 2000; 406:747–752.

9. Coop A, Dressman M, Lavedan C, et al. Correlation of immunohistochemistry (IHC) and gene microarray analysis of breast biopsies from a preoperative endocrine therapy trial. Proc Am Soc Clin Oncol 2001; 20:342.

10. Hamm T J, Allegra JC. Loss of hormonal responsiveness in cancer. In: Stoll BA, ed. Endocrine Management of Cancer—Biological Cases. Basel: Karger, 1988:61–71.

11. Hawkins RA, Tesdale AL, Anderson EDC, et al. Does the estrogen receptor concentrations of a breast cancer change during systemic therapy? Br J Cancer 1990; 6:877–880.

14

Mechanisms of Resistance
to Endocrine Therapy

Nancy E. Hynes
Friedrich Miescher Institute for Biomedical Research
Basel, Switzerland

I. ABSTRACT

The ErbB family of receptors have an important role to play in the development of human breast cancer. There are four members of this receptor tyrosine kinase family that are selectively activated in various homo- and heterodimer combinations by a large family of peptides known as the epidermal growth factor (EGF)–related peptides. ErbB1 and ErbB2, in particular, have been extensively analyzed in human breast carcinomas, as they are often constitutively activated either by autocrine production of ligands or for ErbB2, in particular, by overexpression. The ErbB family of receptors and their ligands have been intensely studied in the past to understand their role in breast cancer malignancy and as potential targets for breast cancer therapy. More recently, ErbB receptors are coming under scrutiny for their potential roles in the development of endocrine resistance.

II. INTRODUCTION

In normal cells the activation of receptor tyrosine kinases (RTKs) is tightly controlled, allowing the correct integration of external signals with internal signal transduction pathways. In contrast, owing to numerous molecular alterations arising during the course of malignancy, tumors are characterized by an abnormal response to external signals, which allows cancer cells to bypass the normal mechanisms controlling cellular proliferation. It has been known for over 15 years that uncontrolled expression of the RTKs epidermal growth factor (EGF) receptor (ErbB1) and ErbB2 are involved in the malignancy of breast cancer. Indeed, one of the earliest identified consistent genetic alterations associated with breast tumors was a c-ErbB2 gene amplification [1]. More recently, a considerable amount of data have become available on the EGF (ErbB) family of receptors in terms of characterizing their role in the normal development, proliferation, and differentiation in cells of epithelial, mesenchymal, and neuronal tissues and of their uncontrolled expression that has been implicated in the malignancy of several types of human cancer [2]. The aim of this chapter is to provide an overview of the ErbB family of receptors and describe the available data on their role in breast cancer, and potential role in resistance to endocrine therapy, with a view to identifying future therapeutic strategies for treatment.

III. ErbB FAMILY OF RECEPTORS

There are four members of the ErbB RTK family: ErbB1 (EGF receptor, HER-1), ErbB2 (HER-2, Neu), ErbB3 (HER-3), and ErbB4 (HER-4). Evidence from *Caenorhabitalis elegans* and *Drosophila* indicate that this receptor family has evolved from a single ligand-receptor combination in basic multicellular organisms to a more complex situation, with four ErbB receptors, which bind multiple ligands as found in many vertebrate species.

Receptor activity is directly regulated by a range of diverse polypeptide ligands (all of which contain a 6-kDa domain homologous to EGF), which bind to the extracellular domain of the receptors [3–5] (Fig. 1). Ligand binding leads to receptor dimerization, kinase activation, and phosphorylation of specific tyrosine residues in the carboxy-terminal domains of these receptors. The phosphorylated residues, in turn, serve as docking sites for cytoplasmic proteins, which couple the activated receptors to diverse intracellular signaling pathways, including the major phosphatidyl-inositol 3' kinase (PI3K)–protein kinase B (PKB) and Ras-mitogen activated protein kinase (MAPK) pathways (reviewed in Ref. 2).

The polypeptide ligands that bind ErbB RTKs fall into three groups: EGF, transforming growth factor-α (TGF-α), and amphiregulin (AR) bind ErbB1; while betacellulin (BTC), heparin-binding EGF (HB-EGF), and epiregulin (EPR) exhibit dual specificity in that they bind ErbB1 and ErbB4. The neuregulins (NRG) make up the third family: NRG-1 and NRG-2 both bind ErbB3 and ErbB4, whereas NRG-3 and NRG-4 bind ErbB4 only (reviewed in Refs. 2 and 3).

Ligand-dependent activation of the ErbB family of receptors is mediated by the formation of receptor homo- and heterodimers [3,4,6]. Furthermore, al-

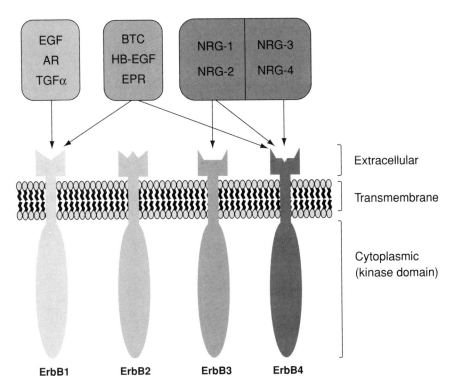

Figure 1 ErbB tyrosine kinase receptor family.

though no specific soluble ErbB2 ligand has been found, all of the EGF-related peptides induce its tyrosine phosphorylation by the process of heterodimerization and cross-phosphorylation [7,8]. For example, in cells expressing ErbB1 and ErbB2, any of the EGF agonists induce formation of ErbB1-ErbB2 heterodimers as well as ErbB1 homodimers. This type of cross-activation extends to most of the receptor combinations. Despite the fact that ErbB2 has no soluble ligand, there is increasing evidence suggesting that its major role is as a coreceptor [4,9]. Results from our lab have shown that the ErbB2 receptor is not only the preferred heterodimerization partner for the other activated ErbB receptors, providing high-affinity binding sites for their ligands [9,10], but also plays a crucial role in lateral transmission of signals between other ErbB receptors [8]. In summary, ErbB2 has a central role to play in the ErbB receptor family and ErbB2-containing heterodimers are responsible for the potent activation of intracellular signaling pathways regulating several fundamental biological responses.

Phenotypes of the ErbB receptor knockout mice are the most striking evidence of the importance of ErbB2-containing heterodimers. For example, mice individually null for ErbB2, ErbB4, or NRG-1 each demonstrate a lack of trabecular formation in the heart, showing that the ErbB2/4 heterodimer is an important signaling moiety in the myocardium and is activated by the paracrine factor NRG-1 [11–13]. These phenotypes clearly demonstrate that NRG-1–induced ErbB4 homodimers cannot replace this function of the ErbB2/4 heterodimer in ErbB2 null mice. ErbB2/3 heterodimers have also been described and shown to have an important role in neuronal development. Mice mutant for ErbB2, ErbB3, or NRG-1 have impaired neural crest formation, leading to aberrant formation of the sympathetic nervous system [14]. It is clear that ErbB receptors have a number of roles to play in several developmental processes. Further, the formation of ErbB heterodimers is vital to their function in many of these situations—a fact perhaps reflective of the requirement for exquisite signaling control during development and diversification of signals provided by the ErbB receptor combinations.

IV. ESTROGENS AND ErbB RECEPTORS IN THE MAMMARY GLAND

A. Expression of ErbB Receptors

The female mammary gland undergoes extensive postnatal development under the influence of systemic hormones, specifically at puberty and during pregnancy. Estradiol is one of the major regulators of mammary epithelial cell proliferation. The biological effects of estrogens are mediated through the estrogen receptor (ER), a member of the superfamily of nuclear receptors. The importance of this steroid/receptor pair is strikingly evident in mice that lack ERα—so-called ERKO mice. In the adult ERKO female, the mammary gland is underdeveloped and consists of a rudimentary ductal structure limited to the nipple area [15]. The effects of estrogens are not direct, since it is known that the division-competent cells in the gland are adjacent to the ER-positive cells [16]. Furthermore, using tissue recombinant technology, Cuhna and colleagues were able to show that the initial requirement for ERα is in the stromal compartment of the gland [17]. These results suggest that ERα-positive cells in the stroma, either fibroblasts or adipocytes, respond to estrogens in pubertal females and secrete paracrine factors that transmit the signal to the epithelial compartment, leading to ductal growth during puberty.

The concept that the ER-positive cells act as "sensors" of circulating steroids also arises from work with human breast cells. Anderson and colleagues have developed an elegant system to study this interaction after implantation of normal human tissue obtained from reduction mammoplasty into athymic nude mice. To examine the effects of estradiol on the proliferation of human breast cells, the mice were implanted with slow-release pellets of estradiol calibrated to deliver serum levels approximating those in the human menstrual cycle. By staining the cells with ER-specific antibodies and with the Ki67 antibody, which detects proliferating cells, they drew two important conclusions. First, approximately 18% of the cells were ER-positive, and they were dispersed throughout the tissue. Second, the ER-positive cells did not stain for Ki67 and therefore were not proliferating [18,19]. Thus, as in the rodent gland, the ER-positive cells respond to estrogens and secrete a paracrine factor that signals the neighboring cells to proliferate—a finding with important implications for breast cancer Since the majority of newly diagnosed tumors are ER-positive and proliferate, one of the early alterations in tumor development must be a switch of the ER-positive cells from a nonproliferative to a proliferative phenotype [20]. It is possible that the ErbB family of receptors and their ligands play a role in this process, particularly since they are known to be transcriptionally activated upon estrogen addition to breast cells [5], something to be more closely examined in the future.

B. ErbB Receptors and Ligands in Normal Mammary Development

During postnatal development of the mammary gland, many peptide factors, including the EGF family ligands, act under the control of systemic hormones to mediate mammary development [21]. In light of the role of the ER-positive cells as sensors mediating ductal growth of the rodent gland and proliferation of human epithelial cells, it is interesting to consider the possibility that the ErbB RTK family and one or more of their ligands have a role downstream of the ER in development of the mammary gland. Various lines of experimental data suggest that this is in fact the case (reviewed in Ref. 20). The role of the ErbB receptors in development of the gland has been studied in various rodent models. It has been shown that all four ErbB receptors are expressed in the mammary glands of adult females while ErbB1 and ErbB2 are preferentially expressed in young females, suggesting an important role for these receptors during mammary gland development [22–24]. At puberty, the mammary ducts become elongated and extend throughout the fatty mesenchyme. During this process, ErbB1 and ErbB2 are present in the stroma and epithelium and are tyrosine phosphorylated, indicating signaling activity [22,24]. Expression of a dominant-negative ErbB1 receptor has been shown to impair ductal morphogenesis in a mouse model [25]. Furthermore, wa-2 mice, which harbor a mutation in the ErbB1 kinase domain, exhibit sparse development of the mammary gland, indicative of defective ductal growth [23].

Turning to the ligands, multiple ErbB1 ligands and NRG-1 are coexpressed at various developmental stages [26,27]. Mice with individual targeted disruption of EGF, AR, and TGF-α as well as triple null mice have been generated to investigate the role of these ligands during development of the gland [24]. Of the three ligands, AR expression is highest in the developing ducts, and only AR deficiency is associated with impaired ductal growth [24].

During pregnancy, a second wave of tyrosine phosphorylation can be observed in the ErbB receptors in mammary tissue [22,27]. This activation of ErbB receptors occurs after the major period of proliferation during pregnancy and after parturition. Studies using dominant-negative ErbB2 and ErbB4 transgenes have demonstrated that these receptors have an important role to play in lobuloalveolar development and milk protein production, which is consistent with the ability of NRG-activated ErbB2 to drive mammary differentiation in various in vitro culture models of the gland [26,28–30]

V. ErbB RECEPTORS AND BREAST CANCER

There is a wealth of clinical data demonstrating the importance of ErbB receptors, in particular ErbB1 and ErbB2 in the development and malignancy of human breast cancer (reviewed in Refs. 1, 5, 31, and 32). ErbB1 gene amplification is rarely seen in breast cancer. However, expression of one or more of the ErbB1 ligands occurs in many tumors, suggesting that ErbB1 is constitutively activated by an autocrine route [5]. The gene encoding ErbB2 is amplified in approximately 25% of breast tumors, which leads to a dramatic overexpression of the protein [1,31,32]. ErbB2 has a concentration-dependent propensity to dimerize, and overexpression of ErbB2 leads to its constitutive activation, as shown by high levels of phosphotyrosine in these tumors. Elevated levels of ErbB3 protein, but not gene amplification, have also been reported in breast cancers [33–35]. Interestingly, many of the tumors that overexpress ErbB2 also have high levels of phosphorylated ErbB3 [36], leading to the hypothesis that the ErbB2/3 heterodimer is important in the development of these tumors—something we are currently testing. ErbB4 is not commonly overexpressed in breast carcinomas [37,38], suggesting that this receptor is either unimportant in breast cancer or may even antagonize carcinogenesis—a hypothesis supported by evidence that ErbB4 expression is associated with positive prognostic factors in breast cancer [39,40].

VI. DOES THE ErbB RECEPTOR/LIGAND NETWORK HAVE A ROLE IN ENDOCRINE RESISTANCE?

The ER is well established as one of the most important predictive and prognostic markers in human breast cancer. ER signaling has a vital role to play in the carcinogenesis of ER-positive tumors, and the ER has been the target for many successful endocrine therapies in recent years. However, it is well documented that many patients develop resistance to the widely used antiestrogen tamoxifen

[41]. Considering the importance of the ErbB RTKs and their ligands in breast cancer, it is interesting to consider the possibility that this family can play a role in endocrine resistance. Endocrine resistance is categorized as de novo or acquired during the course of treatment with antiestrogens. Concerning de novo resistance, there is a general consensus that an inverse relationship exists between elevated expression of the ErbB receptors and endocrine sensitivity in breast cancer patients [42,43]. This suggests that these receptors might interfere with the antiestrogenic effect of tamoxifen. In the breast, tamoxifen is a total ER antagonist. In fact, it has been shown that the nuclear receptor corepressor (N-CoR) can be found in a complex with the tamoxifen bound ER, providing a mechanism for the negative effects of tamoxifen on transcription [44]. Importantly, N-CoR is displaced from the tamoxifen-bound ER complex upon activation of ErbB1, which is due to MAPK-mediated phosphorylation of the ER [44]. This clearly shows that activation of signaling pathways initiated by the ErbB receptors can impinge upon the ER, causing the tamoxifen-bound receptor to switch from a transcriptionally repressed to an activated state. ER modification of this type might contribute to de novo antiestrogen insensitivity.

It is also interesting to consider that activation of ErbB receptors in breast tumors might make their normal ER dependency redundant. In fact, ER and oncogenic overexpressed ErbB2 impinge upon similar cell-cycle regulators, including the transcription factor, myc, and cyclinE/cdk2. MCF7 breast tumor cells, which are growth-arrested with tamoxifen, have low levels of myc expression [45] and low cyclinE/cdk2 activity owing to high expression of the cyclin kinase inhibitors (CKIs) p21 and p27 [46]. Upon reentry into the cell cycle after tamoxifen withdrawal and estrogen addition, there is a rapid increase in myc expression [45]. CyclinE/cdk2 activity also increases owing to loss of the CKIs, and the cells enter S phase [46]. In ErbB2 overexpressing breast tumor cells, we have observed that proliferation of the cells is driven by high activity of cyclinE/cdk2, which occurs even in the presence of relatively high levels of the CKI p27.

Interestingly, oncogenic ErbB2 employs essentially the same cell-cycle effectors as the ER. We have downregulated oncogenic ErbB2 activity either by treatment with 4D5/Herceptin [47], a growth-inhibitory antibody, or by intracellular expression of an ErbB2 specific single-chain antibody that inactivates the receptor functionally [48]. These experiments revealed that oncogenic ErbB2 maintains high levels of cyclinE/cdk2 activity via sequestration of p27 away from the cyclinE/cdk2 complex. This is accomplished by maintaining high levels of myc and other cell-cycle regulators involved in the sequestration of p27 from cyclinE/cdk2 [47,48]. These observations suggest a model whereby p27 is required for normal cell-cycle control. Overexpression of ErbB2 results in the sequestration of p27, thereby activating the cyclinE/cdk2 complex, which leads to uncontrolled cellular proliferation. Since the ligand-activated ER uses the same cell-cycle effectors as oncogenic ErbB2, one could postulate that with high levels of ErbB2 activity, the estrogen-mediated pathway may become redundant. Clearly this is one mechanism that could lead to tamoxifen resistance.

Turning to acquired endocrine resistance, the fact that tumors often respond to other endocrine therapies, such as aromatase inhibitors, shows that loss of ER cannot explain tumor progression on an antiestrogen [49]. It is not yet clear from clinical analyses of primary breast tumor material whether overexpression of the ErbB family has a role in acquired in vivo resistance. Intriguingly, using the MCF7 breast tumor cell model, it has been possible to characterize a role for these receptors. Nicholson and colleagues have found that a tamoxifen-resistant variant of the MCF7 cells that proliferates in the presence of the antiestrogen shows an increased level of ErbB1 and constitutively expresses several ligands for the receptor. Furthermore, these tamoxifen-resistant cells cease to proliferate in response to an ErbB1-selective tyrosine kinase inhibitor, clearly demonstrating the importance of the apparently autocrine-activated receptor and its downstream pathways in the development of tamoxifen resistance [50]. Overexpression of ErbB2 has also been implicated in the emergence of estrogen-independent MCF7 cell growth. Introduction of an ErbB2 expression vector into MCF7 cells followed by selection for high expressors produced an MCF7 subline that was insensitive to tamoxifen [51].

In addition to the published in vitro evidence, data from recent clinical studies in breast cancer suggest that patients with tumors that overexpress ErbB2 are more resistant to endocrine (tamoxifen) therapy (see Chap. 12). Sound molecular data supports this hypothesis. For instance, one could postulate that the proliferating cells can switch from requiring estrogens for growth and being blocked by tamoxifen to a situation where overexpressed ErbB2 substitutes for the estrogen-dependent response to drive the cell cycle and continue proliferation.

VII. SUMMARY

Considerable evidence exists implicating the ErbB family of receptors and ErbB2, in particular in carcinogenesis in human breast cells and potentially in the development of endocrine-resistant tumors. Furthermore, there are in vitro data showing that ErbB and ER mediate their effects on the cell cycle via some of the same effector molecules. When these data are taken together and considered from a clinical perspective, they suggest that, in the future, compounds targeted to one or more of the ErbB receptor family tyrosine kinases given together with aromatase inhibitors or tamoxifen may well be the best way to proceed in the clinic.

REFERENCES

1. Slamon D J, Clark GM, Wong SG, et al. Human breast cancer: Correlation of relapse and survival with amplification of the HER2/Neu oncegene. Science 1987; 235:177–182.

2. Olayioye MA, Neve RM, Lane HA, Hynes NE. The ErbB signaling network: Receptor heterodimerization in development and cancer. EMBO J 2000; 19(13): 3159–3167.

3. Riese DJ, Stern DF. Specificity within the EGF/ErbB receptor family signaling network. BioEssays 1998; 20:41–48.

4. Klapper L, Glathe S, Vaisman N, et al. The ErbB-2/Her2 oncoprotein of human carcinomas may function solely as a shared coreceptor for multiple stroma-derived growth factors. Proc Natl Acad Sci USA 1999; 96:4995–5000.

5. Slamon DJ, Brandt R, Ciardello F, Normanno N. Epidermal growth factor-related peptides and their receptors in human malignancies. Crit Rev Oncol Hematol 1995; 19:183–232.

6. Riese DJ, van Raaij TM, Plowman GD, et al. Cellular response to neuregulins is governed by complex interactions of the ErbB receptor family. Mol Cell Biol 1995; 15:5770–5776.

7. Beerli RR, Hynes NE. Epidermal growth factor-related peptides activate distinct subsets of ErbB receptors and differ in their biological activities. J Biol Chem 1996; 271(11):6071–6076.

8. Graus-Porta D, Beerli RR, Daly JM, Hynes NE. ErbB-2, the preferred heterodimerization partner of all ErbB receptors, is a mediator of lateral signaling. EMBO J 1997; 16(7):1647–1655.

9. Karunagaran D, Tzahar E, Beedi R, et al. ErbB2 is a common auxilliary subunit of NDF and EGF receptors: Implications for breast cancer. EMBO J 1996; 15: 254–264.

10. Tzahar E, Waterman H, Chen X, et al. Yarden Y. A heirarchical network of inter-receptor interactions determines signal transduction by neu differentiation factor/neuregulin and epidermal growth factor. Mol Cell Biol 1996; 16:5276–5287.

11. Gassmann M, Casagranda F, Orioli D, et al. Aberrant neural and cardiac development in mice lacking the ErbB4 neuregulin receptor. Nature 1995; 378(6555):390–394.

12. Lee KF, Simon H, Chen H, et al. Requirement for neuregulin receptor erbB2 in neural and cardiac development. Nature 1995; 378(6555):394–398.

13. Meyer D, Birchmeier C. Multiple essential functions of neuregulin in development. Nature 1995; 378(6555):386–390.

14. Britsch S, Li L, Kirchhoff S, et al. The ErbB2 and ErbB3 receptors and their ligands, neuregulin-1, are essential for development of the sympathetic nervous system. Genes Dev 1998; 12:1825–1836.

15. Bocchinfuso WA, Korach KS. Mammary Gland development and tumorigenesis in estrogen receptor knockout mice. J Mamm Gland Biol Neopl 1997; 2:323–334.

16. Zeps N, Bentel JM, Papadimitriou JM, et al. Estrogen receptor–negative epithelial cells in mouse mammary gland development and growth. Differentiation 1998; 62(5):221–226.

17. Cunha GR, Young P, Hom YK, et al. Elucidation of a role of stromal steroid hormone receptors in mammary gland growth and development by tissue recombination experiments. J Mamm Gland Biol Neopl 1997; 2:393–402.

18. Clarke RB, Howell A, Potten CS, Anderson E. Dissociation between steroid receptor expression and cell proliferation in the human breast. Cancer Res 1997; 57(22):4987–4991.

19. Anderson E, Clark RB, Howell A. Estrogen responsiveness and control of normal breast proliferation. J Mamm Gland Biol Neopl 1998; 3:23–25.

20. Shoker BS, Jarvis C, Clarke RB, et al. Abnormal regulation of the oestrogen receptor in benign breast lesions. J Clin Pathol 2000; 53(10):778–783.

21. Fendrick JL, Raafat AM, Haslam SZ. Mammary gland growth and development from the postnatal period to postmenopause: Ovarian steroid receptor ontogeny and regulation in the mouse. J Mamm Gland Biol Neopl 1998; 3:7–21.

22. Sebastian J, Richards RG, Walker MP, et al. Activation and function of the epidermal growth factor receptor and ErbB-2 during mammary gland morphogenesis. Cell Growth Differ 1998; 9:777–785.

23. Fowler KJ, Walker F, Alexander W, et al. A mutation in the epidermal growth factor receptor in waved-2 mice has a profound effect on receptor biochemistry that results in impaired lactation. Proc Natl Acad Sci USA 1995; 92(5):1465–1469.

24. Luetteke NC, Qui TH, Fenton SE, et al. Targeted inactivation of the EGF and amphiregulin genes reveals distinct roles for EGF receptor ligands in mouse mammary gland development. Development 1999; 126:2739–2750.

25. Xie W, Paterson A, Chin E, et al. Targeted expression of a dominant negative epidermal growth factor receptor in the mammary gland of transgenic mice inhibits pubertal mammary duct development. Mol Endocrinol 1997; 1:1766–1781.

26. Yang Y, Spitzer E, Meyer D, et al. Birchmeier C, Birchmeier W. Sequential requirement of hepatocyte growth factor and neuregulin in the morphogenesis and differentiation of the mammary gland. J Cell Biol 1995; 131:215–226.

27. Schroeder JA, Lee DC. Dynamic expression and activation of ErbB receptors in the developing mouse mammary gland. Cell Growth Differ 1998; 9:451–464.

28. Jones F, Stern D. Expression of dominant negative ErbB2 in the mammary gland of transgenic mice reveals a role in lobuloalveolar development and lactation. Oncogene 1999; 18:3481–3490.

29. Jones F, Weite T, Fu X-Y, Stern D. ErbB4 signalling in the mammary gland is required for lobuloalveolar development and Stat5 activation during lactation. J Cell Biol 1999; 147:77–88.

30. Niemann C, Brinkmann V, Spitzer E, et al. Birchmeier W. Reconstitution of mammary gland development in vitro: requirement of c-met and c-ErbB2 signaling for branching and alveolar morphogenesis. J Cell Biol 1998; 143:533–545.

31. Hynes NE, Stern DF. The biology of ErbB-2/neu/HER-2 and its role in cancer. Biochim Biophys Acta 1994; 1198(2–3):165–184.

32. Tang CK, Lippmann ME. EGF family receptors and their ligands in human cancer. In O'Malley BW, ed. Hormones and Signaling. Vol 1. San Diego, CA: Academic Press, 1999:113–165.

33. Travis A, Pinder S, Robertson J, et al. C-ErbB-3 in human breast carcinoma: Expression and relation to prognosis and established prognostic indicators. Br J Cancer 1996; 74:229–233.

34. Seigel P, Ryan E, Cardiff R, Muller W. Elevated expression of activated forms of Neu/ErbB-2 and ErbB-3 are involved in the induction of mammary tumors in transgenic mice: Implications for human breast cancer. EMBO J 1999; 18:49–64.

35. Lemoine NR, Barnes DM, Hollywood DP, et al. Expression of the ERBB3 gene product in breast cancer. Br J Cancer 1992; 66:1116–1121.

36. Alimandi M, Romano A, Curia MC, et al. Cooperative signaling of ErbB3 and ErbB2 in neoplastic transformation and human mammary carcinomas. Oncogene 1995; 10(9):1813–1821.

37. Srinivasan R, Poulsom R, Hurst H, Gullick W. Expression of the c-ErbB-4/HER4 protein and mRNA in normal human fetal and adult tissues and in a survey of nine solid tumor types. J Pathol 1997; 185:236–245.

38. Vogt U, Bielawski K, Schlotter CM, et al. Amplification of erbB-4 oncogene occurs less frequently than that of ErbB-2 in primary human breast cancer. Gene 1998, 223:375–380.

39. Bacus SS, Cin D, Zelnick CR, Stern DF. Type 1 receptor tyrosine kinases are differentially phosphorylated in mammary carcinoma and differentially associated with steroid receptors. Am J Pathol 1998; 148:549–558.

40. Knowlden J, Gee J, Seery L, et al. C-ErbB3 and c-ErbB4 expression is a feature of the endocrine responsive phenotype in clinical breast cancer. Oncogene 1998; 17:1949–1957.

41. Osborne CK, Boldt DH, Clark GM, Trent JM. Effects of tamoxifen on human breast cancer cell cycle kinetics: Accumulation of cells in early G1 phase. Cancer Res 1983; 43(8):3583–3585.

42. Klijn J, Berns P, Schmitz P, Foekens J. The clinical significance of of epidermal growth factor receptor (EGF-R) in human breast cancer: a review on 5232 patients. Endocr Rev 1992; 13:3–17.

43. Nicholson R, McClelland RA, Finaly P, et al. Relationship between EGF-R, c-ErbB-2 protein expression and Ki67 immunostaining in breast cancer and hormone sensitivity. Eur J Cancer 1993; 29A(7):1018–1023.

44. Lavinsky RM, Jepsen K, Heinzel T, et al. Diverse signaling pathways modulate nuclear receptor recruitment of N-CoR and SMRT complexes. Proc Natl Acad Sci USA 1998; 95(6):2920–2925.

45. Dubik D, Shiu RP. Mechanism of estrogen activation of c-myc oncogene expression. Oncogene 1992; 7(8):1587–1594.

46. Cariou S, Donovan JCH, Flanagan WM, et al. Down-regulation of p21 WAF1/CIP1 or p27 Kip1 abrogates antiestrogen-mediated cell cycle arrest in human breast cancer cells. Proc Natl Acad Sci USA 2000; 97(16):9042–9046.

47. Lane HA, Beuvink I, Motoyama AB, et al. ErbB2 potentiates breast tumor proliferation through modulation of p27[Kip1]-Cdk2 complex formation: Receptor overexpression does not determine growth dependency. Mol Cell Biol 2000; 20:3210–3223.

48. Neve RM, Sutterluty H, Pullen N, et al. Effects of oncogenic ErbB2 on G1 cell cycle regulators in breast tumor cells. Oncogene 2000; 19:1647–1656.

49. Robertson JF. Oestrogen receptor: a stable phenotype in breast cancer. Br J Cancer 1996; 73(1):5–12.

50. Nicholson RI, Gee JMW, Barrow D, et al. (abstr). Clin Cancer Res 1999; 5(suppl).

51. Pietras RJ, Arboleda J, Reese DM, et al. HER-2 tyrosine kinase pathway targets estrogen receptor and promotes hormone-independent growth in human breast cancer cells. Oncogene 1995; 10:2435–2448.

Panel Discussion 3

Neoadjuvant Therapy

James N. Ingle and Ian E. Smith, *Chairmen*
Tuesday, June 26, 2001

J. Ingle: There are several general areas for discussion. Let's discuss the markers, because being able to predict the outcome of the tumor is one of the advantages of neoadjuvant or preoperative therapy. We can talk about the definition of terms. *Neoadjuvant,* at least to me, implies something like Matt Ellis's protocol, where there is therapeutic intent over a period of time. *Preoperative* may be considered where you give it for a short period of time to a woman, maybe with a smaller tumor, who is going to have surgery in a couple of weeks. That raises the issue of markers. Bill (Miller) was talking about early markers. Maybe I can open this up to a discussion of the optimal or potential candidates for early markers in this setting. Bill, can you start and then we'll open it up to the floor.

W. Miller: I don't know that I can really contribute at the moment. The last slide I showed on this was largely blank. There was a little strip of results down the left-hand side, and I think until we actually get some of these arrays fully analyzed with sufficient numbers so that we can make some meaningful correlations, it is just crystal ball gazing. Perhaps some others around this table are better able to do this.

M. Dowsett: We focused specifically on apoptosis and proliferation on the basis that if we are going to have a shrinkage or a change in the growth, you need to have some effect on at least one of those processes. I was particularly interested to hear Dr. Sasano's presentation, that in their early microarray data, the genes that are affected are largely related to proliferation or apoptosis. I would be very keen for him to expand on that a little.

H. Sasano: What we have done are cell culture studies. Therefore I believe that the next important step is a comparison with surgical pathology specimens of before and after therapy. It is, however, important to note that breast cancer tissue is composed of stromal cells and epithelial cells. In order to provide any biologically significant data, laser capture microscopy is required to separate the stromal and epithelial components. Fibroblasts and inflammatory cells also overexpress the genes related to proliferation and apoptosis, and apoptosis of inflammatory cells is well known to occur at the sites of invasion. Therefore, the next step that we have to take is use laser capture microscopy for visual dissection of the proliferative components in the specimen before and after therapy.

P. Lønning: I can add some comments on the use of microarrays. The *Nature* paper that we published last year has extended the number of samples, so we have now analyzed more than 80 breast cancer tumors with this method. When you look at the pre- and posttreatment samples under chemotherapy, there is a remarkable similarity in gene expression profiles between the two samples. We also have some results with primary tumors and with lymph node metastasis, which also show a remarkably similar gene profile. Nobody, as far as I know, has been able to analyze micrometastasis, because the number of cells is simply too few to analyze the mRNA and do the microarrays at this stage. A final remark is that having a similar profile in the two samples does not exclude a certain limited number of critical genes to be altered (between the two situations), because this is a hierarchical clustering of all genes that change in expression by more than fourfold across the tumor samples. Also, if you have different alterations between responders versus nonresponders, you may be able to correlate it to the expression in the primary sample, because that is the reason why there is already a difference in the primary sample.

C. Benz: Yesterday, I asked Mitch (Dowsett) about the importance of the two time points that he looked at, which were 24 h and 21 days after treatment. Now we are hearing from Bill (Miller) that he's looking at 10 to 14 days and comparing it to data collected 3 months after treatment. It boggles my mind to think of all the variables that are changing between these different time points. It has been mentioned that we can have changes in cell compartments, maybe insignificant within the first 24 hours or even several days, but certainly changing weeks or months after a single treatment. I think we must take into account, that tumor sampling at different time points may catch treatment sensitive cells early on and more resistant populations later on. Let me also relate one other cautionary observation that my UCSF colleagues have recently made studying breast tumor xenografts by expression array analysis at these early time points. We have simply been taking our human xenograft models in nude mice and core needle biopsying them at hours, days, and weeks after a control injection. We have found that within the first 24–48 h after routine handling and/or IP injection of saline, significant changes can be detected in hundreds of genes analyzed on an 8K expression array.

W. Miller: Maybe I could comment. Chris (Benz) you point out a very important problem that one should not minimize in doing these studies. Very clearly, in order to get a pretreatment biopsy, we are undertaking, in terms of the tumor anyway, a major surgical procedure. So we are going to have reactive changes from the very fact of doing a biopsy. It does worry me that if you take very early time points you will not pick up markers of response to a drug but markers of manipulating a tumor. One has to be very careful about that and it is one of the reasons why we have not examined very early time points. We have been pragmatic (like Mitch Dowsett) about the actual time of taking 10–14 days, as that tends to correspond to a convenient time in patient management. But it does obviate, hopefully, the initial changes that may have occurred as a result of doing a biopsy on the tumor. I think you're also right (and I doubt that we are ever going to be able to sort this out very easily), to draw attention to the variation between individual patients in the time it takes to respond for individual markers. I think Mitch (Dowsett) has data and David Cameron presented data—the reference was on Hironobu

(Sasano)'s slide—on the type of study that you have just described, in which animals bearing MCF-7 xenografts were biopsied and the time courses of the increase in apoptotic bodies and the decrease in proliferation, following exposure to tamoxifen were monitored. It is very clear that providing you have studied sufficient animals (and there is variation between individual animals) even though it is the same clonal MCF-7 cell line, the changes in apoptotic bodies do precede those of proliferation. We need sampling to cover both. I don't underestimate the difficulties, but unless we start to do the studies, we're not going to address the problem.

M. Dowsett: You are right when we were looking at the MCF-7 xenografts, the apoptotic changes did precede the changes in Ki67. However, when we went back and looked at S phase, the S-phase effects were much earlier than those on Ki67. This is, I think, a reflection of the index that we were using for assessing proliferation as opposed to what actually was occurring with proliferation. But I would really like to come back to Hironobu (Sasano)'s point and relate some of the data that you showed with those of Per (Lønning). That is, when we treat these patients with, in Per (Lønning)'s case, chemotherapy and in your (H. Sasano) case endocrine therapy and in data that Trevor (Powles) and ourselves have generated with chemotherapy, the treated/pretreatment sample in these hierarchical clustering analyses come together, almost always, as the first line of clustering. But to what extent is this because we are not doing the dissection that you (H. Sasano) are requesting? We are getting genes involved with vasculature, fibroblasts, etcetera, that we might not expect to change as much as the malignant cells themselves.

H. Sasano: I think that the important thing about xenografts is that the handling and surgical procedure can change the profile of gene expression. It may be because of the lymphocytes or other inflammatory cells that are associated with proliferation and apoptosis can frequently be seen even in the specimens after the therapy. But it is carcinoma cells in which cell proliferation and/or apoptosis should be examined. Some cytokines or some factors that are produced in lymphocytes are additionally important in causing apoptosis in carcinoma cells. Therefore in looking at the DNA abnormalities and/or expression of c-ErbB2 or EGF-R, you may not need microdissection. However, in this case—i.e., dealing with the gene associated with proliferation and apoptosis—I believe that it is necessary to separate epithelial cells. If you would really like to obtain the biologically relevant data, separation is very important regardless of the quality of the microarray.

M. Ellis: We are planning to focus on estrogen-regulated genes and the ER cluster, which are genes whose expression is essentially limited to the epithelial components of ER tumors. I agree that if you are going to do a complete fishing expedition or you are looking at general factors say those associated with proliferation—microdissection may be mandatory. But if you are looking for genes that are selectively and highly overexpressed by malignant epithelial cells, you might be able to get away without it.

H. Sasano: I agree with you, but the purpose of microarray *is* fishing and something unexpected might pop out. But there are also some controversies that ER-β is present in inflammatory cells, so I'm not that confident that ER-related genes are expressed only in epithelial cells. But I am not that expert in that field.

A. Howell: Returning to the issue of the timing of the biopsy, a lot of experiments have been done on patients by taking a biopsy then giving the agent of interest and then taking the primary tumor at operation. That's a 2–3 week period and it is very hard to change that. If you go back to Bill (Miller)'s point, it may be that the appropriate timing of biopsy may be different for every patient. I think that is a very important point. I have a question for Chris (Benz). You are trying to find an appropriate time for biopsy—have you got any feel from the experiments that you have done already?

C. Benz: No, it's too early; but I will say that we don't think that the gene expression changes noted early after tumor xenograft treatment are due to any inflammatory or infiltrative change in the tumor's cellular component. One concern is the potential effect on tumor gene expression by altering the host animal's cardiovascular system. If you look at in vivo tumor blood flow in such experimental models, nutrient and oxygen delivery is marginal at the tumor's most rapidly growing edge, and it does not take much of a drop in tumor blood flow to dramatically, and perhaps only transiently, alter tumor cell metabolism and gene expression in these rapidly growing cells. We are looking for a time point that will reflect an early chemotherapy or endocrine response that is also beyond the treatment-induced stress response produced in the host.

I. Smith: It seems to me that what we are all saying is that ideally we would like to standardize the timing of serial biopsies, but we don't know what the optimal time might be. There are certainly pragmatic issues to do with patients, but these are not insuperable. I think, if you say that we have got to do the biopsy 3 days later at midnight, we could do that. So it is fundamentally a scientific question of what are the key things we think we should be looking for and what would be the optimal time to do that given all the variables and unmeasurables.

R. Nicholson: As an alternative to using clinical material to identify genes involved in breast cancer progression, cDNA arrays may be very gainfully employed on model systems that are less heterogeneous and more amenable to the study of time-dependent transitions. Following this approach, identified changes in gene expression, which have been observed in the model systems, may then be easily confirmed/refuted in clinical samples.

M. Dixon: First of all, it takes a week to get adequate blood levels of letrozole, so one of the reason why we have chosen 10–14 days is that by then we have reasonable blood levels of letrozole, and by 2 weeks we also will have satisfactory levels of tamoxifen. So there are other reasons why you might choose a time point other than that it happens to coincide with an effect in animals. Animals are different; they metabolize drugs differently. The other issue is how you get the biopsy and how much material you need. We have just invested in a mammotome. The standard method of getting a biopsy is a 14-gauge core biopsy; this gives about 7 mg or so of tissue. An 11-gauge mammotome will get you about 30–40 mg and an 8-gauge mammotome gets you 100 mg. These are different ways of sampling the tumor that are not more traumatic to the patient but give bigger samples. This will help get over some of the problems with tumor heterogeneity. If you are going to do the biopsy, you must make sure you remove an adequate sample. This is nontherapeutic research; you are asking patients to submit themselves to biopsy from which they will get no benefit whatsoever.

M. Dowsett: I would just like to comment on the potential for using MCF-7 cells, in particular, as a model system, that I have a couple of specific worries about. I showed yesterday, in the xenograft studies, that apoptosis is enhanced about fourfold on the withdrawal of estrogen from the animals, and this replicates entirely the data Kyprianou published several years ago. Yet when we look clinically, in the short-term, if anything, apoptosis goes down. This is a somewhat bizarre finding in vorozole-treated patients (and we seem to be confirming this in the IMPACT study). It may be due to the greater effect these agents have on proliferation, thus shunting cells out of cell cycle and possibly restricting apoptosis. This is quite different from the time dependent effects in MCF-7 cells. The other point, which is perhaps even more worrying, is that when we look in the tumor samples, ER levels go down with aromatase inhibitors, yet all of us find that when we withdraw estrogen from MCF-7 cells in the culture situation, the ER levels go up quite substantially. This has to be quite a fundamental difference between these.

R. Nicholson: I would like to suggest that the differences in ER that Mitch (Dowsett) has identified between the model and the clinical material might indicate that changes in ER are not that central to the estrogen withdrawal response mechanism. With respect to the involvement of apoptosis and response. I believe that this complex and time-dependent process is much better studied in models than in clinical material.

J. Forbes: To follow up and support Mike Dixon's comment that the mammotome is much less traumatic than a gun that is fired, we have used it for a long time and have seen a lot of pathology specimens that have been done after it, and there is less inflammatory response. You can also instill a marker quite precisely from where the sample was taken, which is a little bit better than just looking at the needle tract. Thirdly, if you wanted to do so, you can instill an agent precisely into the internal part of the tumor if you had an appropriate solution that you are prepared to do that for. This opens up a host of different ways of monitoring this.

I. Smith: Could you John (Forbes) or Mike (Dixon) just comment on hematoma afterwards? That's a big problem with the bigger needles.

J. Forbes: After the mammotome, the hematoma rate in our hands has been about one patient in a thousand. There is minimal skin discoloration and 98–99% of the patients describe it as an interesting procedure of no fuss.

W. Miller: I would support Bob (Nicholson) in a way. It is important that if you are really looking for candidate genes, not just to do the fishing exercise, I think that you can identify candidate genes from the model systems. However, I am in the fortunate position of having patient data, and when you have access to patient material that can be well-characterized, then you are in the position to do translational research. I wonder also whether there are not alternatives to tumor excision and microarrays. One of the ways forward that would obviate doing a biopsy is to think about in situ measurements. Imaging of the tumor using position emission tomography (PET) or looking at angiogenesis by a noninvasive methodology are attractive options. Just as technology is racing ahead in molecular biology, so also are imaging techniques moving forward.

J. Ingle: Let me just summarize a few things. Clearly clinical trials will proceed and I think they will proceed with greater enthusiasm with the recent publication of the study Matt (Ellis) presented. The standardization of techniques is going to be very important, especially in terms of tissue banks and specimen handling. The issue of the timing of the biopsy will be very important also. Does anyone want to summarize any issues with respect to standardization and timing?

G. Kelloff: I doubt that there will be a unifying answer for this timing. In the stromal sarcoma situation, where we're using a tyrosine kinase inhibitor to KIT, we see tumors becoming completely silent metabolically after 7 h. That's 7 h after exposure. That physiological change predicts for clinical responses that occur 6–10 months later. So, for in vivo imaging, there are many new strategies, there are in vivo approaches to monitoring apoptosis now (imaging strategies) at least in animals. I think this is an area to pay attention to, because that would be a remarkable step in terms of targeting some of the issues that we are talking about here. Otherwise, it is going to be very complicated. There are so many parameters, as Tony (Howell) pointed out yesterday.

J. Ingle: There was an article in the most recent issue of the *Journal of Clinical Oncology* suggesting that PET scanning could be a predictor of response to endocrine therapy. Imaging will become increasingly important, but obtaining tissue will continue to be a crucial part of the neoadjuvant approach.

A. Bhatnagar: I would just like to try and connect up with yesterday afternoon, when perhaps we didn't have enough time for discussion. There is a fundamental discussion that one needs to have. We have seen here that the number of markers and the number of things that one can do with the tumor that one takes in the neoadjuvant setting are limitless. One can discuss all afternoon which markers one should measure and how we should do it and at what time. But I think that one of the most important things that I would like to have is an answer to the question raised in the discussion between Drs. Senn and Dowsett. That is, do these neoadjuvant setting studies really allow us to get information that is of help in, for example, designing fewer but better-controlled adjuvant studies in phase III? Obviously it will bring us tremendous amounts of information on the molecular biology of breast cancer and mechanisms of resistance and mechanisms of proliferation. But, at the end of the day, in the next 5–10 years, one of the things that we will have to deal with is the situation where there are many new drugs coming down the line and they are all candidates for testing in the adjuvant situation. Do we test them all or do we use the neoadjuvant setting as a first triage step to see which ones should be tested in large, well-controlled trials in the adjuvant setting? That's the discussion I would like.

M. Ellis: That is probably why the P024 study is so important, because it predicts, in an early setting, that letrozole will be more effective that tamoxifen. Since we have done the adjuvant study, we will soon be able to see if the connection between the neoadjuvant and adjuvant settings can been made. If this is the case, we can set evidence of improved efficacy in the neoadjuvant setting as a prerequisite to be met before committing thousands of women's lives to adjuvant trials. If you look at the current generation adjuvant trials, it is shocking how little preliminary data there are that favor one arm over the other. Paclitaxel versus docetaxel would be an example. There is no evidence in the metastatic setting or neoadjuvant setting that there is superiority for one drug over the other. So I think we need to move beyond so-called "pragmatic" trial designs into an era where we can make sensible decisions based on biological data.

A. Howell: The study that Matt (Ellis) has presented is of the highest importance and what you are going to do now is to get array data that will tell us the genes related to letrozole responsiveness. Per (Lønning), you have probably got genes that are related to Adriamycin responsiveness. Now when we know these we will be tending to go back to what Ajay (Bhatnagar) was asking; do a biopsy, treat with something, and then take the tumor out. And we will have an answer to some of these questions within 14 days. That's what we need to move toward.

J. Forbes: There are two issues here that we need to distinguish. One is the biological information that we can learn, which has been well discussed. The second is the trial design. One of the problems is that we may assume that the tumor that we can see and feel and sample will have the same parameters and behavior and response to therapy as micrometastases. Now a tumor in the breast is not a fatal illness per se, it is of course the occult disease that is the problem, and we may or may not learn much about that from the biological studies. In terms of trial design, the correct strategy, if you want to see if a new strategy produces a different outcome, needs to be modified from what Matthew (Ellis) put up. To remind you, his concept was to randomize, in the neoadjuvant setting for chemotherapy and letrozole, for potentially responding patients and then, after that, all the chemotherapy patients got the aromatase inhibitor, letrozole, for 5 years. But the other group was divided by response category: if they responded they also got letrozole for 5 years, and the ones who didn't had chemotherapy added. Now, the correct comparison for that is *all* of the patients who got letrozole versus all of the patients who got chemotherapy up front. Otherwise, we may just select out a group of patients who, because they have red hair or were short in stature, actually had a better outcome, rather than because of the treatment. I would suggest that what needs to be discussed is a design where both groups are actually randomized according to their response category. So you are comparing a strategy that is dependent on the response after neoadjuvant therapy versus a strategy where you are not relying on the measurement of response for adjuvant therapy. That is different from the biological studies and may well take us forward with a new trial design.

M. Ellis: Actually what I am suggesting is very close to what you suggest. The trial would be powered and examined on the basis of the initial randomization. The hypothesis is that overall clinical outcomes (disease-free and overall survival) for the standard practice arm of chemotherapy/surgery/letrozole is the same as letrozole/surgery/chemotherapy unless there is an excellent response to letrozole/letrozole.

J. Forbes: The analysis has to be the patients initially randomized for chemotherapy versus the patients initially (all of them) randomized for letrozole. You would have to pool together those who got the response and had letrozole added and those who did not have chemotherapy added as the total population to be compared with the so-called control arm.

Just to reiterate. What is the control arm? When you say chemotherapy followed by letrozole, is that in the adjuvant setting or is that in the primary tumor?

M. Ellis: To reiterate the study is designed as an equivalency trial. So if the two approaches lead to the same disease-free and overall survival, there is a clear advantage for the experimental arm because the use of chemotherapy is reduced. That's going to be a major advance for patients.

B. Groner: I would like to encourage you to take the insights that have been gained by the molecular biologists seriously. Nancy (Hynes) pointed out very nicely what kind of components and parameters you have to look out for. If our concepts of ER action really hold—that is, that estrogen deprivation induced by aromatase inhibitors really prevent ER from inducing target genes—we know which downstream events we have to examine. The idea of microarrays as deus ex machina, where we look at 36,000 genes arranged on a single high-density Affymetrics chip, is all nice and fine, but why don't we look first at things which seem more straightforward and obvious? An important example has been pointed out by Nancy (Hynes). She explained that blockade of the ER causes a block in cell-cycle progression. We know most of the crucial components of the cell cycle, we know how these components are regulated, we know which ones are transcriptionally regulated—e.g., the D-cyclins. We know which ones are important but would never show up on a microarray analysis, because their mechanism of regulation is not at the transcriptional level. An example is the subcellular localization or the complex formation of p27. My plea is look at the known pathways. Think of the mechanism of action of drugs in terms of interference with signal transduction pathways. A prerequisite is, of course, that you know the pathways. This is not always trivial. However, there is only a relatively small number that you really have to study. The pathways involved in cell-cycle regulation related to the action of p53 and Rb in the regulation of E2F transcription factor activity, pathways related to growth factors action and the effects of the MAP kinase, PI-3 kinase and the phosphatase PP2A, which is not so well understood, and pathways that relate to telomerase action, the regulator of the generation clock. So, instead of analyzing microarrays and all the genes that happen to be changed in their level of expression, we should try to fit the knowledge of essential pathways into the framework of drug action. In this case the target genes of the ER, including the mechanism of action of the ER, should be integrated into the pathways known to drive cellular transformation. In this context, we also have to view coactivators and corepressors and the histone code which these coactivators and corepressors actually modulate. These types of approaches should be discussed.

J. Ingle: I had hoped that we could focus this; we have gone down two pathways. I think that first we would talk about the general expression arrays, then get into the specific markers and then get into some trial designs. So maybe what we could do is hold off on the trial design just for a minute and follow up on the specific marker that would be targeted at this point in time. You (B. Groner) have mentioned a number of these, the Erb pathway, MAP kinase, PI-3-kinase, and did you want to add any others?

B. Groner: My suggestion is to take the mechanism of action of transcriptional regulation through the ER into consideration and link them to the cellular signal transduction pathways that are known to underlie cellular proliferation and transformation.

P. Lønning: I want to add some comments based on the microarray experiments, because Tony (A. Howell) said that we probably had predictors for the outcome with chemotherapy. We don't have them yet, but we are currently working on the problem. That also illustrates the question that always comes up: should we use the microarray to generate a hypothesis, or should we use a hypothesis to generate a microarray? Well, we have to answer that in our experience, you need both. We have our hypothesis based on our previous p53 findings, but on the other hand, I can tell you that some of these tumors that do not express p53 mutations come up with a remarkably similar design in the microarrays. So you can go both ways. In relation to the micrometastasis question, what we are doing in our current neoadjuvant studies is that, in addition to doing the presurgical biopsies and the sampling at surgery, we are also obtaining bone marrow specimens before therapy and after the 3 months of chemotherapy (and these are all locally advanced breast cancers—meaning that a high number of them would have the micrometastases), so at least we can correlate the eradication of micrometastases to the molecular pathways of the tumors.

B. Groner: Testing hypotheses and formulating new hypotheses are not mutually exclusive. If you think of mechanisms by which aromatase inhibitors should work, they should inhibit the cell-cycle progression. And this is something you can easily test. If you want to formulate new hypotheses, of course you have to know about global expression patterns of target genes. These are not things that preclude each other, but if we want to have quick and clean answer to questions like "Does chemotherapy give a benefit in neo-adjuvant treatment?" and "Does aromatase inhibition give you a benefit in this type of setting?" then you know what you have to look at initially.

C. Benz: One way to reconcile this issue is to be sure that if you are going to do microarray analyses, that the genes involved in the pathways of interest are all present on your 7, 10, or 14K arrays. I think the Norwegian/Stanford breast cancer expression array study is a case in point here, as it identified at least two different luminal subtypes of breast cancer, each expressing ER, yet the PgR clone was not on their arrays. Thus characterizing these different ER expressing tumor subtypes by PgR expression was not possible.

W. Miller: I think we are arguing about something we shouldn't be arguing about. We agree there are pathways that are clear favorites—

i.e., endpoints of estrogen action. We must go for those genes and, as Chris (Benz) says, we must ensure that all the relevant genes are included on microarrays. That's the logical way forward. But one can't help being seduced by the possibility that there may be markers that we don't know about, and we have the possibility of looking for these. I think we can do both.

W. Eiermann: I have quick question for Matt Ellis: Did you look at aromatase in your cell probes? With the new antibody? This is a very easy question. It's a very easy marker.

M. Ellis: I will make a general point and a specific point about that. The general point is that we are convening the Correlative Science Committee for the second round of correlative science, so I am listening very carefully to what people are saying and please communicate your suggestions soon because there's a limited amount of material and I have to work out exactly what we should do with it. Secondly, I'll let Dr. Miller answer the question of aromatase antibodies.

W. Miller: Maybe I could address two things. I think it is an assumption that antibodies against aromatase will be useful for predicting for response to an aromatase inhibitor. The data we have, at this point in time, do not totally substantiate this. Angela Brodie has data, and I showed data in Port Douglas that there are tumors with aromatase that do not respond to aromatase inhibitors. There are also tumors that do not have aromatase and yet respond to aromatase inhibitors—that's because you are inhibiting the peripheral aromatase. So the absolute correlation will not be there. The question that we need to ask therefore is: "Are those tumors that have high levels of aromatase more likely to respond to an aromatase inhibitor, than say an antiestrogen?" That's a project that is worth doing. But to do it you have to have an antibody (if you're going to use archival material) that actually picks up the protein, and we must make the assumption that when you measure the protein, you measure activity (which isn't necessarily true). Furthermore the antibody must measure the protein in levels that are present in breast cancers, and they are roughly 10,000-fold lower than levels in placenta. We have got plenty of antibodies, which measure placental aromatase, but what we want is an antibody that will go down

10,000-fold lower and at the same time be quantitative. While there are quite a lot of antibodies around, I have not seen one whose characterization has been done at the level of tumors. So I would like an antibody that is well characterized and clearly measures aromatase in breast tumors; then I think we can go forward. To update you on the antibody project: we have established with Novartis a team of pathologists who will use antibodies which have been generated by Dean Edwards and characterize them on breast tumors. At the moment, we have some lead antibodies that do stain breast cancers, but we do not know whether this relates to aromatase activity.

D. Hayes: Are there polymorphisms in germline aromatase genes? And does that predict whether or not the specific aromatase inhibitors will or will not bind? In other words, can one look at germline polymorphisms in the aromatases of individuals and predict benefit or not?

J. Ingle: There are polymorphisms, but they are very unusual. There is about a 1% incidence (of the variant allele) in the population in whites.

D. Hayes: So for practical purposes, we are pretty much homogeneous?

J. Ingle: Is there anyone in the room who does not think that the neoadjuvant setting is absolutely vital setting with many opportunities that we should exploit? Is there anyone that doesn't think this is very important? [No response]

Given that we've been asked by Dr. Bhatnagar to make comments on research over the next five years, we will spend some more time this afternoon with that. But I would like to take a few minutes to start it now. We have actually had two proposals that we could use to stimulate discussion. The first was in women who were ER-positive; HER-1– or HER-2–positive and patients were randomized in a classic phase III study to tamoxifen or letrozole.

M. Dowsett: Before answering that, I would like to make a couple of general points, since I think Ajay (Bhatnagar) was thinking of strategy as much as specifics for how these fit together. I've taken part in a lot of different meetings of this type and smaller meetings discussing how we can use the neoadjuvant or the presurgical setting, which you distinguished earlier on. I think there are important distinctions when we think about how we can use these scenarios for drug development. In the true neoadjuvant setting, where we are treating to downstage, it's a therapeutic situation: we can't go in there with single experimental agents; we need to have some therapeutic confidence that we are giving the patient something useful in those circumstances. You can clearly begin to think about adding in a new agent to something you already know to be effective, so perhaps in a scenario like this, you might be thinking of letrozole or tamoxifen plus or minus Herceptin or plus or minus a tyrosine kinase inhibitor or whatever. So that is a scenario that I think can be very useful. The other situation in the short-term presurgical setting is, in many ways I think, a more useful setting for very early drug development. The classical demonstration of this was one of the first studies that was done in this area, that Tony (Howell) was intimately involved in setting up, and that was the Faslodex study. That particular study took place in the 7 days prior to surgery. No woman up until that time had actually received repeat doses of Faslodex. Now that has some ethical dilemmas, in that you are essentially using those patients for phase I development in terms of tolerability as well. So I think that was perhaps stretching things a little bit. But for these studies to be really useful, we need to use them very early in the development of a compound. In the meetings I described, what has tended to be the case is that the pharmaceutical company people have listened but backed off. They haven't used it and then they have come back at a later stage, and effectively the data that have been developed from the study have been one-tenth of the use that it would have been if we had been using the information to instruct our clinical development. That is my view of the potential strategies for the use of these scenarios in drug development.

J. Ingle: I think you are right. In our developmental therapeutics program, a number of the small molecules are going into the neoadjuvant but prechemotherapy portion of the neoadjuvant treatment. There you have some early markers or markers of action—the farnesyl transferase inhibitors, for instance. Here the problem is what kind of markers can you use with confidence, whether you give the hormone for a week and then start chemotherapy, or you give a small molecule with a hormone. This is more a first approximation neoadjuvant study that has been put forward. I think you are absolutely right Mitch (Dowsett), a variety of designs can be used. This is going to be an ideal place to study new small molecules.

M. Dixon: First of all there is already another neoadjuvant study that many of you know about, called IMPACT, which compares tamoxifen, anastrozole, or the two together. So we will get an answer as to whether HER-2/neu impacts on response. We are already having ethical problems with that study because letrozole has been shown to be better than tamoxifen.

I. Smith: I don't think we are at the stage of designing neoadjuvant trials to determine clinical practice. I wish we were, but I don't think we are. What we need, as we have already said, is the correlation between the surrogate endpoint from the neoadjuvant whether the clinical response (whether it be biological markers) with long-term outcome. The letrozole neoadjuvant trial is very encouraging, but it does not tell us anything until we see the adjuvant trial. The IMPACT trial is designed entirely to mirror the ATAC adjuvant trial. Again, we don't have results from either yet, so we need to be very careful about designing trials at this stage that determine clinical practice. I don't think we are there yet. I think what we need to be doing is continuing to design trials that will help us to answer specific questions. Can we actually define surrogate markers that predict for outcome? The one other point we need to be careful about is that we are looking at biological surrogate markers that correlate with response, but we don't know whether response will predict for outcome in these trials. I was quite encouraged to see Bill (Miller) actually presenting, pretty well for the first time that I have seen, biological endpoints that correlate with longer-term outcome.

M. Gnant: I would like to raise another clinical issue when thinking about neoadjuvant trials, and that is the issue of breast conservation. It has been shown that with preoperative chemotherapy, the actual response rate depends on what regimen you use, but there is literally no progressive disease. In all the preoperative endocrine treatment reports, there are between 15 and 25% of patients with progressive disease while on preoperative treatment. That concerns me. Most of these data have been derived from patient cohorts who are not suitable for adequately dosed preoperative chemotherapy. But if we now go into the head-to-head comparison letrozole versus chemotherapy, for example, I believe we have to be careful and need to prove that we actually don't subject patients to the potential of progressive disease before surgery, which is literally absent in the anthracyclin- and taxane-containing preoperative chemotherapy regimen.

M. Ellis: I have to respond to that. First of all, if you look at the data on confirmed ER-positive tumors, the local progression rate to letrozole was 8%, not 20% or 30%. Whichever series you look at, some patients progress on neoadjuvant chemotherapy with a rate that is around 5%. So you are looking at 5% versus 8%. In the end, the argument would be settled by a randomized trial along the lines of what we discussed. I understand your reservations, but I think that they are somewhat mitigated by new data from the letrozole 024 study.

J. Klijn: I have a question for Dr. Ellis in relation to the greater efficacy of letrozole in tumors with high ErbB2 expression. We know that ductal carcinoma in situ (DCIS) has a much higher frequency with respect to overexpression of HER-2/neu and that patients with invasive tumors with an extensive intraductal component do worse in general on breast-conserving treatment. So my question is: "In your trial, in both arms after surgery (after extirpation of the primary tumor) how was the incidence of the extensive intraductal component in the two arms?"

M. Ellis: We didn't look at it. That is an interesting point, but I think it is going to be difficult to sort out because preoperatively or in the pretreatment situation, we have just got core needle biopsies. So it is difficult to determine how much of the tumor is DCIS and how much is invasive. All of the predictive marker studies I showed you are based on an exclusive examination of the invasive component of the tumor. So we were not scoring the DCIS component. It might be possible to go back and look at the surgical specimens (if we could get them) to consider that issue. But I don't have any direct answer for you.

D. Hayes: I would like to reiterate what Jim Ingle has said. There are two reasons to do neoadjuvant trials. First, to use them as phase II testing grounds for new drugs or new ideas with old drugs. I am also concerned about moving really new drugs into the adjuvant setting, because without some clinical toxicity data in patients in whom we traditionally do phase I and II trials (patients with metastatic disease for whom the stakes are not quite so high), I think it is risky business. For example, to move some of the tyrosine kinase inhibitors into a group of patients who have a very good chance of being cured is premature. We have no idea what these things do long term. I think there must be some caution there, although I am enthusiastic about these agents and novel trial design.

The second reason to do neoadjuvant studies is to choose (what Ian Smith talked about yesterday) to use clinical response to pick the patients most likely to benefit rather than using molecular markers (and I am all for molecular markers, since I made my career, more or less on that). There was a comment made yesterday that adjuvant chemotherapy had little or no benefit in post-menopausal women. I would take exception to that. SWOG have just rereported their data at ASCO in ER-positive, node-positive postmenopausal women who were randomized to tamoxifen versus cyclophosphamide/Adriamycin/fluorouracil (CAF) plus tamoxifen. There is a statistically significant, although small, survival benefit. That means there must be a small group of postmenopausal ER-positive women who benefited. Peter Ravdin has suggested that they are the HER-2 positive group, although I am not sure that is the case. A trial like that suggested by Matthew Ellis (although I wouldn't do it exactly like this), would allow you perhaps to select the women most likely to benefit from chemotherapy by first of all identifying the women who benefit from hormone therapy. I'm guessing it's the women who benefit from hormone therapy who are less likely to benefit from chemotherapy, and also, given that it is the women who look like they should benefit from hormone therapy because they are ER-positive but who turn out not to, who benefit from chemotherapy. I think that one could use a trial design like Matthew Ellis's to actually allow us now to select, in this case, postmenopausal women who are ER-positive and who are most likely to benefit from chemotherapy. Again, I personally wouldn't design it exactly like Matthew has, but he and I have spent several lunches (before he left our program) discussing it. I think something like this should come out of the cooperative groups. I really think this is the way of the future.

W. Eiermann: My concern is the relatively low rate of pathologically complete response with endocrine neoadjuvant treatment. We use the pathological complete response (PCR) as a surrogate marker in neoadjuvant chemotherapy for the outcome of the patients. That has been our method in NSABP18, the ECTA trial, and the Milan trial, and so on. They all have the surrogate marker for pathological complete response. We have a very low rate with endocrine therapy, which is beyond 2%, and the best chemotherapies show PCR of up to 20–25%. My questions are: "Is there another biology with the endocrine therapies that we have to compare first? Is the outcome with endocrine neoadjuvant therapy the same as chemotherapy in postmenopausal patients?"

D. Hayes: That is a critical question, I think, for this second trial design. Matthew (Ellis), if we use the M.D. Anderson pathological 1, 2, and 3 response criteria, what percentage were pathological response 1 in your trial, or in whichever trial?

M. Ellis: There were just a handful.

D. Hayes: What about if you look at response 1 or 2 then?

M. Ellis: We didn't really apply that kind of analysis, although we can maybe go back and try that. The way that posttreatment samples were obtained was by core biopsy. We didn't have all the pathological specimens for general pathological review. The reason was that for many for countries involved, sending the blocks was problematic.

D. Hayes: I have been involved in trials where you treat for a while and then, if something happens, you do something else (randomized). If the criteria for "if" are not very strict, it is a mess, especially in multicenter studies. I think we would have to have very careful pathological criteria. If it's pathological stage 1, then you randomize, and if it's not, then you don't, and everyone has to be trained and agree what those are.

M. Ellis: The point is that chemotherapy and hormonal therapy have very different mechanisms of action. I don't ever dream that the response rate to hormones is going to be greater than the response to chemotherapy in the neoadjuvant phase. The point of this trial is to show that preoperative endocrine therapy provides a benefit to the patient in the form of tumor triage to separate endocrine therapy responders who don't need chemotherapy, which would represent a great step forward. It is true that you get a more pathologically complete response with chemotherapy, but in the end we do not do very much with that information. You just tell the patient that she is going to do great or she is not going to do so great because of the presence of positive nodes postchemotherapy. There's no therapeutic decision based on that information, although there could be. No one has ever designed a trial to look at that, although maybe people will now.

The design is intended to address the conundrum generated by the data concerning chemotherapy in postmenopausal women with ER-positive disease. Are the benefits of chemotherapy large enough to warrant widespread application of chemotherapy to postmenopausal women with ER-positive disease? In the United States, post-SWOG 8814 and the ASCO presentation, huge numbers of women are going to be receiving chemotherapy where perhaps they weren't before. So I think that this is a very good design to address the problem of overtreatment of older patients with breast cancer.

I. Smith: I would like to underline one little practical point that I like about this trial. What is there in neoadjuvant therapy for patients? Mainly we are doing these studies at present to look at biological markers predicting long-term outcomes. The only thing that is currently in it for patients is downstaging to avoid mastectomy, and that doesn't necessarily involve that many patients. The attractive thing about this trial is the potential that patients might be able to avoid chemotherapy. One of the difficulties is going to be explaining this trial to patients. Although we understand what it is about, it is not going to be the easiest thing to explain.

D. Hayes: As I was saying, I might design a slightly different trial, but we can discuss that later.

I. Smith: Why don't you tell us what that might be?

D. Hayes: Well, what I would do is what Matthew (Ellis) originally proposed when he first came up with the letrozole versus tamoxifen study. So, I'm stealing his ideas, but it would be letrozole for 4 months and at the end of 4 months, some criteria should be assessed for pathological response. Those patients that you consider poor, let's say pathological response 3 using the M.D. Anderson criteria, would get chemotherapy followed by more letrozole. Those that you consider good, say pathological responses 1 and 2, would then be randomly assigned to ongoing letrozole versus chemotherapy followed by letrozole. I think that would allow you to select out the small group of patients who are likely to benefit from chemotherapy (i.e., those for whom letrozole was not adequately effective) and a large group of patients who probably don't need chemotherapy.

M. Ellis: The problem is that that doesn't get to the core of the matter, which is that the standard of care throughout the world for preoperative therapy currently is chemotherapy.

D. Hayes: I agree that it would take a Bernie Fisher–type of personality to get people to drop their biases and do something really innovative, at least in the United States.

M. Dixon: I think that Ian (Smith) has always insisted that one of the virtues of neoadjuvant therapy is that you can predict response to the drug and therefore it gives you an option, if the drug doesn't work, to change to something else. One of the problems with this study is that we are giving letrozole for 3–4 months, we're showing it is not doing any good to the tumor, and then we're giving it for another 5 years just to reinforce the fact that we know it is no good for the patient. That strikes me as not being a sensible use of the information you have, and I would favor letrozole for 3–4 months. Then, if there's no response, give chemotherapy and switch to another endocrine agent—for example, tamoxifen. People are saying that there is no evidence that response of the primary tumor relates to outcome, but I showed that for a 12- to 15-year follow-up, if you take the patients who have reduced their volume by 50% within a 3-month period, they have a significantly better survival than patients whose tumor volume is not halved within the first 3 months. I presented these data earlier today with long-term follow-up, showing that response in the primary tumor does predict in relation to eventual outcome.

M. Ellis: The problem is that we can't have more than one major experimental difference in the two treatment arms or we end up in a mess. There are a few leaps of faith there in what you say, which are very reasonable leaps of faith of course, but as yet unproven. I think there is a window of time in which we can do this, and it is as soon as we are comfortable with aromatase inhibitors in the adjuvant setting.

Part V

CHEMOPREVENTION

15

Epidemiological Basis of Hormonal Chemoprevention of Breast Cancer

Malcolm C. Pike, John R. Daniels, and Darcy V. Spicer
University of Southern California Keck School of Medicine
Norris Cancer Center
Los Angeles, California

I. ABSTRACT

All three of the major female cancers (breast, endometrium, and ovary) have been demonstrated to be preventable—i.e., their incidence can be significantly reduced by a hormonal chemopreventive approach. Oral contraceptive (OC) use significantly reduces the incidence of both ovarian and endometrial cancer, and use of the SERM tamoxifen has been shown to yield an equally impressive reduction in the incidence of breast cancer. The task now is to work out how best to combine these chemopreventive approaches to maximize the benefits and reduce the risks associated with their use.

In this chapter we have concentrated on two major issues concerning hormonal chemoprevention of breast cancer: hormone replacement therapy (HRT) and hormonal contraception. HRT is not usually considered in the context of the chemoprevention of breast cancer, but HRT with the use of an estrogen and a progestin is a major cause of breast cancer, and there is an urgent need to change current prescribing practices of HRT so as to minimize its harmful effects on the breast.

The second issue is the challenge of designing a hormonal contraceptive regimen that will be chemopreventive for breast cancer while maintaining the chemopreventive effect of OCs against cancer of the ovary (and hopefully against endometrial cancer). For hormonal chemoprevention of breast cancer to have its maximal effect, it should start at a young age. For this to occur, the chemoprevention regimen must have other benefits as well, so that young women will use the regimen for reasons not associated, for them, with the remote, far-in-the-future risk of breast cancer. A contraceptive chemopreventive regimen that is as effective a contraceptive as OCs will satisfy this need.

II. INTRODUCTION

Hormonal chemoprevention of ovarian cancer was first demonstrated in the late 1970s. The chemopreventive agent was the oral contraceptive (OC or "the pill"). The protection achieved was highly significant and duration of use–dependent; 5 years of OC use provides a long-term reduction in risk of around 32%, and 10 years of use a reduction of around 54% [1]. Hormonal chemoprevention of endometrial cancer was first demonstrated in the early 1980s. The chemopreventive agent was again OCs. The protection was again highly significant and duration of use–dependent; 5 years of OC use provides a long-term reduction in risk of around 46%, and 10 years of use a reduction of around 71% [1]. These chemopreventive effects of OCs do not extend to breast cancer for reasons that are now clear (see below).

However, hormonal chemoprevention of breast cancer is now an established fact. The selective estrogen receptor modulator (SERM) tamoxifen has been proven to substantially reduce breast cancer risk in the short term [2]. This is an extraordinary milestone in our fight against this disease. The SERM raloxifene is likely to be as effective a chemopreventive agent against breast cancer as tamoxifen [3].

All three of the major female cancers are thus preventable (i.e., their incidence can be significantly reduced) by a hormonal chemopreventive approach. Our task now is to work out how best to combine these chemopreventive approaches to maximize the benefits and reduce the risks associated with their use. Efforts to decrease the risks associated with use of OCs led to reduced doses of both the estrogen and progestin content of OCs, and the overall health benefits of current OC use clearly outweigh the associated increased risks [4]. As one would expect, with the more recent introduction of tamoxifen as a chemopreventive agent, the risk-benefit picture is not so clear [5]; but concentrated investigation of the mechanisms causing the added risks of stroke, pulmonary embolism, and deep venous thrombosis and the likely possibility of improved SERMs should lead to continuing improvement in the risk-benefit equation associated with SERM use.

In this chapter, we concentrate on two major issues concerning hormonal chemoprevention of breast cancer: hormone replacement therapy (HRT) and hormonal contraception. The first issue, HRT, is not usually considered in the context of the chemoprevention of breast cancer, but HRT as currently prescribed, with the use of an estrogen and a progestin, is a major cause of breast cancer. There is an urgent need to change current prescribing practices of HRT so as to minimize its harmful effects on the breast [6,7].

The second issue, that of hormonal contraception, poses the challenge of improving on the risk-benefit equation associated with OCs by finding a hormonal contraceptive regimen that will be chemopreventive for breast cancer. For hormonal chemoprevention of breast cancer to have its maximal effect, it should start at a young age. For this to occur, the chemoprevention regimen must have other benefits, so that young women will use the regimen for reasons not associated, for them, with the remote, far-in-the-future risk of breast cancer. A contraceptive chemopreventive regimen that is as effective a contraceptive as OCs will satisfy this need.

III. CRITICAL OBSERVATIONS

The essential elements of the etiology of breast cancer are well understood. The incidence of breast cancer can be largely explained by reference to the exposure of the breast to endogenous estrogens and progesterone and exogenous estrogens and progestins. This explains the age incidence of breast cancer, the increasing risk associated with younger age at menarche and older age at menopause, the increasing risk associated with increasing postmenopausal weight, the small increased risk associated with postmenopausal estrogen replacement therapy (ERT) and the much larger increased risk associated with postmenopausal estrogen-plus-progestin replacement therapy (EPRT), and—most impressively—the much lower rates of breast cancer in "traditional" Asian women. The only major factor (excluding major genetic factors such as BRCA1) requiring additional special explanation is the long-term protective effect of early first full-term pregnancy.

The incidence of most non-hormone-dependent cancers rises continuously and increasingly rapidly with age, and a plot of the logarithm of incidence against the logarithm of age produces a straight line, as predicted by the multistage theory of carcinogenesis and confirmed by modern molecular biological studies (Fig. 1) [8]. In contrast, the age-incidence curve of cancer of the breast shows a distinct slowing of the rate of rise at the age of menopause (Figure 2). (Note: The breast cancer age-incidence curve around 1970 shown in Figure 2 more truly reflects the biology of breast cancer than more recent age-incidence curves, as the latter are significantly affected by mammographic screening, which increases detected cancer rates in the postmenopausal period. A significant proportion of such cancers might not, without mammography, have been diagnosed for many years.) Important etiological elements are, therefore, present in premenopausal women and are reduced following menopause.

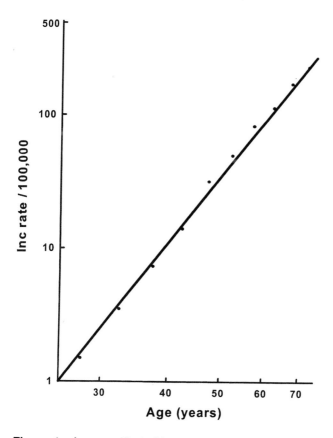

Figure 1 Age-specific incidence rates for colorectal cancer in U.S. white females, 1969–1971 [60].

Figure 2 strongly suggests that early menopause will reduce a woman's breast cancer risk, and epidemiological case-control and cohort studies have confirmed this [9–11]. The younger the age at natural menopause, the greater the protection achieved. That the protection is directly due to the curtailment of ovarian function is shown by studies demonstrating the same protection with bilateral oophorectomy. Age at menopause is a major risk factor: e.g., if women continued to ovulate until age 70, breast cancer risk would be increased some sixfold over present rates. If bilateral oophorectomy occurs before age 40, breast cancer incidence is reduced by as much as two-thirds. The protection afforded by early menopause, whether it is natural or occurs through bilateral oophorectomy, is the key epidemiological observation regarding the etiology and chemoprevention of breast cancer.

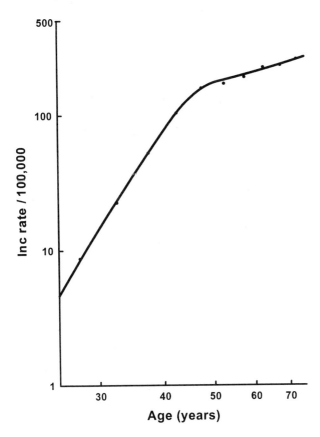

Figure 2 Age-specific incidence rates for breast cancer in U.S. white females, 1969–1971 [60].

Breast cancer risk was also found to increase with earlier age at menarche, and these observations of increasing risk with later menopause and earlier menarche, as well as critical experimental and clinical studies, concentrated attention on ovarian function as a major, if not *the* major, influence on breast cancer risk. Estrogen was the focus of interest. Many other epidemiological observations as well as experimental and clinical studies supported this focus on estrogen. Increasing weight during the postmenopausal years was found to increase risk, in agreement with the known increasing bioavailable endogenous estrogen levels with increasing weight in postmenopausal women [12], and use of postmenopausal ERT was found to increase breast cancer risk [13,14].

Subsequently, in addition to estrogen, a major etiological role for progestins was strongly suggested by the observation that the use of postmenopausal

EPRT increases breast cancer risk substantially more than does the use of ERT. This is consistent with the estrogen-progestin hypothesis for breast cancer: i.e., that both estrogens and progestins increase breast cancer risk. This hypothesis had first been suggested by the observation that, during the menstrual cycle, breast-cell proliferation is lowest during the follicular phase and then increases some twofold in the luteal phase (bottom graph in Fig. 3) [15,16]. In addition to providing an explanation of the greater increased risk from EPRT than ERT, this hypothesis also provides an explanation of the *decreased* risk found in obese premenopausal women. Premenopausal obesity is associated with increased anovulation, which decreases breast exposure to progesterone. After menopause, the decreased risk associated with premenopausal obesity is gradually eliminated and an increased risk finally achieved by the increased bioavailable estrogen levels associated with postmenopausal obesity. The reason that risk is only slightly increased by ERT is the relatively low dose of estrogen used in postmenopausal ERT and the absence of a progestin [17]. The addition of a relatively high-dose progestin to ERT is predicted to increase the risk substantially; this is precisely what is observed (see below).

Studies of OC use and breast cancer have found either no effect or a slight increase in risk [18]. This is entirely consistent with the estrogen-progestin hypothesis. OCs contain an estrogen and a progestin. OCs inhibit gonadotropin secretion, thus reducing ovarian steroidogenesis to very low levels, but the ovarian steroid loss is compensated for by the synthetic estrogen and progestin of the OC. One would predict that breast-cell proliferation in women taking OCs would be less than, equal to, or greater than that observed during a normal menstrual cycle, depending on the dose of estrogen and progestin in the particular OC. Direct observational studies of breast-cell proliferation in women taking OCs show that the total breast-cell proliferation is very similar over an OC cycle and a normal menstrual cycle [15,16,19]. These results predict that breast cancer risk should not be substantially affected by OC use, as is observed [18].

IV. MODELING BREAST CANCER INCIDENCE

To use the estrogen-progestin hypothesis to predict the long-term effects of hormonal chemoprevention regimens on breast cancer risk, it is necessary to be more quantitative than we have been in the above discussion.

As illustrated in Figure 1, for most non-hormone-dependent cancers, the relationship between incidence, I, and age, t, can be represented by the equation: $log[I(t)] = constant + k \times log(t)$, where k is the slope of the line shown in the figure. Expressing this on the usual arithmetic scale, we find that incidence is a power function of age:

$$I(t) = a \times t^k, \tag{1}$$

where a is a constant.

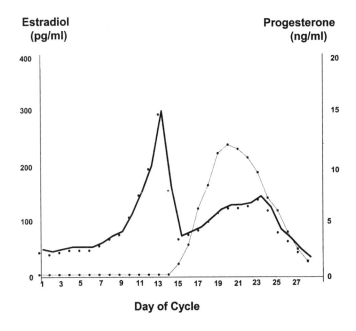

Day of Cycle

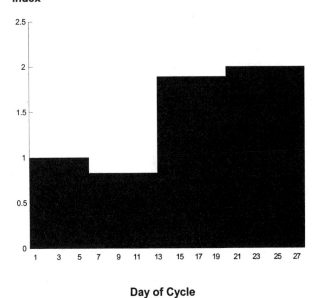

Day of Cycle

Figure 3 (Top) Serum concentrations of estradiol and progesterone by day of cycle [61]. (Bottom) Breast-cell labeling index (mitotic rate) by day of cycle in parous women [15].

273

Equation (1) may be generalized to cover a broader range of situations if we express incidence as

$$I(t) = a \times [d(t)]^k \tag{2}$$

where $d(t)$ is the relevant "intensity-weighted duration of exposure" of the tissue up to age t[20]. For example, for lung cancer at a constant cigarette consumption, expressing $d(t)$ as duration of smoking to age t gives a very accurate description of the age incidence of the disease [8,21].

The female hormone–associated cancers (breast, endometrium, and ovary) can similarly be reconciled with a linear log-log plot if we define $d(t)$ as the cumulative "effective mitotic rate" of the relevant tissues. The fundamental notion here is that the "aging" of a tissue relates directly to its cell kinetics: while the tissue is not undergoing cell division, its rate of aging is close to zero; while it is aging at a maximal rate when the mitotic rate of the cells is maximal. This notion can be justified simply in terms of its success in describing the known epidemiology of these tumors; it does, however, also have a basis in the known biology of carcinogenesis.

For breast cancer, k is estimated to be 4.5 and a simple definition of $d(t)$ that incorporates the known effects of menarche, first full-term pregnancy (FFTP), and menopause assumes that $d(t)$ increases steadily at rate 1 from menarche to FFTP (this is a relative rate, so setting it to 1 is only setting a value for other rates to be compared), then slows to rate 0.70 until menopause, when it slows further to 0.105 [20]. This simple definition needs to be modified slightly to account for the fact that late FFTP is associated with an increased risk of breast cancer (relative to nulliparous women) and to take account of the perimenopausal period. The effect of late FFTP is accommodated by incorporating a constant, b, to represent a one-time increase in $d(t)$ associated with FFTP. To account for the perimenopause, we incorporate a decline in the rate of breast tissue aging starting around age 40 and ending at the last menstrual period. These modifications agree broadly with what we know about breast tissue mitotic rates and with data on changes in hormonal profiles with age. The model so modified provides an excellent fit to the known effects of menarche, FFTP, and menopause. It explains why late age at FFTP increases breast cancer risk and predicts that, at young ages, parous women will have a higher risk of breast cancer than nulliparous women—a prediction borne out by direct epidemiological observation [22,23].

A. Explaining "Traditional" Japanese Breast Cancer Rates

If the estrogen-progestin hypothesis is correct and the model described by Equation (2) holds, then one should be able to explain the sixfold increase in breast cancer rates in the United States compared to "traditional" Japan around 1970 on this basis. The two risk factors that clearly have a major role in breast cancer etiology and differ greatly between the U.S. and traditional Japan are age at menarche (about 2 years later in Japan) and postmenopausal weight (approximately 50 kg in Japan compared with approximately 67 kg in the United States around 1970 [24,25]). The much reduced weight of postmenopausal Japanese women will lead to very low postmenopausal estrogen levels and therefore to a near zero breast-cell mitotic rate. At ages 65 to 69, the 1970 U.S. rate was sixfold greater than the Japanese rate [26]; the model-predicted combined effect of a two-year delay in menarche and a near zero postmenopausal mitotic rate in the Japanese reduces the difference to 3.1-fold. The differences in age at FFTP had only a very small effect on the differences in rates, and this ratio would appear to hold at all ages for this generation of women. This excess can be accounted for by a lower breast-cell mitotic rate in the premenopausal period among the traditional Japanese than among U.S. women [20]. The magnitude of the difference in breast-cell mitotic rates is predicted by the model (Eq. 2) to be an approximately 22% reduction in the Japanese breast-cell mitotic rate compared to the U.S. breast-cell mitotic rate. This is calculated as follows: Let the U.S. relative premenopausal mitotic rate be 1.0 and the Japanese rate be r. Then, with the same age at menarche and FFTP, the Japanese $d(t)$, which we denote $d_J(t)$, is r times the U.S. $d(t)$, which we denote $d_{US}(t)$: i.e., $d_J(t) = r \times d_{US}(t)$. The relative incidence of breast cancer is thus

$$I_{US}(t)/I_J(t) = \{a \times [d_{US}(t)]^{4.5}\}/\{a \times [d_J(t)]^{4.5}\}$$
$$= [d_{US}(t)]^{4.5}/[d_J(t)]^{4.5}$$
$$= [d_{US}(t)]^{4.5}/[r \times d_{US}(t)]^{4.5}$$
$$= 1/r^{4.5}$$

Setting this equal to 3.1, the ratio of incidence rates after allowing for menarche and postmenopausal weight, produces an estimated r of 0.78; i.e., the traditional Japanese effective breast-cell mitotic rate is calculated to be approximately 22% lower than the U.S. effective breast-cell mitotic rate.

There are no data on relative breast-cell mitotic rates in U.S. and traditional Japanese women, but there is ample evidence that serum estradiol levels were lower in the Japanese women. Studies done in the early 1970s showed that urinary conjugated estrone, estradiol, and estriol were much reduced in Japanese compared to U.S. women, both in the follicular phase and in the luteal phase [27,28]. Similarly, almost all studies that have compared serum estradiol concentrations in Caucasians and Asians and that paid special attention to obtaining samples from Asian women who were maintaining a lifestyle like that of the women enjoying a low breast cancer rate in 1970 show clearly reduced serum estradiol in the Asian women [29–31]. The average reduction found in serum estradiol levels in the Asian women was around 20 to 25%—i.e., very close to the reduction in breast-cell mitotic rate predicted to be necessary to explain their very low breast cancer rates. There is no direct evidence that an approximately 20% reduction in serum estradiol will lead to a similar reduction in breast-cell mitotic rate, but this is a very reasonable assumption. In U.K. and U.S. women, breast-cell proliferation is maximal during the luteal phase of the menstrual cycle, decreases during the follicular phase, and decreases further after menopause. Thus, over this range of hormonal values, breast-cell proliferation decreases with lower hormonal exposure, and the decrease in serum estradiol of the Japanese women will thus almost certainly have resulted in lower breast-cell proliferation compared to that in U.S. women.

The estrogen-progestin hypothesis, therefore, provides a very satisfactory explanation of even the large difference between traditional Japanese and U.S. breast cancer rates, and we can confidently use this model to predict long-term effects of hormonal chemopreventive regimens.

V. HORMONE REPLACEMENT THERAPY

Postmenopausal ERT at the dose usually administered in the United States increases breast cancer risk approximately 2% per year of use (relative risk, RR, of ~1.02 per year of use [13, 14]). Five years of ERT use increases risk by approximately five times this amount (RR ~1.10 per 5 years of ERT use), and longer use increases the risk proportionately. ERT is associated with much greater increased relative risks for endometrial cancer (RR ~2.0 per 5 years of ERT use [32,33]). The endometrial cancer risks were established in the mid-1970s, and, in response to the greatly increased risks, progestins were added to ERT (estrogen-progestin replacement therapy; EPRT). The progestin is either added for 10 to 12 days per month in a sequential fashion (sequential estrogen-progestin replacement therapy, or SEPRT), or estrogen and a lower dose of progestin are always taken together (continuous-combined estrogen-progestin replacement therapy, or CCEPRT).

As we have noted, EPRT use increases breast cancer risk to a much greater extent than ERT use [34–36]. These studies suggest that the relative risk per year of EPRT use is approximately three times that associated with ERT use: i.e., RR ~1.06 per year of EPRT use. Five years of EPRT use increases risk by approximately five times this amount (RR ~1.30 per 5 years of EPRT use), and longer use increases the risk proportionately. Evidence that these effects are directly due to EPRT use comes from the randomized PEPI trial which showed substantial increases in mammographic densities in women taking EPRT (including use of micronized progesterone), much greater increases than were seen in the ERT arm of the trial [37]. Further evidence comes from the finding of greatly increased breast-cell proliferation in women using EPRT [38]. In our case-control study, the risk with SEPRT was greater than that with CCEPRT, but the difference was not statistically significant, and no such difference was seen in the study of Magnusson et al. [34]. Furthermore, the increase in mammographic densities reported by Greendale et al. [37] was the same for SEPRT and for CCEPRT, and the EPRT regimen reported on by Hofseth et al. [38] was CCEPRT. There is thus little basis to currently distinguish between these regimens on the basis of breast cancer risk. It should be noted that the total dose of both estrogen and progestin is very nearly equal in SEPRT and CCEPRT regimens.

Progestins clearly must be given to protect the endometrium from the carcinogenic effects of ERT. They must be delivered to the endometrium in a manner that will have minimal effect on the breast. There is good evidence that this can be accomplished by using a direct endometrial route of administration with an intrauterine device (IUD) containing progesterone (Progestasert® [39]), which was designed as an intrauterine contraceptive device (IUCD). Use of this device is associated with a very low serum progesterone concentration of <1.5 nmol/L (no more than the level in the follicular phase of the menstrual cycle). The levonorgestrel-containing IUCD (Mirena®) will also provide endometrial protection with probably very little effect on the breast, although that is yet to be demonstrated [40]. Alternatively, it may be possible to administer micronized progesterone by an intravaginal tablet at a dose that will provide adequate endometrial progestin levels with low blood levels, so that the effects of the progesterone on the breast should be small [41,42]. If these routes of administration are unacceptable to a woman, then giving progestins for 10 days every 3 to 4 months should provide satisfactory protection of the endometrium with much less effect on the breast than current forms of EPRT. Two clinical trials of 10 mg per day of medroxyprogesterone acetate (MPA) given for 14 days every 3 months have been published, in which the dose of estrogen was conjugated estrogens at 0.625 mg/day [43,44]. These two studies suggest that this approach may be satisfactory, in that the extent of associated endometrial hyperplasia was minimal. A further trial did not show satisfactory control of hyperplasia, but in this trial a much higher dose of estrogen was given [45]. A full discussion of this issue is given in Pike and Ross [6].

The standard by which current and future generation progestins are judged, and the methods and regimens for their delivery, needs to be changed. The burden of proof should no longer be on epidemiologists and other investigators to demonstrate that such agents (or regimens) significantly increase the risk of breast cancer; rather, it should shift to the proponents of systemic use of such agents to demonstrate that they do not. All currently prescribed regimens, including those using the new generation of progestins, need to be evaluated for breast cancer risk by using mammographic densities or other biomarkers of action on the breast. Proponents of new EPRT regimens should, at minimum, have to show that they are not more harmful to the breast than the standard regimens based on conjugated estrogens and MPA.

VI. PREMENOPAUSAL CHEMOPREVENTION

Tamoxifen use significantly reduces the incidence of premenopausal as well as postmenopausal breast cancer [2], but the hormonal effects of tamoxifen in premenopausal women differ from those seen in postmenopausal women. In premenopausal women, estradiol and progesterone levels are increased significantly by tamoxifen, and levels of follicle-stimulating hormone and luteinizing hormone remain normal or increase slightly [46–48]. Tamoxifen is structurally similar to clomiphene, and it is equivalent to clomiphene for induction of ovulation [49]. The raised hormone levels have been suggested to be due to maturation of multiple ovarian follicles. These effects may cause an increase in ovarian cancer [50]. For this reason and to achieve an actual significant reduction in ovarian cancer incidence, the approach currently being favored is to add a gonadotropin-releasing hormone agonist (Gn-RHA) to block ovarian function to tamoxifen for chemoprevention in premenopausal women. We had earlier suggested the use of a Gn-RHA with add-back low-dose estrogen-progestin as a chemopreventive regimen for breast and ovarian cancer [51,52], and the use of a Gn-RHA with raloxifene or tibolone has recently also been proposed.

A. Gn-RHA Alone

The use of a Gn-RHA alone will lead to very significant reductions in breast cancer incidence, since Gn-RHAs are given in sufficiently high doses to not only block ovulation but also to reduce ovarian steroid production to very low levels. This medical bilateral oophorectomy should have close to the same protective effect on breast cancer as surgical oophorectomy. Using our model of breast cancer incidence, the chemoprotective effect can readily be estimated. Some predicted reductions in breast cancer incidence from use of a Gn-RHA are shown in Table 1. If a Gn-RHA is used from age 35, the lifetime risk (cumulative incidence to age 75) of breast cancer should be reduced by around 70%. If a Gn-RHA is used from age 25, the risk should be reduced by approximately 96%—i.e., the risk of breast cancer is predicted to be reduced to 4% of "normal" so that 24 of 25 current breast cancer cases would be prevented. Some predicted effects on breast cancer risk of using a Gn-RHA for a limited length of time and then stopping are shown in Table 2. Life-

Table 1 Predicted Reduction in Cumulative Breast Cancer Risk to Age 75 with Continuous Chemoprevention

Chemoprevention Starting at Age	Gn-RHA Alone	Gn-RHA + Add-Back EP
25	96%	87%
35	70%	54%

Table 2 Predicted Reduction in Cumulative Breast Cancer Risk to Age 75 with Shorter-Term Chemoprevention Starting at Age 25

Length of chemoprevention	Gn-RHA alone	Gn-RHA + add-back EP
5 years	47%	39%
10 years	75%	64%
15 years	89%	80%

time breast cancer risk is predicted to be reduced by about 47% if the regimen is used for 5 years, by about 75% if used for 10 years, and by about 89% if used for 15 years. The reason why these figures may appear larger than one would naively predict on the basis of the figures given in Table 1 is that this use of Gn-RHA all occurs before the perimenopausal period, with its associated declining levels of ovarian estrogen and progesterone. These chemopreventive effects appear likely to be directly applicable to carriers of BRCA1 mutations [53].

Although it may be objected that the figures given in Tables 1 and 2 were calculated from a mathematical model, they can be seen to be likely to be close to correct by comparing the figure for starting Gn-RHA alone at age 35 to the known effects of early oophorectomy. Epidemiological studies have found that early surgical menopause around age 35 with no HRT is associated with a 60 to 75% reduction in breast cancer risk [9–11]. Our presumption that Gn-RHA use is equivalent to oophorectomy is strongly supported by the results of the ZIPP randomized trial [54]. In this trial the Gn-RHA depot Zoladex® was given to premenopausal breast cancer patients and a 40% reduction in contralateral disease was observed.

B. Gn-RHA Plus Add-Back Estrogen-Progestin

Gn-RHA alone is thus a most effective agent for chemoprevention of breast cancer. Use of a Gn-RHA alone is, however, unacceptable except for brief periods because of the associated side effects, including hot flushes, dyspareunia, and loss of bone mineral density (BMD). These side effects and others that have been reported in some women reflect the hypoestrogenic state induced by the Gn-RHA as well as the low levels of androgens induced by the Gn-RHA (see below); they can be prevented in the main by add-back low-dose estrogen treatment. With add-back estrogen, it is also necessary to use add-back progestin to protect the endometrium from the estrogen treatment; we have assumed that progestin is given for 10 days in every 3-month period (i.e., ERT for 2 months followed by SEPRT for 1 month). To estimate the effect on breast cancer risk of use of such a Gn-RHA + estrogen-progestin (GEP) regimen, we have assumed that the Gn-RHA use will induce a reversible medical oophorectomy and that the effect of the estrogen and progestin will be the same as that observed in postmenopausal HRT users (see Sec. V above)—i.e., a small effect in the months that ERT is given and a larger effect in the month that SEPRT is given. The regimen for which we calculated the results, shown in the right hand columns of Tables 1 and 2, assumes that the estrogen dose is as commonly given in HRT regimens (0.625 mg/day of conjugated estrogen or "equivalent") and the progestin is given as 5 mg/day of MPA for 10 days in every period of 3 months [6]. The predicted reductions in breast cancer incidence are, of course, less than with Gn-RHA alone, but they remain very substantial. If the GEP regimen is used from age 35 until menopause, the lifetime risk of breast cancer should be reduced by about 54% (Table 1). If the regimen is used from age 25, the risk of breast cancer should be reduced by about 87%—i.e., more than 6 of every 7 current breast cancers would be prevented. The predicted effect on breast cancer risk of using the GEP regimen for a limited length of time and then stopping is illustrated in Table 2. Lifetime breast cancer risk is predicted to be reduced by about 39% if the regimen is used for 5 years, by about 64% if used for 10 years, and by about 80% if used for 15 years.

We have tested a prototype GEP regimen in a pilot clinical trial [55,56]. Mammographic densities of women on the GEP regimen were quite dramatically decreased after 1 year on the regimen [56]. This is precisely what happens at menopause, and, as we have noted, early menopause is associated with a much reduced risk of breast cancer. The statistically highly significant reductions in mammographic density at 1 year suggest that the aim of the regimen to reduce breast cancer risk has been accomplished.

Women on the GEP regimen had significantly fewer symptoms on the regimen than before they started it [55]. However, despite the use of an estrogen dose that is known to prevent loss of BMD in normally postmenopausal women, a small (~2%) loss of spinal BMD was seen in the women on the GEP regimen at 1 year. The reason for this loss of BMD appears to be inhibition of ovarian androgen production by the Gn-RHA. Women on the GEP regimen had a 62% drop in non-sex-hormone-binding globulin-bound testosterone. In contrast, during the early naturally postmenopausal period, testosterone levels are stable. The addition to the regimen of just sufficient testosterone to replace that lost by the action of the Gn-RHA should eliminate this problem, and our preliminary findings with the addition of a small amount of methyltestosterone supports this conjecture.

The likely improvement in efficacy of screening mammography to be gained from use of such a GEP-based regimen in premenopausal women has been emphasized by Feig [57], and this possibility is strongly supported by the studies of the effects of EPRT on mammographic screening, in which EPRT use led to an increased incidence of interval cancers between screening mammograms [58,59].

B. Gn-RHA Plus Tamoxifen

A Gn-RHA plus tamoxifen (GTam) regimen is very likely to be more chemopreventive against breast cancer than a GEP regimen, and it is likely that such a regimen will also be more chemopreventive against breast cancer than a Gn-RHA–alone regimen. The essential question that needs answering is not whether a GTam regimen will prevent breast cancer but rather how acceptable to women such a regimen will be and whether the negative side effects of such a regimen are clearly outweighed by its benefits. The latter will clearly vary depending on the individual woman's underlying risk of breast (and ovarian) cancer and her risks of negative consequences.

C. Gn-RHA and Reduction in Ovarian Cancer Risk

The suppression of ovulation and ovarian function by any Gn-RHA–based regimen should protect against ovarian cancer to at least the same extent as has been found to occur with use of OCs. If the Gn-RHA regimen is used from age 35, the subsequent risk of ovarian cancer is calculated to be reduced by 84% [51]. Use for 5 years is predicted to reduce the lifetime risk of ovarian cancer by 41%. These are very substantial chemopreventive effects.

VII. FUTURE DEVELOPMENTS

In order to make a GEP with replacement testosterone regimen practical, it will be necessary to make its administration simple and to produce it at a reasonable cost. The latter does not appear to be a major issue in the long term. We are currently in clinical trial with the development of such a regimen based on using a Gn-RHA administered by intranasal spray. The clinical trials comprise the treatment of uterine fibroids and endometriosis; there is considerable evidence that such a regimen can successfully treat both conditions.

This is a most optimistic time for breast cancer chemoprevention. Proof of principle has clearly been established and, with a number of different approaches being tested, we can confidently look forward to making significant inroads into reducing the incidence of the disease in the foreseeable future.

ACKNOWLEDGMENTS

Drs. Pike, Daniels, and Spicer are associated with Balance Pharmaceuticals, Inc., a company set up to develop the Gn-RHA plus low-dose estrogen-progestin regimen discussed here.

REFERENCES

1. Pike MC, Spicer DV. Oral contraceptives and cancer. In Shoupe D, Haseltine F, eds. Contraception. New York: Springer-Verlag, 1993:67–84.
2. Fisher B, Constantino JP, Wickerham DL, et al. Tamoxifen for prevention of breast cancer: Report of the National Surgical Adjuvant Breast and Bowel Project P-1 Study. J Natl Cancer Inst 1998; 90:1371–1388.
3. Cummings SR, Eckert S, Krueger KA, et al. The effect of raloxifene on risk of breast cancer in postmenopausal women: Results from the MORE randomized trial. JAMA 1999; 281:2189–2197.
4. Vessey MP. An overview of the benefits and risk of combined oral contraceptives. In Mann RD, ed. Oral Contraceptives and Breast Cancer. Carnforth, UK: Parthenon, 1990:121–135.
5. Gail MH, Constantino JP, Bryant J, et al. Weighing the risks and benefits of tamoxifen treatment for preventing breast cancer. J Natl Cancer Inst 1999; 91:1829–1846.
6. Pike MC, Ross RK. Progestins and menopause: Epidemiological studies of risks of endometrial and breast cancer. Steroids 2000; 65:659–664.
7. Pike MC, Ross RK. Response to "Re: Effect of hormone replacement therapy on breast cancer risk: Estrogen versus estrogen plus progestin." J Natl Cancer Inst 2000; 92:1950–1952.
8. Doll R. The age distribution of cancer: implications for models of carcinogenesis. J R Stat Soc Series A 1971; 134:133–166.
9. Hirayama T, Wynder EL. A study of the epidemiology of cancer of the breast. II. The influence of hysterectomy. Cancer 1962; 15:28–38.
10. Feinleib M. Breast cancer and artificial menopause: A cohort study. J Natl Cancer Inst 1968; 41:315–329.
11. Trichopoulos D, MacMahon B, Cole P. Menopause and breast cancer risk. J Natl Cancer Inst 1972; 48:605–613.
12. Grodin JM, Siiteri PK, MacDonald PC. Source of estrogen production in postmenopausal women. J Clin Endocrinol Metab 1973; 36:207–214.
13. Steinberg KK, Thacker SB, Smith SJ, et al. A meta-analysis of the effect of estrogen replacement therapy on the risk of breast cancer. JAMA 1991; 265:1985–1990.
14. Collaborative Group on Hormonal Factors in Breast Cancer. Breast cancer and hormone replacement therapy: collaborative reanalysis of data from 51 epidemiological studies of 52,705 women with breast cancer and 108,411 women without breast cancer. Lancet 1997; 350:1047–1059.
15. Anderson TJ, Battersby S, King RJB, et al. Oral contraceptive use influences resting breast proliferation. Hum Pathol 1989; 20:1139–1144.
16. Pike MC, Spicer DV, Dahmoush L, Press MF. Estrogens, progestogens, normal breast cell proliferation, and breast cancer risk. Epidemiol Rev 1993; 15:17–35.
17. Key TJA, Pike MC. The role of estrogens and progestogens in the epidemiology and prevention of breast cancer. Eur J Cancer Clin Oncol 1988; 24:29–43.
18. Collaborative Group on Hormonal Factors in Breast Cancer. Breast cancer and hormonal contraceptives: collaborative reanalysis of individual data on 53,297 women with breast cancer and 100,239 women without breast cancer from 54 epidemiological studies. Lancet 1996; 347:1713–1727.

19. Williams G, Anderson E, Howell A, et al. Oral contraceptive (OCP) use increases proliferation and decreases oestrogen receptor content of epithelial cells in the normal human breast. Int J Cancer 1991; 48:206–210.

20. Pike MC, Krailo MD, Henderson BE, et al. "Hormonal" risk factors, 'breast tissue age' and the age-incidence of breast cancer. Nature 1983; 303:767–770.

21. Doll R, Peto R. Cigarette smoking and bronchial carcinoma: dose and time relationships among regular smokers and lifelong non-smokers. Epidemiol Comm Health 1978; 32:303–313.

22. Janerich DT. Pregnancy, breast-cancer risk, and maternal-fetal genetics. Lancet 1979; 1240–1241.

23. Kelsey JL, Gammon MD, John M. Reproductive factors and breast cancer. Epidemiol Rev 1993; 15:36–47.

24. De Waard F, Poortman J, Collette HJA. Relationship of weight to the promotion of breast cancer after menopause. Nutrition Cancer 1981: 2:237–240.

25. Hoel DG, Wakabayashi T, Pike MC. Secular trends in the distributions of the breast cancer risk factors—menarche, first birth, menopause, and weight—in Hiroshima and Nagasaki, Japan. Am J Epidemiol 1983; 118:78–89.

26. Waterhouse J, Muir C, Correa P, Powell J, eds. Cancer Incidence in Five Continents. Vol. 3. IARC Scientific Publication No. 15. Lyon, France: International Agency for Cancer Research, 1976.

27. MacMahon B, Cole P, Brown JB, et al. Oestrogen profiles of Asian and North American women. Lancet 1971; 2:900–902.

28. MacMahon B, Cole P, Brown JB, et al. Urine oestrogen profiles of Asian and North American women. Int J Cancer 1974; 14:161–167.

29. Goldin BR, Adlercreutz H, Gorbach SL, et al. The relationship between estrogen levels and diets of Caucasian American and Oriental immigrant women. Am J Clin Nutr 1986; 44:945–953.

30. Key TJA, Chen J, Wang DY, et al. Sex hormones in women in rural China and in Britain. Br J Cancer 1990; 62:631–636.

31. Bernstein L, Yuan JM, Ross RK, et al. Serum hormones levels in premenopausal Chinese women in Shanghai and white women in Los Angeles. Cancer Causes Control 1990; 1:51–58.

32. Grady D, Gebretsadik T, Kerlikowske K, et al. Hormone replacement therapy and endometrial cancer risk: A meta-analysis. Obstet Gynecol 1995; 85:304–313.

33. Pike MC. Peters RK, Cozen W, et al. Estrogen-progestin replacement therapy and endometrial cancer. J Natl Cancer Inst 1997; 89:1110–1116.

34. Magnusson C, Baron JA, Correia N, et al. Breast-cancer risk following long-term oestrogen- and oestrogen-progestin-replacement therapy. Int J Cancer 1999; 81:339–344.

35. Ross RK, Paganini-Hill A, Wan PC, Pike MC. Estrogen versus estrogen-progestin hormone replacement therapy: Effect on breast cancer risk. J Natl Cancer Inst 2000; 92:328–332.

36. Schairer C, Lubin J, Troisi R, et al. Menopausal estrogen and estrogen-progestin replacement therapy and breast cancer risk. JAMA 2000; 283:485–491.

37. Greendale GA, Reboussin BA, Sie A, et al. Effects of estrogen and estrogen-progestin on mammographic parenchymal density. Ann Intern Med 1999; 130:262–269.

38. Hofseth LJ, Raafat AM, Osuch JR, et al. Hormone replacement therapy with estrogen or estrogen plus medroxyprogesterone acetate is associated with increased epithelial proliferation in the normal postmenopausal breast. J Clin Endocrinol Metab 1999; 84:4559–4565.

39. Shoupe D, Meme D, Mezrow G, Lobo RA. Prevention of endometrial hyperplasia in postmenopausal women with intrauterine progesterone. N Engl J Med 1991; 325:1811–1812.

40. Sivin I, Stern J, Coutinho E, et al. Prolonged intrauterine contraception: A seven-year randomized study of the levonorgestrel 20 mcg/day (LNg 20) and the copper T380 Ag IUDs. Contraception 1991; 44:473–480.

41. Miles RA, Paulson RJ, Lobo RA, et al. Pharmacokinetics and endometrial tissue levels of progesterone after administration by intramuscular and vaginal routes: A comparative study. Fertil Steril 1994; 62:485–490.

42. Fanchin R, de Ziegler D, Bergeron C, et al. Transvaginal administration of progesterone. Obstet Gynecol 1997; 90:396–401.

43. Ettinger B, Selby J, Citron JT, et al. Cyclic hormone replacement therapy using quarterly progestin. Obstet Gynecol 1994; 83:693–700.

44. Williams DB, Voigt BJ, Fu YS, et al. Assessment of less than monthly progestin therapy in postmenopausal women given estrogen replacement. Obstet Gynecol 1994; 84:787–793.

45. Cerin A, Heldaas K, Moeller B. Adverse endometrial effects of long-cycle estrogen and progestogen replacement therapy. N Engl J Med 1996; 334:668–669.

46. Groom GV, Griffiths K. Effect of the anti-estrogen tamoxifen on plasma levels of luteinizing hormone, follicle-stimulating hormone, prolactin, estradiol and progesterone in normal premenopausal women. J Endocrinol 1976; 70:421–428.

47. Sherman BM, Chapler FK, Crikard K, Wycoff D. Endocrine consequences of continuous antiestrogen therapy with tamoxifen in premenopausal women. J Clin Invest 1979; 64:398–404.

48. Manni A, Pearson OH. Antiestrogen-induced remissions in premenopausal women with stage IV breast cancer: Effects on ovarian function. Cancer Treat Rep 1980; 64:779–785.

49. Messinis IE, Nillius SJ. Comparison between tamoxifen and clomiphene for induction of ovulation. Acta Obstet Gynecol Scand 1982; 61:377–379.

50. Spicer DV, Pike MC, Henderson BE. Ovarian cancer and long-term tamoxifen in premenopausal women. Lancet 1991; 337:1414.

51. Pike MC, Ross RK, Lobo RA, et al. LHRH agonists and the prevention of breast and ovarian cancer. Br J Cancer 1989; 60:142–148.

52. Spicer D, Shoupe D, Pike MC. GnRH agonists as contraceptive agents: Predicted significantly reduced risk of breast cancer. Contraception 1991; 44:289–310.

53. Rebbeck TR, Levin AM, Eisen A, et al. Breast cancer risk after bilateral prophylactic oophorectomy in BRCA1 mutation carriers. J Natl Cancer Inst 1999; 91:1475–1479.

54. Baum M. Adjuvant treatment of premenopausal breast cancer with zoladex and tamoxifen: Results from the ZIPP trial organized by the Cancer Research Campaign (CRC) Breast Cancer Trials Group (abstr). Breast Cancer Res Treat 1999; 57:30.

55. Spicer DV, Pike MC, Pike A, et al. Pilot trial of a gonadotropin hormone agonist with replacement hormones as a prototype contraceptive to prevent breast cancer. Contraception 1993; 47:427–444.
56. Spicer D, Ursin G, Parisky YR, et al. Changes in mammographic densities induced by a hormonal contraceptive designed to reduce breast cancer risk. J Natl Cancer Inst 1994; 86:431–436.
57. Feig SA. Hormonal reduction of mammographic densities: Potential effects on breast cancer risk and performance of diagnostic and screening mammography. J Natl Cancer Inst 1994; 86:408–409.
58. Kavanagh AM, Mitchell H, Giles GG. Hormone replacement therapy and accuracy of mammography screening. Lancet 2000; 355:270–274.
59. Mandelson MT, Oestreicher N, Porter PL, et al. Breast density as a predictor of mammographic detection: comparison of interval- and screen-detected cancers. J Natl Cancer Inst 2000; 92:1081–1087.
60. Cutler S J, Young JL. Third National Cancer Survey: Incidence Data. National Cancer Institute Monograph 41. 1975.
61. Goebelsmann U, Mishell DR. The menstrual cycle. In Mishell DR, Davajan V, eds. Reproductive Endocrinology, Infertility and Contraception. Philadelphia: Davis, 1979: 67–89.

16

Breast Carcinogenesis and Its Prevention by Inhibition of Estrogen Genotoxicity

Joachim G. Liehr
Stehlin Foundation for Cancer Research
Houston, Texas

I. ABSTRACT

The elevated breast cancer risk associated with prolonged use of estrogen medications has previously been proposed to be based on uncontrolled stimulation of estrogen receptor (ER)–mediated cell proliferation. More recent evidence from human and animal studies points to an additional role of estrogen as precursor of genotoxic metabolites causing DNA damage. From these more recent data, it has been concluded that the natural hormone estradiol is a weak carcinogen and mutagen and induces tumors, including human breast cancer, by a complex interaction of genotoxic and hormonal effects. This mechanistic possibility of breast cancer induction points to several novel pathways of breast cancer prevention by inhibition of the metabolic activation of estrogen to DNA-reactive intermediates. Breast cancer prevention by modulation of estrogen metabolism remains to be explored in future studies.

II. CAUSES OF MAMMARY CARCINOGENESIS

The natural hormones estrone and estradiol (E_2) are generally accepted as carcinogens based on studies in laboratory rodents and in humans [1,2]. In mice or rats, E_2 increases the incidence of tumors of the mammary or pituitary glands, uterus, cervix, vagina, testes, lymphoid system or bone [3–9], whereas in hamsters, estrogens elicit a high incidence of kidney tumors [10]. In humans, a chronic intake of estrogen medications unopposed by progestin has long been accepted by epidemiologists as a risk factor of endometrial adenocarcinoma [11–13]. More recent epidemiological results relating estrogen use to breast cancer have been reviewed by Pike (see Chap. 15). Strong evidence relates breast cancer risk to lifetime exposure to estrogen or elevated plasma or urinary estrogen levels [14–16]. A similar increase in relative breast cancer risk as that obtained by Pike has been identified by a recent meta-analysis of more than 50 studies of hormone replacement therapy and breast cancer risk [17]. Estrogen and progestin combinations are also carcinogenic to humans [2,18].

In summary, the laboratory data document that estrogens, including the natural hormones E_2 and estrone, are carcinogens. In humans, high plasma levels of estrogen elevated either by hormone medications or by an increased endogenous estrogen production raise breast or uterine cancer risk. In contrast to more powerful carcinogens used in laboratory experiments, such as benzo[a]pyrene or 7,12-dimethylbenzanthracene, estrogens may have only weak carcinogenic activity. The weak carcinogenicity of estrogens is indicated by the rather modest 30% increase in relative breast cancer risk after taking estrogen replacement therapy for 5–10 years [16,17]. Various risk factors of breast cancer have been investigated by researchers. A careful examination of the results suggests that steroidal hormones appear to be the only realistic risk factors for the majority of breast cancers. Aromatic hydrocarbon carcinogens, such as 7,12-dimethylbenzanthracene, are environmental pollutants that induce mammary tumors in animals [19–21] at high doses (50–100 mg/kg body weight); thus these compounds do not realistically cause breast cancer in humans. Moreover, although cigarette smoke is a rich source of such aromatic hydrocarbon carcinogens and leads to tumor development in many organ sites of smokers, it does not appear to increase breast cancer risk [22].

Other researchers have focused on organochlorines such as 1,1-dichloro-2,1-bis(p-chlorophenyl)ethylene (DDE) and other pesticides as well as on the polychlorinated biphenyls, which have weak hormonal estrogenic activity and have been implicated as risk factors for breast cancer [23]. However, in a recent meta-analysis of five epidemiological studies, Laden et al., demonstrate that DDE and polychlorinated biphenyls do not increase the risk of human breast cancer [24]. Finally, radiation exposure is a known risk factor for breast cancer [25]. The dose response is linear, and risk is inversely related to age at the time of exposure. However, most women in Europe and North America do not appear to have been exposed to the doses required for tumor induction. Thus, the following text focuses entirely on the mechanism of induction of breast cancer by estrogens rather than by other potential breast cancer–causing agents. It is now well established—from studies in animals, cells in culture, cell-free systems, and epidemiological studies—that estrogen can cause cancer; moreover, estrogen genotoxicity combined with hormone action appears to be the most plausible cause of the epidemic of breast cancer in western countries.

III. DUAL ACTION OF ESTROGEN AS HORMONE AND CARCINOGEN

The failure of estrogens to induce mutations in bacterial or mammalian systems [26–29] has resulted in the classification of estrogens as epigenetic carcinogens, which function mainly by stimulating cancer cell proliferation via receptor-mediated mechanisms [30–33]. Although this view is widely supported, other investigators have obtained experimental evidence incompatible with this generally accepted endocrine mechanism of breast carcinogenesis. Moreover, various types of DNA damage have been induced by catecholestrogen (CE) metabolites in cell-free systems, in cells in culture, or by parent hormones in vivo [34–51] and have been postulated to play a role in carcinogenesis.

The primary evidence contradicting the view that breast cancers develop solely from the stimulation of cell proliferation mediated by estrogen is that the ER is expressed in many primary breast cancers and cancer cell lines but in only a few types of normal human mammary epithelial cells [52]. Moreover, ER protein cannot be detected in proliferating normal human mammary epithelium, which expresses the proliferation marker Ki67 [53,54]. On the other hand, cells containing ER do not express Ki67. These data clearly point to a more complex mechanism of mammary carcinogenesis than previously proposed [30–33].

Genetic experiments have also been carried out to determine the role of the ER in mammary carcinogenesis. For this purpose, ER knockout (ERKO) mice have been cross-bred with mice overexpressing the Wnt-1 gene, because the latter strain develops mammary tumors within a few months after birth [55]. In the cross-bred ERKO/Wnt-1 animals, the onset of mammary tumorigenesis was delayed but not eliminated. Therefore, Wnt-1 protooncogene expression in these animals induces mammary tumors independent of ER status. Moreover, ovariectomy of these ERKO/Wnt-1 animals reduced circulating estrogen levels and also tumor induction. These data point to a role of estrogen in mammary carcinogenesis not mediated by ER and are consistent with E_2 genotoxicity.

Other evidence was obtained by experiments in Syrian hamster, where estrogens induce a nearly 100% incidence of kidney tumors [10]. This incidence of renal tumors is reduced by inhibitors of estrogen metabolism, such as α-naph-thoflavone, or by free radical scavengers such as ascorbic acid (vitamin C) or butylated hydroxyanisol (BHA) [56–58]. In addition, several synthetic estrogens have been identified, such as 2-fluoroestradiol or 17α-ethinylestradiol, which are poorly carcinogenic in this model system compared with the high incidence induced by E_2, despite a high hormonal potency of the synthetic estrogens comparable with that of the natural hormone [10,59,60]. When the metabolism of the modified estrogens was examined in the hope of detecting the reasons for the differing carcinogenic activities, a decreased CE formation was detected from 2-fluoroestradiol and 17α-ethinylestradiol compared with rates of aromatic hydroxylation observed with the parent hormone [61–63]. From these data, it has been concluded that metabolic activation of estrogens to catechol metabolites and further to genotoxic reactive intermediates played an important part in the carcinogenic process [64,65]. Hormonal activity of estrogens via receptor-mediated pathways may be necessary but not sufficient for tumor induction.

IV. MECHANISMS OF TUMOR INITIATION BY E_2

Estrogen-induced genotoxicity and tumor initiation have been examined mainly for CE metabolites because, as discussed above, metabolism studies implicate CE as mediators in the carcinogenesis process and because these metabolites are hydroquinones and therefore easily oxidized to chemically reactive semiquinones and quinones [66]. Specifically, the 4-hydroxylated catechols, 4-hydroxyestradiol and 4-hydroxyestrone, have been proposed to be metabolic intermediates in hormone-induced cancer [64,65], because 4-hydroxyestradiol is as carcinogenic as E_2 in the hamster kidney tumor model [28,67] and nine times as carcinogenic as E_2 in a mouse model of uterine adenocarcinoma [68]. 2-Hydroxyestradiol was less carcinogenic in the mouse uterus and did not induce any tumors in the hamster, most likely due to the rapid methylation (inactivation) of this estrogen metabolite [69]. In the following text, there is a discussion of the metabolic activation of estrogens to CE and specifically to 4-hydroxyestrogens and further to semiquinones and quinones and of the various types of DNA damage and mutations induced by these reactive estrogen intermediates.

The specific conversion of E_2 to 4-hydroxyestradiol has been observed in those organs of rats and mice [70–73] where estrogens induce tumors, such as in the mouse uterus [68], the rat pituitary [74], and in the hamster kidney [10]. In humans, the predominant 4-hydroxylation of E_2 has been detected in uterine myometrium and fibroids [75], in benign and malignant mammary tumors, and in normal mammary tissue [76]. This specific conversion to 4-hydroxylated estrogens is catalyzed by cytochrome P450 1B1 [77] (Fig. 1), whereas the major hepatic and extrahepatic metabolism of E_2 is catalyzed by cytochromes P450 3A

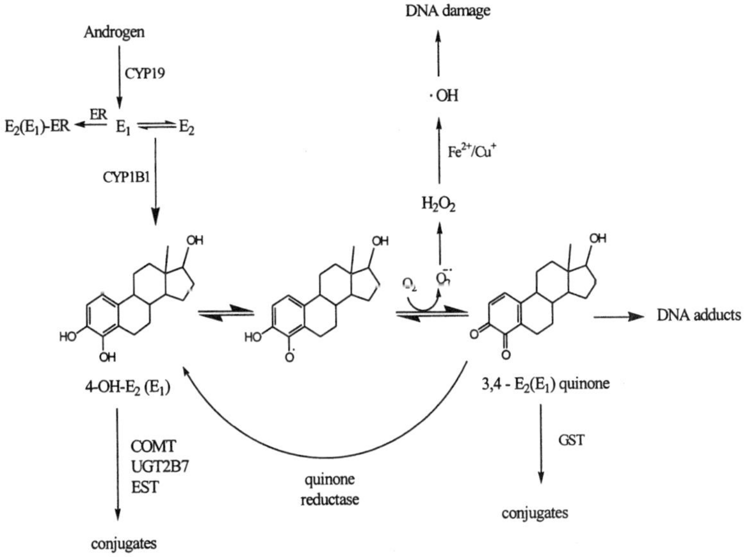

Figure 1 Proposed mechanism of estrogen-induced genotoxicity. Aromatase [CYP19] catalyzes the metabolic conversion of androgen to estrone [E_1]. E_1 or E_2 initiates hormone action by binding to the ER and thus forming an estrogen receptor complex [$E_2(E_1)$-ER]. E_1 or E_2 undergoes 4-hydroxylation catalyzed by CYP1B1. Thus 4-hydroxestradiol (structure shown) or 4-hydroxyestrone [4-OH-$E_2(E_1)$] may undergo metabolic redox cycling by lipid hydroperoxide-dependent oxidation to 3,4-estradiol quinone (structure shown) or 3,4-estrone quinone, respectively [3,4-$E_2(E_1)$ quinone], and subsequently reduction of these quinones back to the catechols catalyzed by NADPH-dependent CYP reductase or other reductase may occur. The estrogen semiquinone radical (structure shown) is an intermediate in each of these one-electron oxidations/reductions and may react with molecular oxygen to form superoxide O_2^-. DNA damage may be induced by hydroxy radicals formed by Fe^{2+}- or Cu^+-mediated reduction of hydrogen peroxide, a product of superoxide. Alternatively, estrogen quinone metabolic intermediates may covalently bind to DNA and form DNA adducts. Detoxification reactions include phase II conjugation of the 4-hydroxylated estrogens 4-OH-$E_2(E_1)$ catalyzed by COMT, UDP glucuronosyl transferase, UGT2B7, or estrogen sulfotransferase (EST), or conjugation of the quinone intermediates 3,4-$E_2(E_1)$ quinone by glutathione transferases (GST). All these conjugation reactions inactivate estrogen metabolites by removing the substrates for metabolic redox cycling. In addition, NADH-dependent quinone reductase inactivates reactive quinone intermediates by two-electron reduction to corresponding CE, bypassing the reactive semiquinone radicals.

and/or 1A enzymes and mainly forms 2-hydroxylated estrogens [78–81]. Based on these data, it has been concluded that the predominant 4-hydroxylation of E_2 occurs in organs or cells prone to estrogen-associated cancer in animals or humans and may lead to high local concentrations of this metabolite to facilitate DNA damage and mutations [64,65], as outlined in Figure 1.

Metabolic redox cycling is a process of activation of CE including 4-hydroxylated estrogens to reactive semiquinone and quinone [66,82]. CEs are oxidized to quinone catalyzed by organic hydroperoxide-dependent cytochrome P450 1A enzymes or by other peroxidases. The reduction of quinone to CE is catalyzed by cytochrome P450 reductase or other reductases. The semiquinone free radical is a reactive intermediate in each of these oxidation/reduction reactions, because these reactions are one-electron oxidations/reductions [82]. In contrast, the reduction of estrogen quinone to CE by NADH-dependent quinone reductase (Fig. 1) is a two-electron reduction reaction, which bypasses the semiquinone intermediate and thus represents a detoxification mechanism [83]. The semiquinone free radical may react with molecular oxygen and produce superoxide and other oxygen radicals by further reduction [82]. Free radicals are also generated by a second nonenzymatic mechanism of redox couples between CE and copper ions [34,39].

V. ESTROGEN-INDUCED DNA DAMAGE AND MUTATIONS

Several classes of estrogen-induced DNA damage have been detected in cell-free systems, in cells in culture, and/or in vivo and have been established by investigations in various laboratories. Metabolic redox cycling of CE, mediated by enzymes or by metal ions, produces oxygen radicals, which subsequently generate the many different types of DNA damage established for oxygen radicals, including single-strand breakage of DNA, 8-hydroxylation of guanine bases, and free radical–mediated lesions arising from the decomposition of lipid hydroperoxides, which generate reactive aldehydes including malondialdehyde [34–42]. This last type of DNA damage and also 8-hydroxyguanine and other oxygen radical–modified bases of DNA have also been detected in human mammary DNA of breast cancer patients [43–45]. It is noteworthy that radiation also generates oxygen radicals and oxygen radical–induced DNA damage. Thus, breast cancer risk may be enhanced by radiation exposure [25] and may result in the same oxygen radical–induced genotoxicity and mutations that are the molecular basis of estrogen-induced genetic lesions. Direct estrogen-DNA adducts have also been described and have been obtained in vitro by incubating DNA with 3,4-estrone quinone or 3,4-estradiol quinone or with a CE and an enzymatic activating system [46–51]. In preliminary experiments, such estrogen-DNA adducts have also been detected in laboratory rodent models [47]. The various types of estrogen-induced genotoxicity have been reviewed in more detail by Liehr [64,65].

Estrogens, including the natural hormone E_2, initially failed to induce point mutations in a series of bacterial and mammalian gene mutation assays such as the *Salmonella typhimurium* (Ames) assay or mutations of the *hprt* gene of V79 Chinese hamster cells [26–29]. However, estrogens generated various types of genetic lesions other than point mutations [84–91], which have been recognized to contribute to genetic instability resulting in the development of tumors [92]. These lesions include alterations in the number of chromosomes (aneuploidy), structural chromosomal translocations, gene amplification, and microsatellite instability [84–91]. More recently, subtle changes in DNA sequence resulting from estrogen exposure have been reexamined, because estrogens have been shown to introduce a low frequency of transformation of Syrian hamster embryo (SHE) cells [91] or MCF-10F human mammary epithelial cells [93] and of mutations in *hprt* gene of V79 and SHE cells [91,94]. Subsequent sequence analyses identified base substitutions (point mutations), deletions, or insertions in the V79 mutant clones [94] and microsatellite instability in MCF-10F cells [93]. In summary, estrogens induce a variety of genetic lesions in cells in culture or in estrogen-induced tumors of rodents (reviewed in more detail by Liehr in Refs. 64 and 65). It is noteworthy that E_2 appears to be a weak mutagen inducing a low frequency of *hprt* gene mutations of V79 cells [94]. This weak mutagenic activity of E_2 may well be the reason for the apparent failure of estrogens to induce mutations in bacterial or mammalian cells reported previously [26–29]. An increased mutagenic activity of CE over that of the parent hormone E_2 has been detected in those experiments, where mutagenicities of estrogen metabolites and of E_2 have been compared [91,95], consistent with the proposed mechanism of E_2 genotoxicity mediated by CE metabolites as shown in Figure 1.

VI. STRATEGIES FOR BREAST CANCER PREVENTION

The proposed mechanism of mammary carcinogenesis is complex and consists of an interplay of both hormonal and carcinogenic effects of estrogens. Tumors may arise from cells transformed by estrogen genotoxicity and mutations and then stimulated to proliferate via receptor-mediated pathways. Mechanistic details of tumor initiation by estrogens are outlined in Figure 1. Tumor promotion and growth by ER-mediated pathways are better known and are thus not reviewed here. The positive aspect of this complexity of breast cancer development is that prevention of cancer may be possible by a larger variety of tools than are thought to be available today. At present, breast cancer prevention is focused almost entirely on modulating the hormonal effects of estrogens. For instance, selective estrogen receptor modulators (SERMs) are designed to inhibit estrogen binding to the ER and thus to inhibit ER-mediated cell proliferation. Tamoxifen has been approved for use as a cancer-preventing agent (see Chap. 20). Raloxifene is undergoing clinical trials to examine its efficacy for cancer treatment and prevention.

Another approach to estrogen-induced and estrogen-dependent breast cancer prevention is the use of an aromatase inhibitor for this purpose (see Chap. 21). Letrozole inhibits the conversion of androgen to estrone and thus lowers concentrations of tumor-inducing and tumor-promoting estrogen. The decrease in endogenous estrogen concentrations by letrozole, while beneficial from the viewpoint of cancer prevention, may, however, be accompanied by undesirable side effects such as increased risk of osteoporosis, hot flushes, and other conditions normally alleviated by circulating estrogen.

A superior approach to breast cancer prevention may consist of inhibiting only the deleterious, genotoxic effects of estrogen metabolites outlined above without altering parent hormone concentrations and the normal hormonal balance. In this way, breast cancer could be prevented and, at the same time, women would not be denied the beneficial effects of estrogens. An inhibition of the genotoxicity of estrogen metabolites potentially may be achieved either by inhibition of the metabolic activation of estrogens to DNA-reactive intermediates or by stimulation of phase II metabolism of the CE.

The inhibition of hepatic estrogen conversion to CE metabolites (CYP3A and/or CYP1A) may not be effective for breast cancer control [78–81]. Although the largest amounts of CE in the body are formed by liver enzymes, these metabolites most likely are further converted to conjugates by hepatic phase II enzymes and excreted [96]. Therefore, for effective breast cancer prevention, it may be necessary to inhibit the local formation in mammary tissue of 4-hydroxyestradiol by CYP1B1 [77]. Unfortunately, inhibitors of this CYP isoform have not yet been described and need to be identified by future research. An elevated breast cancer risk has indeed been identified in women homozygous for the *Leu* allele of CYP1B1, which points to differences in aromatic hydroxylation of estrogens as a risk-determining factor [97].

Another possibility is the induction of quinone reductase to decrease concentrations of DNA-reactive quinone intermediates. Inducers of this enzyme, such as, for instance, Oltipraz, are known but have not yet been tested for the prevention of mammary tumors [98,99]. Quinones may also be scavenged nonenzymatically by sulfur-containing compounds or by ascorbic acid (vitamin C), which reduces quinones to the respective catechol forms [57]. Vitamin C has been shown to inhibit E2-induced tumorigenesis in hamsters [56]. Elevated vitamin C intake has also been reported to lower the risk of breast cancer in humans [100].

The stimulation of phase II enzymes may result in an increased conjugation of CE metabolites, thus decreasing concentrations of the substrates for redox cycling and cancer risk. The inhibition of catechol-O-methyl transferase (COMT) increases the severity of E_2-induced tumors in hamsters [101] and points to a critical role of this enzyme in estrogen inactivation. Moreover, expression of the low-activity allele of COMT in humans is a known risk factor for breast cancer [102]. Unfortunately, inducers of COMT are not known and need to be identified in future studies.

Another approach to reduce the risk of estrogen-induced breast cancer might be to increase the sulfation or glucuronidation of CE. A candidate enzyme for estrogen metabolite conjugation may be UGT2B7, which specifically conjugates 4-hydroxyestrone and 4-hydroxyestradiol [103]. Enzyme inducers such as phenobarbital may activate the glucuronidation and sulfation of CE by UGT2B7 and EST, respectively, and the glutathione conjugation of estrogen quinone metabolites by glutathione transferases (GST), but such inducers have not been explored as preventing agents for breast cancer. Moreover, phase II enzyme inducers with a better side-effect profile will have to be identified to be useful as breast cancer–preventing agents.

VII. CONCLUSION

The studies reviewed above clearly demonstrate the carcinogenic activity of steroidal estrogens in laboratory animals. In humans, exposure to estrogen medications or elevated endogenous production of this hormone is a risk factor for breast cancer. The mechanism of carcinogenesis by estrogens is more complex than previously proposed and involves an interplay of hormonal and genotoxic events. The genotoxicity of estrogens is indicated by the various types of chromosomal and genetic damage and by the slightly elevated yet significant frequency of gene mutations in several test systems. All these studies point to E_2 as a weak carcinogen and weak mutagen. The prevention of mammary carcinogenesis has been explored using SERMs and inhibitors of estrogen biosynthesis (CYP19). Although these approaches to breast cancer prevention may be feasible and useful, they also deprive women of the beneficial effects of estrogens. A superior approach to prevention of estrogen-induced mammary carcinogenesis may be the inhibition of only the deleterious action of estrogen—i.e., the metabolic activation of estrogen metabolites (CE) to DNA reactive metabolic intermediates. Concentrations of estrogen quinone metabolites may be decreased by reducing the quinones to the CE by scavenging the quinones using reducing agents or sulfur-containing compounds. In addition, concentrations of the CE precursor metabolites may be decreased by inhibiting their formation (CYP1B1) or enhancing their phase II conjugation. Unfortunately, these avenues of tumor prevention have not yet been explored and require future studies.

ACKNOWLEDGMENTS

The author wishes to thank Constantine Markides for the drawing of the figure and Carlos Velasquez for the preparation of the manuscript. Studies in the author's laboratory have been funded by the National Cancer Institute, NIH (CA74971).

REFERENCES

1. International Agency for Research on Cancer. Monographs on the Evaluation of Carcinogenic Risks to Humans. Lyon, France: IARC, 1987; 7:280–285.
2. International Agency for Research on Cancer. Monographs on the Evaluation of Carcinogenic Risks to Humans: Hormonal Contraception and Postmenopausal Hormone Therapy. Lyon, France: IARC, 1999;72:288–294.
3. Huseby RA. Demonstration of a direct carcinogenic effect of estradiol on Leydig cells of the mouse. Cancer Res 1980; 40:1006–1013.
4. Highman B, Roth SI, Greenman DL. Osseous changes and osteosarcomas in mice continuously fed diets containing diethylstilbestrol or 17β-estradiol. J Natl Cancer Inst 1987; 67:653–662.
5. Highman B, Greenman DL, Norvell MJ, et al. Neoplastic and preneoplastic lesions induced in female C3H mice by diets containing diethylstilbestrol or 17β-estradiol. J Environ Pathol Toxicol 1980; 4:81–95.
6. Nagasawa H, Mori T, Nakajima Y. Long-term effects of progesterone or diethylstilbestrol with or without estrogen after maturity on mammary tumorigenesis in mice. Eur J Cancer 1980; 16:1583–1589.
7. Inoh A, Kamiah K, Fujii Y, Yokoro K. Protective effects of progesterone and tamoxifen in estrogen-induced mammary carcinogenesis in ovariectomized W/Fu rats. Jpn J Cancer Res 1985; 76:699–704.
8. Noble RL, Hochachka BC, King D. Spontaneous and estrogen-produced tumors in Nb rats and their behaviour after transplantation. Cancer Res 1975; 35:766–780.
9. Shull JD, Spady TJ, Snyder MC, et al. Ovary intact, but not ovariectomized female ACI rats treated with 17β-estradiol rapidly develop mammary carcinoma. Carcinogenesis 1997; 18:1595–1601.
10. Kirkman H. Estrogen-induced tumors of the kidney. III. Growth characteristics in the Syrian hamster. Natl Cancer Inst Monogr 1959; 1:1–57.
11. Greenwald P, Caputo TA, Wolfgang PE. Endometrial cancer after menopausal use of estrogens. Obstet Gynecol 1977; 50:239–243.
12. Key TJA, Pike MC. The dose-effect relationship between "unopposed" estrogens and endometrial mitotic rate: its central role in explaining and predicting endometrial cancer risk. Br J Cancer 1988; 57:205–212.
13. Weiderpass E, Adami H-O, Baron JA, et al. Risk of endometrial cancer following estrogen replacement with and without progestins. J. Natl Cancer Inst 1999; 91:1131–1137.
14. Toniolo PG, Levitz M, Zeleniuch-Jacquotte A, et al. A prospective study of endogeneous estrogens and breast cancer in postmenopausal women. J Natl Cancer Inst 1995; 86:1076–1082.
15. Adlercreutz H, Gorbach SL, Goldin BR, et al. Estrogen metabolism and excretion in Oriental and Caucasian women. J Natl Cancer Inst 1994; 86:1076–1082.
16. Pike M, Bernstein L, Spicer D. Exogenous hormones and breast cancer risk. In Neiderhuber J, ed. Current Therapy in Oncology. St. Louis: Decker, 1993: 292–302.
17. Collaborative group on hormonal factors in breast cancer and hormone replacement therapy: Collaborative reanalysis of data from 51 epidemiological studies of

52,705 women with breast cancer and 108,411 women without breast cancer. Lancet 1997; 350:1047–1059.

18. Ross RK, Paganini-Hill A, Wan PC, Pike MC. Effect of hormone replacement therapy on breast cancer risk: Estrogen vs. estrogen plus progestin. J. Natl Cancer Inst 2000; 16:328–332.

19. Huggins C, Grand LC, Brillantes FP. Critical significance of breast structure in the induction of mammary cancer in the rat. Proc Natl Acad Sci USA 1959; 45:1294–1300.

20. Huggins C, Briziarelli G, Sutton H. Rapid induction of mammary carcinoma in the rat and the influence of hormones on the tumors. J. Exp Med 1959; 109:25–42.

21. Huggins C, Yan NC. Induction and extinction of mammary cancer. Science 1962; 137:257–262.

22. Palmer JR, Rosenberg L. Cigarette smoking and the risk of breast cancer. Epidemiol Rev 1993; 15:145–156.

23. Davis DL, Bradlow HL, Wolff M, et al. Medical Hypothesis: Xenoestrogens as preventable causes of breast cancer. Environ Health Perspect 1993; 101: 372–377.

24. Laden F, Collman G, Iwamoto K, et al. 1,1-Dichloro-2,2-bis(p-chlorophenyl) ethylene and polychlorinated biphenyls and breast cancer: Combined analysis of five U.S. studies. J Nat Cancer Institute 2001; 93:768–775.

25. Boice JD. Radiation and breast carcinogenesis. Med Pediatr Oncol 2001; 36:508–513.

26. Lang R, Redmann U. Non-mutagenicity of some sex hormones in the Salmonella/microsome test. Mutat Res 1979; 67:361–365.

27. Lang R. Reiman R. Studies for a genotoxic potential of some endogenous and exogenous sex steroids. I. Communication: Examination for the induction of gene mutations using the Ames Salmonella/microsome test and the HGPRT test in V79 cells. Environ Mol Mutagen 1993; 21:272–304.

28. Liehr JG, Fang WF, Sirbasku DA, Ari-Ulubelen A. Carcinogenicity of catechol estrogens in Syrian hamsters. J Steroid Biochem 1986; 24:353–356.

29. Drevon C, Piccoli C, Montesano R. Mutagenicity assays of estrogenic hormones in mammalian cells. Mutation Res 1981; 89:83–90.

30. Furth J. Hormones as etiological agents in neoplasia. In Becker FF, ed. Cancer. A Comprehensive Treatise. 1. Etiology: Chemical and Physical Carcinogenesis. New York: Plenum Press, 1982:89–134.

31. Feigelson HS, Henderson BE. Estrogens and breast cancer. Carcinogenesis 1996; 17:2279–2284.

32. Li JJ, Li SA. Estrogen carcinogenesis in hamster tissues: A critical review. Endocr Rev 1990; 11:524–531.

33. Li JJ. Estrogen carcinogenesis in hamster tissues: Update. Endocr Rev 1993; 1:94–95.

34. Li Y, Trush MA, Yager JD. DNA damage caused by reactive oxygen species originating from a copper-dependent oxidation of the 2-hydroxy catechol of estradiol. Carcinogenesis 1994; 15:1421–1427.

35. Ho S-M, Roy D. Sex hormone-induced nuclear DNA damage and lipid peroxidation in the dorsolateral prostates of Noble rats. Cancer Lett 1994; 84:155–162.

36. Han X, Liehr JG. DNA single strand breaks in kidneys of Syrian hamsters treated with steroidal estrogens. Hormone-induced free radical damage preceding renal malignancy. Carcinogenesis 1994; 15:977–1000.

37. Han X, Liehr JG. 8-Hydroxylation of guanine bases in kidney and liver DNA of hamsters treated with estradiol: Role of free radicals in estrogen-induced carcinogenesis. Cancer Res 1994; 54:5515–5517.

38. Han X, Liehr JG. Microsome-mediated 8-hydroxylation of guanine bases of DNA by steroid estrogens: Correlation of DNA damage by free radicals with metabolic activation to quinones. Carcinogenesis 1995; 16:2571–2574.

39. Mobley JA, Bhat AS, Brueggemeier RW. Measurement of oxidative DNA damage by catechol estrogens and analogues in vitro. Chem Res Toxicol 1999; 12:270–277.

40. Nutter LM, Ngo EO, Abul-Hajj YY. Characterization of DNA damage induced by 3,4-estrone-o-quinone in human cells. J Biol Chem 1991; 226:16380–16386.

41. Nutter LM, Wu YY, Ngo EO, et al. An o-quinone form of estrogen produces free radicals in human breast cancer cells: Correlation with DNA damage. Chem Res Toxicol 1994; 7:23–28.

42. Wang MY, Liehr JG. Lipid hydroperoxide-induced endogenous DNA adducts in hamsters: Possible mechanism of lipid hydroperoxide-mediated carcinogenesis. Arch Biochem Biophys 1995; 316:38–46.

43. Malins DC, Holmes EH, Polissar NL, Gunselman SJ. The etiology of breast cancer. Characteristic alteration in hydroxyl radical-induced DNA base lesions during oncogenesis with potential for evaluating incidence risk. Cancer 1993; 71:3036–3043.

44. Malins DC, Polissar NL, Nishikida K, et al. The etiology and prediction of breast cancer. Cancer 1995; 75:503–516.

45. Wang MY, Dhingra K, Hittelman WN, et al. Lipid peroxidation-induced putative malondialdehyde-DNA adducts in human breast tissues. Cancer Epidemiol Biomarkers Prev 1996; 5:705–710.

46. Abul-Hajj YJ, Tabakovic K, Tabakovic I. An estrogen-nucleic acid adduct. Electroreductive inter-molecular coupling of 3,4-estrone-o-quinone and adenine. J Am Chem Soc 1995; 117:6144–6145.

47. Cavalieri EL, Stack DE, Devanesan PD, et al. Molecular origin of cancer: Catechol estrogen-3,4-quinones as endogenous tumor initiators. Proc Natl Acad Sci USA 1997; 94:10937–10942.

48. Roy D. Abul-Hajj YJ. Estrogen-nucleic acid adducts: Guanine is a major site for interaction between 3,4-estrone quinone and CO III gene. Carcinogenesis 1997; 18:1247–1249.

49. Shen L, Qiu S, van Breemen RB, et al. Reaction of the Premarin metabolite 4-hydroxyequilin semiquinone radical with 2′-deoxyguanosine: Formation of unusual cyclic adducts. J Am Chem Soc 1997; 119:11126–11127.

50. Shen L, Qiu S, Chen Y, et al. Alkylation of 2′-deoxynucleosides and DNA by the Premarin metabolite 4-hydroxyequilenin semiquinone radical. Chem Res Toxicol 1998; 11:94–104.

51. Stack DE, Byun J, Gross ML, et al. Molecular characteristics of catechol estrogen quinones in reactions with deoxyribonucleosides. Chem Res Toxicol 1996; 9:851–859.

52. Shoker BS, Jarivs C, Sibson DR, et al. Oestrogen receptor expression in the normal and pre-cancerous breast. J Pathol 1999; 188:237–244.

53. Clarke RB, Howell A, Potten CS, Anderson E. Dissociation between steroid receptor expression and cell proliferation in human breast. Cancer Res 1997; 57:4987–4991.

54. Russo J, Ao X, Grill C, Russo IH. Pattern of distribution of cells positive for estrogen receptor α and progesterone receptor in relation to proliferating cells in the mammary gland. Breast Cancer Res Treat 1999; 53:217–227.

55. Bocchinfuso WP, Hively WP, Couse JF, et al. A mouse mammary tumor virus-Wnt-1 transgene induces mammary gland hyperplasia and tumorigenesis in mice lacking estrogen receptor-α. Cancer Res 1999; 59:1869–1876.

56. Liehr JG, Wheeler WJ. Inhibition of estrogen-induced renal carcinoma in Syrian hamsters by vitamin C. Cancer Res 1983; 43:4638–4642.

57. Liehr JG, Roy D, Gladek A. Mechanism of inhibition of estrogen-induced renal carcinogenesis in male Syrian hamsters by vitamin C. Carcinogenesis 1989; 10:1983–1988.

58. Liehr JG, Gladek A, Macatee T, et al. DNA adduct formation in liver and kidney of male Syrian hamsters treated with estrogen and/or α-naphthoflavone. Carcinogenesis 1991; 12:385–389.

59. Liehr JG. 2-Fluoroestradiol: Separation of estrogenicity from carcinogenicity. Mol Pharmacol 1983; 23:278–281.

60. Liehr JG, Stancel GM, Chorich LP, et al. Hormonal carcinogenesis: Separation of estrogenicity from carcinogenicity. Chem Biol Interact 1986; 59:173–184.

61. Ashburn SP, Han X, Liehr JG. Microsomal hydroxylation of 2- and 4-fluoroestradiol to catechol metabolites and their conversion to methyl ethers: Catechol estrogens as possible mediators of hormonal carcinogenesis. Mol Pharmacol 1993; 43:534–541.

62. Zhu BT, Roy D, Liehr JG. The carcinogenic activity of ethinyl estrogens is determined by both their hormonal characteristics and their conversion to catechol metabolites. Endocrinology 1993; 132:577–583.

63. Stalford AC, Maggs JL, Gilchrist TL, Park BK. Catecholestrogens as mediators of carcinogenesis: Correlation of aromatic hydroxylation of estradiol and its fluorinated analogs with tumor induction in Syrian hamsters. Mol Pharmacol 1994; 45:1259–1267.

64. Liehr JG. Is estradiol a genotoxic mutagenic carcinogen? Endocrinol Rev 2000; 21:40–54.

65. Liehr JG. Genotoxicity of estrogens: A role in cancer development? Hum Reprod Update 2001; 7:1–9.

66. Liehr JG, Ulubelen AA, Strobel HW. Cytochrome P-450–mediated redox cycling of estrogens. J Biol Chem 1986; 261:16865–16870.

67. Li JJ, Li SA. Estrogen carcinogenesis in hamster tissues: Role of metabolism. Fed Proc 1987; 46:1858–1863.

68. Newbold RR, Liehr JG. Induction of uterine adenocarcinoma in CD-1 mice by catechol estrogens. Cancer Res 2000; 60:235–237.

69. Lipsett MB, Merriam GR, Kono S, et al. Metabolic clearance of catechol estrogens. In Merriam GR, ed. Catechol Estrogens. New York: Raven Press, 1983.

70. Liehr JG, Roy D, Ari-Ulubelen A, et al. Effect of estrogen treatment of Syrian hamsters on microsomal enzymes mediating formation of catecholestrogens and their redox cycling: Implications for carcinogenesis. J Steroid Biochem 1990; 35:555–560.

71. Bui QD, Weisz J. Monooxygenase mediating catecholestrogen formation by rat anterior pituitary is an estrogen-4-hydroxylase. Endocrinology 1988; 124:1085–1087.

72. Paria BC, Chakraborty C, Dey SK. Catechol estrogen formation in the mouse uterus and its role in implantation. Mol Cell Endocrinol 1990; 69:25–32.

73. Weisz J, Bui QD, Roy D, Liehr JG. Elevated 4-hydroxylation of estradiol by hamster kidney microsomes: A potential pathway of metabolic activation of estrogens. Endocrinology 1992; 131:655–661.

74. Clifton HK, Meyer RK. Mechanism of anterior pituitary tumor induction by oestrogen. Anat Rec 1956; 125:65–81.

75. Liehr JG, Ricci MJ, Jefcoate CR, et al. 4-Hydroxylation of estradiol by human uterine myometrium and myoma microsomes: Implications for the mechanism of uterine tumorigenesis. Proc Natl Acad Sci USA 1995; 92:9220–9224.

76. Liehr JG, Ricci MJ. 4-Hydroxylation of estrogens as marker of human mammary tumors. Proc Natl Acad Sci USA 1996; 93:3294–3296.

77. Hayes CL, Spink DC, Spink BC, et al. 17β-Estradiol hydroxylation catalyzed by human cytochrome P450 1B1. Proc Natl Acad Sci USA 1996; 93:9776–9781.

78. Guengerich FP. Characterization of human microsomal cytochrome P450 enzymes. Annu Rev Pharmacol Toxicol 1989; 29:241–264.

79. Aoyama T, Korzekwa K, Nagata K, et al. Estradiol metabolism by complementary deoxyribonucleic acid-expressed human cytochrome. Endocrinology 1990; 126: 310–3106.

80. Kerlan V, Dreano Y, Bercovici JP, et al. Nature of cytochrome P450 involved in the 2/4-hydroxylation of estradiol in human liver microsomes. Biochem Pharmacol 1992; 44:174–1756.

81. Hammond DK, Zhu BT, Wang MY, et al. Cytochrome P450 metabolism of estradiol in hamster liver and kidney. Toxicol Appl Pharmacol 1997; 145:54–60.

82. Roy D, Liehr JG. Temporary decrease in renal quinone reductase activity induced by chronic administration of estradiol to male Syrian hamsters. J Biol Chem 1988; 263:3646–3651.

83. Brunmark A, Cadenas E, Lind C, et al. DT-diaphorase-catalyzed two-electron reduction of quinone epoxides. Free Radic Biol Med 1987; 3:181–188.

84. Banerjee SH, Banerjee S, et al. Cytogenetic changes in renal neoplasms and during estrogen-induced carcinogenesis. In Li JJ, Nandi S, Li SA, eds. Hormonal Carcinogenesis. New York: Springer-Verlag, 1992:247–251.

85. Banerjee SK, Banerjee S, Li SA, Li JJ. Induction of chromosome aberrations in Syrian hamster renal cortical cells by various estrogens. Mut Res 1994; 311: 191–197.

86. Tsutsui T, Suzuki N, Fukuda S, et al. 17β-Estradiol-induced cell transformation and aneuploidy of Syrian hamster embryo cells in culture. Carcinogenesis 1987; 8:1715–1719.

87. Tsutsui T, Suzuki N, Maizumi H, Barrett JC. Aneuploidy induction in human fi-

broblasts: Comparison with results in Syrian hamster fibroblasts. Mutation Res 1990; 240:241–249.

88. Tsutsui T, Taguchi S, Tanaka Y, Barrett JC. 17β-Estradiol, diethylstilbestrol, tamoxifen, toremifene, and ICI 164384 induce morphological transformation and aneuploidy in cultured Syrian hamster embryo cells. Int J Cancer 1997; 70: 188–193.

89. Li JJ, Hou X, Banerjee SK, et al. Overexpression and amplification of c-myc in the Syrian hamster kidney during estrogen carcinogenesis: A probable critical role in neoplastic transformation. Cancer Res 1999; 59:2340–2346.

90. Hodgson AV, Ayala-Torres S, Thompson EB, Liehr JG. Estrogen-induced microsatellite DNA alterations are associated with Syrian hamster kidney tumorigenesis. Carcinogenesis 1998; 19:2169–2172.

91. Tsutsui T, Tamura Y, Yagi E, Barrett JC. Involvement of genotoxic effects in the initiation of estrogen-induced cellular transformation: Studies using Syrian hamster embryo cells treated with 17β-estradiol and eight of its metabolites. Int J Cancer 2000; 86:8–14.

92. Lengauer C, Kinzler KW, Vogelstein B. Genetic instabilities in human cancers. Nature 1998; 396:643–649.

93. Russo J, Hu YF, Tahin Q, et al. Carcinogenicty of estrogens in human breast epithelial cells. APMIS 2001; 109:39–52.

94. Kong L-Y, Szaniszlo P, Albrecht T, Liehr JG. Frequency and molecular analysis of HPRT mutations induced by estradiol in Chinese hamster V79 cells. Int J Oncol 2000; 17:1141–1149.

95. Thibodeau PA, Bissonnette N, Bedard SK, et al. Induction by estrogens of methotrexate resistance in MCF-7 breast cancer cells. Carcinogenesis 1998; 19:1545–1552.

96. Raftogianis R, Creveling C, Weinshilboum R, Weisz J. Estrogen metabolism by conjugation. J Natl Cancer Inst Monogr 2000; 27:113–124.

97. Zheng W, Xie DW, Jin F, et al. Genetic polymorphism of cytochrome P450-1B1 and risk of breast cancer. Cancer Epidemiol Biomarkers Prev 2000; 9:147–150.

98. Kensler TW, Groopman JD, Sutter TR, et al. Development of cancer chemopreventive agents: Oltipraz as a paradigm. Chem Res Toxicol 1999; 12:113–126.

99. Benson AM, Barretto PB, Stanley JS. Induction of DT-diaphorase by anticarcinogenic sulfur compounds in mice. J Natl Cancer Inst 1986; 76:467–473.

100. Howe GR, Hirohata R, Hislop TG, et al. Dietary factors and risk of breast cancer: Combined analysis of 12 case-control studies J Natl Cancer Inst 1990; 82:561.

101. Zhu BT, Liehr JG. Quercetin increases the severity of estradiol-induced tumorgenesis in hamster kidney. Toxicol Appl Pharmacol 1994; 125:149–158.

102. Thompson PA, Ambrosone C. Chapter 7: Molecular epidemiology of genetic polymorphisms in estrogen metabolizing enzymes in human breast cancer. J Natl Cancer Inst Monogr 2000; 27:125–134.

103. Ritter JK, Sheen YY, Owens IS. Cloning and expression of human liver UDP-glucuronosyltransferase in COS-1 cells. J Biol Chem 1990; 265:7900–7906.

17

Use of Selective Antiestrogens for the Chemoprevention of Breast Cancer

Trevor J. Powles
Royal Marsden Hospital
Sutton, Surrey, England

I. ABSTRACT

Most breast cancers have a sensitivity to estrogen, which contributes to their progression. Therefore it has been postulated that antiestrogens could be used to chemoprevent breast cancer. Selective estrogen receptor modulators (SERMs) are antiestrogens with some beneficial estrogenic effects, causing a lowering of cholesterol and preservation of bone mineral density in postmenopausal women. This chapter covers the data from trials using SERMs, especially tamoxifen, for the chemoprevention of breast cancer in healthy women.

II. INTRODUCTION

The use of antiestrogenic intervention to chemoprevent breast cancer is an attractive proposition because of the likelihood that most occult breast cancers need estrogen to promote their development into overt clinical tumors. Epidemiological evidence that early ovarian ablation protects against breast cancer and the observed reduction in contralateral breast cancer in women who receive adjuvant tamoxifen after treatment for primary breast cancer [1] encouraged the commencement of randomized, placebo-controlled trials in healthy women. Tamoxifen is a promising candidate for clinical testing owing to its extensive use in over 20 years of clinical practice and established low toxicity in the treatment of women with breast cancer.

In 1986, a feasibility trial of tamoxifen versus placebo was started at the Royal Marsden Hospital (RMH) to evaluate acute toxicity, safety, acceptability, and compliance in healthy women at increased risk of breast cancer because of a family history. In this trial, compliance was excellent and the acute toxicity of tamoxifen was low, indicating that tamoxifen was a suitable agent for large, multicenter chemoprevention trials [2]. Of added benefit, the safety monitoring in this feasibility trial indicated that tamoxifen was a "selective" antiestrogen (or SERM) with some estrogenic effects, causing a lowering of cholesterol and preservation of bone mineral density in postmenopausal women [2,3]. Because of delays in starting a national multicenter trial in the United Kingdom, the feasibility trial continued into a pilot trial, which by 1996 had recruited 2500 women.

Since 1992, several trials—the UK National trial (International Breast Cancer Intervention Study, or IBIS), followed by trials in the United States (National Surgical Adjuvant Breast Project, or NSABP) and in Italy (Italian National Trial, INT)—have provided data on the efficacy of tamoxifen in the chemoprevention of breast cancer.

In addition, in 1994, a trial was initiated to evaluate another SERM, raloxifene, in the prevention of osteoporosis. This trial included mammography to detect a secondary endpoint of breast cancer incidence (Multiple Outcomes of Raloxifene, or MORE).

Other trials with SERMs are proposed or under way with the objective of producing an antiestrogenic agent for the chemoprevention of breast cancer. Some of the tested SERMs may offer more attractive spectra of overall activity than tamoxifen, having multiple health benefits to healthy women, including the prevention of osteoporotic fractures, cardiovascular disease, menopausal symptoms including vasomotor symptoms, and other postmenopausal problems.

III. NSABP P-1 TRIAL

Between June 1992 and September 1993 the NSABP P-1 trial accrued a total of 13,388 women, 6681 randomized to tamoxifen (20 mg per day) and 6707 to placebo for 5 years. Eligibility depended on women having an estimated 5-year risk of breast cancer of about 1.66% (16.6/1000/5 years) as determined by the Gail model, taking into account being 60 years old or, if younger, by having additional risk factors such as a family history, previous benign breast biopsy, nulliparity, or early menarche [4]. Women with a previous history of lobular carcinoma in situ were also eligible.

An interim analysis, published in 1998, after a median follow-up of 54.6 months, showed that the tamoxifen-treated group developed 86 fewer breast cancers than the placebo group, indicating a 49% reduction in the early incidence of breast cancer [5]. Although in this trial assessment of mortality was a primary endpoint, the data monitoring committee considered that the highly significant (p=0.00001) reduction in early incidence of breast cancer at the time of this interim analysis justified the termination and unblinding of the trial before completion of the planned follow-up. Because of this unblinding, no further analyses of this trial for primary endpoints were possible.

Although there were 86 fewer breast cancers in women who received tamoxifen, this interim analysis showed an increase in the frequency of thromboembolic events, endometrial cancer, and cataracts. Without more clinical data, it is not possible to balance these potential long-term hazards against the benefits of a reduced breast cancer incidence, especially because we cannot be sure that the appearance of these cancers was not simply delayed instead of prevented or that they could not have been as easily treated as they occurred rather than treating the whole population of healthy women.

IV. THE ROYAL MARSDEN TRIAL (RMH TRIAL)

The Royal Marsden feasibility trial had shown that it would be possible to perform large multicenter chemoprevention trials of tamoxifen in 1991, but—because of delays in starting the UK National IBIS trial—the feasibility trial extended into a pilot trial in its own right [2]. Prior calculations on the Royal Marsden feasibility trial in 1991 had indicated that if accrual of 2500 women were completed, there would be a 90% chance of detecting a 50% reduction in breast cancer incidence by 1998. Therefore, recruitment was completed at 2500 patients. Between October 1986 and April 1996, a total of 2494 eligible women were randomized to tamoxifen 20 mg per day or placebo. The median age of participants was 47 years and 34% of the women were postmenopausal. Use of hormone replacement therapy (HRT) was allowed either at the time of randomization or subsequently if required. HRT was used during 13% of the tamoxifen medication period. In 1998, the planned interim analysis of this pilot trial showed an identical incidence of breast cancer for women on tamoxifen and placebo [6]. There was no evidence of any negative interaction between HRT and tamoxifen on breast cancer incidence.

It could be argued that this negative result is statistically compatible with the reduction in incidence reported from the NSABP trial. However, it is much more likely that the differences in chemopreventive effects observed between trials relates to the different risk characteristics of the participants in these trials. In the Royal Marsden trial, participants were younger than in the NSABP P-1 trial and were more likely to have inherited a high-penetrance breast cancer–predisposing gene. High-risk benign histology such as lobular carcinoma in situ or atypical hyperplasia was not included in the entry criteria for the Royal Marsden trial. These risk factors were shown to confer the greatest sensitivity to tamoxifen chemoprevention in the NSABP P-1 trial. It is therefore possible that the participants in the Royal Marsden trial are relatively resistant to tamoxifen chemoprevention compared to those in the NSABP P-1 trial.

V. ITALIAN NATIONAL TRIAL (INT)

In this trial, performed between October 1992 and July 1997, a total of 5408 healthy women aged between 35 and 70 were randomized to tamoxifen 20 mg per day or placebo. All participants were hysterectomized (74% of the patients had also had oophorectomy and 14% of the patients were on HRT). An interim analysis of this trial reported in 1998 showed no statistical difference in the incidence of breast cancer between women on tamoxifen and those on placebo [7]. However, it was noted that there was a significant reduction in the incidence of breast cancer for women on HRT who received tamoxifen. This indicated that any chemopreventive effect of tamoxifen might have been compromised by oophorectomy unless the women were also receiving HRT.

VI. IBIS TRIAL

Between 1992 and 2000, over 7000 women were accrued to this trial and randomized to receive tamoxifen 20 mg per day or placebo. A family history of breast cancer and other risk factors, including abnormal benign histology, were required for eligibility, giving an overall increase in the risk of breast cancer of about two- to threefold. No results are available to date from this trial, but the first interim analysis of breast cancer incidence is scheduled for 2002.

VII. RALOXIFENE (MORE AND CORE TRIALS)

Raloxifene, a SERM that is structurally unrelated to tamoxifen, has been shown to be potentially beneficial for the prevention of loss of bone in postmenopausal women. In 1994, a double-blind, randomized trial of raloxifene versus placebo (MORE) was started to evaluate the effect of raloxifene on the prevention of fractures in healthy postmenopausal women with osteoporosis detected by bone mineral density [8]. As a secondary endpoint, annual mammography was offered to all women to screen for breast cancer. After 30 months of follow-up, there was a significant reduction in the incidence of fractures. This was associated with a reduction in the incidence of breast cancer by over 80% for women on raloxifene [8,9]. There was no proliferative effect on the uterus. Raloxifene has now been approved for treatment and prevention of osteoporosis but has not been accepted by the regulatory authorities for licensing for risk reduction of breast cancer because the breast cancer incidence data were only a secondary endpoint in this study. Continued follow-up of the MORE trial (CORE trial) with breast cancer incidence as a primary endpoint has now been agreed on and results from this should be available within the next two years.

VIII. FUTURE TRIALS USING OTHER SERMS

Results of the NSABP P-1 trial and the MORE trial have strongly indicated that in some populations of women, the use of selective antiestrogens can reduce the early incidence of breast cancer. Following the results of these trials, the NSABP started a new trial in postmenopausal women at moderate risk of breast cancer, as determined by the Gail model, to directly compare tamoxifen 20 mg per day with raloxifene 60 mg per day. This trial has no placebo arm and its primary objective is to compare efficacy between tamoxifen and raloxifene on the early incidence of breast cancer and to compare the acute toxicity of the two agents, particularly their effects on other tissues, such as the uterus. This trial will randomize a total of 22,000 women; to date, 8000 women have been randomized. Because of the lack of a placebo control arm, this trial will not show the overall efficacy or clinical benefit of tamoxifen or raloxifene.

Further information regarding efficacy and clinical benefit can only now come from the continued follow-up of the ongoing placebo-controlled trials (RMH, IBIS, INT, and CORE). As other selective antiestrogens are developed, they will be considered for chemoprevention in healthy women, particularly if they have an attractive spectrum of activity. This could include the ability to reduce the incidence of breast cancer, osteoporotic fractures, cardiovascular disease, uterine cancer, vasomotor menopausal symptoms, atrophy of the urogenital tract, and menopausal symptoms. Ideally, such an agent should not increase the risk of thromboembolism, cataract, or cancer. It is possible that such agents already exist; if they are proven to be efficacious for treatment of breast cancer, especially as adjuvant therapy for patients with primary breast cancer, they should be considered as potential chemopreventive agents in healthy women. Within this strategy, it will also become increasingly important to identify which women are likely to gain benefit from selective antiestrogens, so that large numbers of healthy women are not exposed to potential risk unnecessarily.

REFERENCES

1. Cuzick J, Baum M. Tamoxifen and contralateral breast cancer (letter). Lancet 1985; 2:282.
2. Powles T, Hardy J, Ashley S, et al. A pilot trial to evaluate the acute toxicity and feasibility of tamoxifen for prevention of breast cancer. Br J Cancer 1989; 60:126–131.

3. Powles TJ, Hickish T, Kanis JA, et al. Effect of tamoxifen on bone mineral density measured by dual-energy x-ray absorptiometry in health premenopausal and post-menopausal women. J Clin Oncol 1996; 14:78–84.

4. Gail M, Brintom L, Byar D, et al. Projecting individualised probabilities of developing breast cancer for white females who are examined annually. J Natl Cancer Inst 1989; 81:1879–1886.

5. Fisher B, Costantino JP, Wickerham DL, et al. Tamoxifen for prevention of breast cancer: Report of the National Surgical Adjuvant Breast and Bowel Project P-1 Study. J Natl Cancer Inst 1998; 90:1371–1388.

6. Powles T, Eeles R, Ashley S, et al. Interim analysis of the incidence of breast cancer in the Royal Marsden Hospital tamoxifen randomised chemoprevention trial. Lancet 1998; 352:98–101.

7. Veronesi U, Maisonneuve P, Costa A, et al. Prevention of breast cancer with tamoxifen: Preliminary findings from the Italian randomised trial among hysterectomised women. Lancet 1998; 352:93–97.

8. Ettinger B, Black DM, Mitlak BH, et al. Reduction of vertebral fracture risk in post-menopausal women with osteoporosis treated with raloxifene: Results from a 3-year randomised clinical trial. Multiple outcomes of Raloxifene Evaluation (MORE) Investigators. JAMA 1999; 282:637–645.

9. Cummings SR, Eckert S, Krueger KA, et al. Raloxifene reduces the risk of breast cancer and may decrease the risk of endometrial cancer in postmenopausal women. Two-year findings from the multiple outcomes of raloxifene evaluation (MORE) trial. Proc ASCO 1998; 17:2a.

18

Aromatase Inhibitors and Chemoprevention of Breast Cancer

Paul E. Goss
University of Toronto
Princess Margaret Hospital
University Health Network
Toronto, Ontario, Canada

I. ABSTRACT

Epidemiological and experimental evidence strongly supports a role for estrogens in the development and growth of breast tumors. As a result, efforts to decrease estrogen production are being explored as a strategy to reduce breast cancer risk. One method to accomplish this is by inhibiting the enzyme aromatase, which catalyzes the final rate-limiting step in estrogen biosynthesis. The use of biomarkers for breast cancer risk will be essential, not only for selecting women for inclusion in trials of putative chemoprevention agents but also for establishing their efficacy at intermediate time points. Some of the candidate biomarkers are discussed here, along with the rationale for utilizing aromatase inhibitors (AIs) as chemopreventives, and an overview of some of the ongoing chemoprevention trials utilizing AIs are reviewed.

II. INTRODUCTION

The role of estrogens in the initiation and promotion of breast cancer is well established [1]. Since aromatase inhibitors have been shown to reduce tissue levels of estrogen, their role as chemopreventives is of interest. In addition to reducing cell proliferation, their ability to prevent the formation of genotoxic metabolites of estrogens could also be of benefit. Tamoxifen and other selective estrogen receptor modulators (SERMs) are able to antagonize both circulating and locally produced estrogens by blocking the estrogen receptor (ER) on breast epithelial cells. Tamoxifen (20 mg daily) has been shown to reduce preinvasive and invasive breast cancers in the National Surgical Adjuvant Breast and Bowel Project P-1 Trial [2]. This agent was, however, associated with an increase in endometrial cancer and thromboembolism [2]. It is expected that the third-generation aromatase inhibitors via their reduction of both circulating, and locally produced, estrogen should also prevent the proposed carcinogenic effects of hormones without causing the adverse effects of tamoxifen. The excellent tolerability and efficacy of the most recently developed third-generation aromatase inhibitors in the treatment of breast cancer might lead to their use as chemopreventives in healthy women considered to be at risk. Studies are ongoing to evaluate their ability to alter surrogate biomarkers of breast cancer risk.

In the meantime, observations in the reduction of contralateral breast cancer from ongoing adjuvant trials are expected to provide the first evidence that aromatase inhibitors prevent breast cancer. In this chapter, we review useful clinical surrogate biomarkers of breast cancer risk and the use of aromatase inhibitors as chemopreventives.

III.   ESTROGEN AND BREAST CANCER RISK

Estrogens exert both direct and indirect proliferative effects on cultured breast cancer cells from humans and in vivo promote the development of mammary cancer in animal models. Proposed mechanisms by which estrogens are considered carcinogenic to the breast include alkylation of cellular molecules, generation of active radicals, and the potential genotoxicity of some estrogen metabolites (e.g., the catechol estrogens) (see Chap. 19) [3,4].

The risk of breast cancer is increased with early menarche, late first full-term pregnancy, and late menopause. A decreased risk is associated with late menarche, early and multiple pregnancies, and early menopause [5,6]. These observations support the model that cumulative exposure to estrogen plays a role in the risk of breast cancer.

In keeping with this model—that cumulative exposure of estrogen increases the risk of breast cancer—estrogen-replacement therapy has been implicated as a risk factor [7–9]. The increased risk of breast cancer increases even more with the administration of combined estrogen-progestin compared to estrogen alone [10].

IV. ESTROGEN SYNTHESIS

In addition to an increased risk of breast cancer with high levels of circulating estrogen, local estrogen synthesis may play a role in the development of breast cancer [11]. For example, aromatase activity in the breast may contribute to the development of breast cancer. Aromatase overexpression in the breast has thus been hypothesized as an indirect cause of breast cancer [12].

The polymorphism of the CYP19 gene, encoding the P450 aromatase, has been identified in the general population. Genetic variations of this gene may be implicated in an increased risk of breast cancer [13]. Studies are ongoing to confirm this. The reason for the overexpression of the gene might be an increase in enhancers of transcription [14] or the loss of a constitutive silencer acting on the promoter region [15,16]. In this regard, our group is researching the possibility that the aromatase gene could act as an oncogene.

V. BIOMARKERS OF ESTROGEN EXPOSURE AND BREAST CANCER RISK

The Gail model is commonly used to identify the risk of breast cancer. Although it has been validated in a number of clinical settings, it has limitations. For example, it does not fully account for genetic risk factors such as known genetic mutation carrier status (*BRCA1* or *BRCA2*) and does not take into account the age of onset in first-degree relatives with breast cancer. The model also does not accurately predict risk for all subsets of the general population, such as ethnic minorities. Clinical biomarkers—such as bone density, plasma estradiol levels, or breast density—that measure estrogen exposure may be useful additions to assessing the risk for the development of breast cancer.

A. Bone Density

A correlation between early menarche, late menopause, high parity, and bone mineral density supports the theory that bone mineral density may serve as a biomarker to cumulative estrogen exposure [17,18]. This holds factually, as estrogen is a determinant of bone mineral density. In the Framingham study of 1373 women, women with bone density in the highest quartile had an incidence of breast cancer 3.5 times higher than that of women in the lowest quartile [19]. This was one of the first studies to indicate that cumulative estrogen exposure may be ascertained by bone mineral density and related to the risk of breast cancer.

B. Serum Estrogen Concentrations

The most important surrogate biomarker for evaluating the risk of developing breast cancer is the plasma estradiol level. The higher the plasma estradiol level, the greater the risk of breast cancer. In a study conducted by Key, plasma concentrations of estradiol and several other hormones linked to breast cancer were databased and compared among female populations in China and Britain. Higher plasma estradiol levels were associated with a greater risk of developing breast cancer [20].

C. Breast Density

It has also been shown that women who have dense breasts, as detected on an annual screening mammogram, are at a greater risk for breast cancer [21–23]. In one large study, the relative risk of breast cancer was 6.0 (95 percent confidence interval, 2.8 to 12.9) for women in the highest category of breast density compared with those in the lowest category [21]. Breast density as revealed by mammography could prove to be a useful tool for assessing chemopreventive therapies.

VI. PREVENTING THE EFFECTS OF ESTROGENS

A. SERMs and Aromatase Inhibitors

In the National Surgical Adjuvant Breast and Bowel Project P-1 Trial, tamoxifen was shown to reduce the incidence of breast cancer in healthy women who were at increased risk of developing the disease [2]. Tamoxifen and other SERMs are able to antagonize the hormone by blocking both locally produced and circulating estrogen on breast epithelial cells. Aromatase inhibitors can be expected to have the same beneficial effect while having the further potential to reduce carcinogenic catechol metabolites in both compartments. It is possible that the parent estrogen compounds may promote tumor growth, but it is the catechol estrogen metabolites that are responsible for the initiation of the cancer. If this model were accurate, the aromatase inhibitors would be true chemopreventives, whereas the antiestrogens would act as chemosuppressants, blocking tumor progression but not initiation.

B. Nutritional or Nutraceutical Methods

Regarding nutraceuticals or nutrition and the prevention of breast cancer, there are growing epidemiological data to suggest that flaxseed prevents breast and colon cancer [24,25]. Its mechanism of action is not fully understood, but is being actively researched. Flaxseed is an abundant source of plant lignans, which in the body are converted to the mammalian lignans enterodiol and enterolactone. These molecules bear structural homology to tamoxifen and estrogen and have weak antiestrogenic effects (Fig. 1). It seems that they can bind to the ER and inhibit aromatase activity (although much more weakly than the third-generation AIs). It is possible that these compounds might also alter the metabolic

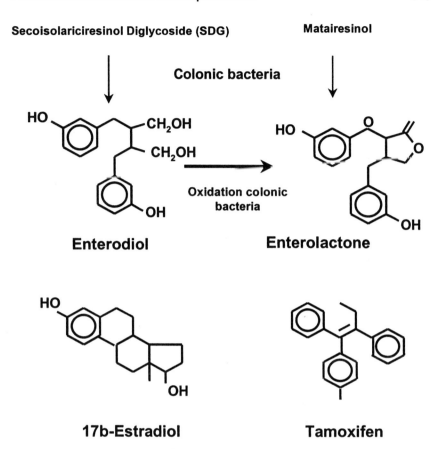

Figure 1 The structure of the active components of flaxseed and their comparison with the structures of estradiol and tamoxifen.

pathway of estrogen. We are seeking to determine whether a change in the ratio of the hydroxylated to methoxylated estrogen metabolites produced by these lignans might reduce cancer risk. In a randomized, double-blind, placebo-controlled study at Princess Margaret Hospital, we examined the effect of flaxseed consumption on preoperative tumor development in 55 women [26]. During the 4–5 week period between initial biopsy and tumor excision, patients consumed daily a muffin containing either 25 g of flaxseed or placebo. Results of this proof-of-principle study demonstrated a 33% reduction in the proliferation marker Ki67 and a statistically significant reduction in the expression of c-ErbB2 ($p=0.04$) (we are currently uncertain about the apoptotic index results; these await confirmation) [26].

C. Our Experience with the Compound Liarozole

Liarozole fumarate is an interesting compound with two separate mechanisms of action (Fig 2). It is a potent aromatase inhibitor (although not completely specific) and a retinomimetic—it blocks the metabolism of retinoic acid, thus allowing it to accumulate in the cell and thereby prolonging its action. The development of this drug has now been discontinued, but phase II studies in postmenopausal patients showed promising results in both ER-positive breast cancer after tamoxifen and in ER-negative tumors [27,28]. A dual mechanism, however, such as that exhibited by liarozole, could be of value in our development of chemopreventive compounds.

Retinoids are known to prevent estrogen stimulation of the uterus, so it was interesting to investigate whether liarozole could prevent the endometrial hypertrophy that is induced by tamoxifen. We found a dose-dependent blockade of the uterine stimulation in the immature rat uterine model. This effect was not seen for the combination of vorozole and tamoxifen, so the result seems to be due to the retinomimetic action of liarozole. Thus, if we could exploit this kind of activity in our search for future drugs, we might find molecules that have more universal applicability—agents that might have a chemoprevention effect for both ER-positive and ER-negative tumors and that could avoid some of the adverse effects that we see today with compounds like tamoxifen.

VII. CHEMOPREVENTIVE TRIALS WITH AROMATASE INHIBITORS

Chemopreventive pilot studies with aromatase inhibitors are in planning or under way in postmenopausal women. The target populations of these studies in-

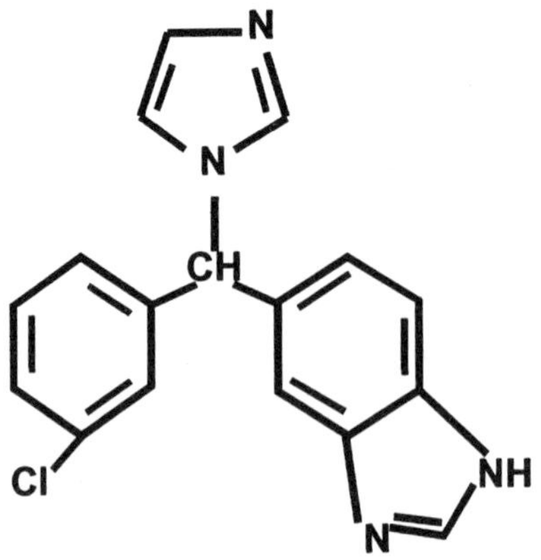

Figure 2 The structure of liarozole.

clude cohorts of women at risk for breast cancer with specific biomarkers such as high breast density, elevated estradiol levels, or premalignant breast lesions.

The National Cancer Institute of Canada is conducting a double-blind, multicenter pilot trial to evaluate the effects of letrozole on breast density in postmenopausal women treated with letrozole or placebo for 1 year. A total of 137 healthy postmenopausal women with high breast density (Norman Boyd's grade of 4–6) are being enrolled to receive either letrozole 2.5 mg every day or placebo. The primary endpoint of the study includes examination of mammographic changes with letrozole; secondary endpoints include examination of bone mineral density, lipid levels, and directed core biopsy for future correlative science studies.

Other chemoprevention pilot trials include a study being conducted by Fabian et al. of high-risk women with atypical hyperplasia or epithelial hyperplasia as assessed by the use of periareolar fine needle aspirates, whether an aromatase inhibitor can reduce the hyperplasia and/or allow for less progression of epithelial hyperplasia to atypical hyperplasia. Lønning et al. have an ongoing study of postmenopausal women with in situ cancer (DCIS) and low-risk invasive cancer T1 and are examining whether aromatase inhibitors decrease proliferative fraction and estrogen receptors and decrease the serum IGF-1. Finally, Dowsett et al. are evaluating aromatase inhibitors and their ability to alter surrogate and biomarkers of breast cancer risk in postmenopausal women with DCIS.

The International Breast Cancer Intervention Study 2 (IBIS-2), a follow-up study to IBIS-1, is planned to investigate the chemopreventive effects of tamoxifen and anastrozole (each alone) and comparing them to placebo in 16,000 patients. Of these 10,000 women are considered at high risk based on their family history and other factors, while 6000 have been diagnosed with ductal carcinoma in situ. This study is planned to begin in late 2001.

VIII. CONCLUSION

The link between estrogen and breast cancer has been well established. Aromatase inhibitors, which inhibit estrogen production, have attracted attention as being potential chemopreventive agents. Future trials will explore the efficacy of aromatase inhibitors in this role along with assessing their long-term safety and effect on quality of life. Although this strategy seems reasonable for ER-positive tumors, it remains much less sure for ER-negative tumors, and we still do not know if these two phenotypes arise from the same precursor tumor cell. The proportion of ER-positive cells within a tumor increases with increasing malignancy risk until one reaches the invasive tumor state, in which the ER-negative cells again form a substantial part. If this turns out to be a conversion of ER-positive to ER-negative cells, then perhaps the strategy of chemoprevention, using compounds that modulate the endocrine environment, will suffice. If, however, they arise through separate mutations, alternative chemotherapeutic agents will have to be developed in tandem. In the meantime, it seems reasonable to expect that postmenopausal women with elevated estrogen levels and increased bone mineral density could beneficially be given small doses of aromatase inhibitors for the prevention of breast cancer.

REFERENCES

1. Beatson GT. On the treatment of inoperable cases of carcinoma of the mamma: Suggestions for a new method of treatment, with illustrative cases. Lancet 1896; 2:104–107.
2. Fisher B, Costantino JP, Wickerham DL, et al. Tamoxifen for prevention of breast cancer: Report of the National Surgical Adjuvant Breast and Bowel Project P-1. J Natl Cancer Inst 1998; 90:1371–1388.
3. Nandi S, Guzman RC, Yang J. Hormones and mammary carcinogenesis in mice, rats, and humans: A unifying hypothesis. Proc Natl Acad Sci USA 1995; 92:3650–3657.
4. Yager JD, Liehr JG. Molecular mechanisms of estrogen carcinogenesis. Annu Rev Pharmacol Toxicol 1996; 36:203–232.
5. Rosner B, Colditz GA. Nurses' health study: log-incidence mathematical model of breast cancer incidence. J Natl Cancer Inst 1996; 88:359–364.
6. Pattenbarger RS Jr, Kampert JB, Chang HG. Characteristics that predict risk of breast cancer before and after menopause. Am J Epidemiol 1980; 112:258–268.
7. Collaborative Group on Hormonal Factors in Breast Cancer. Breast cancer and hormone receptor replacement therapy: collaborative reanalysis of data from 51 epidemiological studies of 52,705 women with breast cancer and 108,411 women without breast cancer. Lancet 1997; 350:1047–1059. [Erratum, Lancet 1997; 350:1484.]
8. Persson I, Weiderpass E, Bergkvist L, et al. Risks of breast and endometrial cancer after estrogen and estrogen-progestin replacement. Cancer Causes Control 1999; 10:253–260.
9. Magnusson C, Baron JA, Carreia N, et al. Breast-cancer risk following long-term oestrogen- and oestrogen-progestin replacement therapy. Int J Cancer 1999; 81:339–344.
10. Schairer C, Lubin J, Troisi R, et al. Menopausal estrogen and estrogen-progestin replacement therapy and breast cancer risk. JAMA 2000; 283:485–491.
11. Clemons M, Goss PE. Estrogen and risk of breast cancer. N Engl J Med 2001; 4:276–285.
12. Harada N. Aberrant expression if aromatase in breast cancer tissues. J Steroid Biochem Mol Biol 1997; 61:175–184.
13. Siegelmann-Danieli N, Buetoa KH. Constitutional genetic variation at the human aromatase gene (Cyp 19) and breast cancer risk. Br J Cancer 1999; 79:456–463.
14. Chen S, Zhou D, Okubo T, et al. Breast tumor aromatase: functional role and transcriptional regulation. Endocr Rel Cancer 1999; 6:149–156.
15. Jin T, Branch DR, Zhang X, et al. Examination of POU homeobox gene expression in human breast cancer cells. Int J Cancer 1999; 81:104–112.

16. Jin T, Zhang X, Li H, Goss PE. Characterization of a novel silencer element in the human aromatase gene PII promoter. Breast Cancer Res Treat 2000; 62:151–159.

17. Cauley JA, Gutai JP, Sandler RB, et al. The relationship of endogenous estrogen to bone density and bone area in normal post-menopausal women. Am J Epidemiol 1986; 124:752–761.

18. Zhang Y, Kiel DP, Kreger BE, et al. Bone mass and the risk of breast cancer among post-menopausal women. N Engl J Med 1997: 336:611–617.

19. Persson I, Adami HO, McLaughlin JK, et al. Reduced risk of breast and endometrial cancer among women with hip fractures (Sweden). Cancer Causes Control 1994; 5:523–528.

20. Key TJ, Chen J, Wang DY, et al. Sex hormones in women in rural China and in Britain. Br J Cancer 1990; 62:631–636.

21. Boyd NF, Byng JW, Jong RA, et al. Quantitative classification of mammographic densities and breast cancer risk: Results from the Canadian National Breast Screening Study. J Natl Cancer Inst 1995; 87:670–675.

22. Brisson J, Sadowsky NJ, Twaddle JA, et al. The relation of mammographic features of the breast to breast cancer risk factors. Am J Epidemiol 1982; 115:438–443.

23. Saftlas AF, Hoover RN, Brinton LA, et al. Mammographic densities and risk of breast cancer. Cancer 1991; 67:2833–2838.

24. Serraino M, Thompson LU. The effect of flaxseed supplementation on early risk markers for mammary carcinogenesis. Cancer Lett 1991; 60:135–142.

25. Haggans CJ, Travelli EJ, Thomas W, et al. The effect of flaxseed and wheat bran consumption on urinary estrogen metabolism in pre-menopausal women. Cancer Epidemiol Biomarkers Prev 2000; 9:719–725.

26. Thompson LU, Goss PE. (abstr 50). Breast Cancer Res Treat 2000; 64:50

27. Goss PE, Oza A, Goel R, et al. Liarozole furmate (R85246): A novel imidazole in the treatment of receptor positive post-menopausal metastatic breast cancer. Breast Cancer Res Treat 2000; 59:55–68.

28. Goss PE, Strasser K, Marques R, et al. Liarozole fumarate (R85246) in the treatment of ER negative, tamoxifen refractory or chemotherapy resistant post-menopausal metastatic breast cancer. Breast Cancer Res Treat 2001; 64:177–188.

Panel Discussion 4

Chemoprevention

Christopher C. Benz and Anthony Howell, *Chairmen*
Tuesday, June 26, 2001

C. Benz: Given the diverse group of speakers we have had this afternoon, I thought it would be helpful to try and introduce our discussion session with a general set of "what, when, who and how" questions pertaining to the use of endocrine agents for the chemoprevention of breast cancer.

What? Obviously it is the breast carcinogenesis process that we want to inhibit. As we have heard this afternoon, chemoprevention approaches to both the initiation and promotion phases of breast carcinogenesis are possible, and these approaches can be quite different, with regard to the endocrine agents employed, their duration of use, and the time point in a woman's life that this intervention is first begun.

When? Should chemoprevention address the process of carcinogenesis initiation or attempt to interrupt the promotion phase? It is my interpretation of both animal studies and clinical models that it might be easier to interrupt the promotion phase of carcinogenesis, recognizing that while this may be an effective strategy, it does not really reverse the underlying genotoxic event(s) initiating carcinogenesis.

Who? Which populations are at greater risk and should be targeted for endocrine chemoprevention? I will expand upon this question in just a moment.

How? What endocrine chemoprevention strategy should we choose? Choosing between an antiestrogen or an antiaromatase agent will also depend upon other factors, such as the menopausal status of the patient.

Defining breast cancer risk: Existing chemoprevention trials were not set up to look specifically at inherited risk, so they are composed of small and variable numbers of women carrying germline mutations in BRCA-1, BRCA-2, or BRCA-X. We don't yet know how these particular inherited-risk subgroups will respond to any endocrine agent. The definition of familial risk is different from that of inherited risk, and risk assessment for the P1 trial was different from that of the Royal Marsden trial. Risk based on previous diagnosis of a preneoplastic lesion is likely to be very different from inherited and familial risk, and we know that many women entered the P1 trial based on a prior diagnosis of atypical ductal hyperplasia (ADH). We haven't really focused much at this meeting on the use of endocrine agents for the treatment of patients diagnosed with ductal carcinoma in situ (DCIS), although we know that tamoxifen not only reduces DCIS recurrence rates when used in conjunction with surgery and radiation therapy but also prevents the development of contralateral breast cancer. Thus we might also want to discuss the potential role of antiaromatase agents in treating DCIS as well as for breast cancer chemoprevention. Last, we have a very large category of patients who have a presumed increased risk for breast cancer, based upon their geographic and/or socioeconomic status, as introduced by Malcolm (Pike), their race and ethnicity, or—as Paul Goss's *New England Journal of Medicine* article has pointed out—both their lifetime estrogen exposure and their current age. There is a 17-fold increase in breast cancer risk during the 5-year interval between ages 60 and 65 years as compared with the interval between ages 30 and 35 years.

Targeted chemoprevention: I think we have already mentioned what tumor markers might best identify patients likeliest to benefit from endocrine therapy. However, are these markers the same in determining who should receive a selective endocrine-receptor modulator (SERM) versus who should receive an aromatase inactivator or inhibitor, whether this be for chemoprevention or adjuvant treatment purposes? Tumor markers like ER and PgR change dramatically with patient age at diagnosis, and the relationship between ER and PgR may also change. To illustrate this let me show you some age-specific incidence curves generated from the National Cancer Institute's SEER database which has also been recording tumor ER and PgR status since 1992. The ER-positive/PgR-positive curve constitutes about 60% of all breast cancers overall, and you can see that it continues to rise quite dramatically even after age 50 years.

The second-largest category of breast cancers is that of ER-negative/PgR-negative tumors, arising in about one-third of all patients. Interestingly, this curve flattens out completely after age 50 years, which suggests that an even more pronounced effect of menopause appears to be on the incidence of this population of breast tumors. Of particular interest to me is the ER-positive/PgR-negative age-specific incidence curve, which continues to rise even more steeply than any of the other curves after age 50, and this observation may have clinical and chemoprevention implications. We know from the early San Antonio studies of Bill McGuire et al., that endocrine (primarily tamoxifen) responsiveness of metastatic disease is quite reduced in the subset of ER-positive/PgR-negative tumors as compared to ER-positive/PgR-positive subset. More recently, Gary Clark has retrospectively evaluated their database of breast tumors formerly assayed for ER and PgR by the same DCC/ligand-binding approach used by McGuire et al. and now shown that patients with ER-positive/PgR-negative primary breast tumors also have at least a 1.6-fold greater risk of recurrence and death despite adjuvant endocrine therapy, as compared with similarly staged and treated patients with ER-positive/PgR-positive breast tumors. Since this adjuvant endocrine therapy was primarily tamoxifen, I would like to remind you, for the purposes of discussion, that we have seen data at this meeting indicating the superior antitumor activity of aromatase inhibitors/inactivators as compared to tamoxifen, and I would thus like to propose that tumor ER-positive/PgR-negative status might represent a tumor marker profile capable of identifying patients likelier to benefit from anti-aromatase agents as compared to an anti-estrogen like tamoxifen.

Establishing goals: Referring back to Malcolm (Pike)'s point that geographically and across all populations, the vast number of patients that are getting breast cancer are those over 50 years of age. In my own mind, we would make great strides if we simply tried to reduce the U.S./Caucasian incidence rates in women over age 50 to the much lower rates seen among Asian women living in Shanghai. For example, with endocrine agents administered later in life, we will probably not only reduce the incidence of ER-positive breast tumors but can also affect the incidence of ER-negative breast cancers by earlier lifestyle changes such as caloric restriction during youth or delaying menarche by either endocrine agents or some other means. We might each share a sense of the expected degree of breast cancer risk reduction we would like to accomplish by one form of endocrine chemoprevention or another, but I wonder if we have really come to grips with the level of toxicity and side effects that otherwise healthy women will consider acceptable to achieve this risk reduction. Trevor Powles pointed out at least 10 different organ systems potentially susceptible to the adverse effects of endocrine chemoprevention, and for each candidate endocrine approach we might advocate, we must better understand their effects on these susceptible organ systems. With this comment, I will now conclude my introductory remarks and open this chemoprevention discussion session for comments and questions from the floor.

M. Dowsett: Can I just go into some of the receptor data that you were talking about there? First, I want to make a slightly cautionary comment about the interpretation of data that we have from the MORE study and P01 study. Matt (Ellis) alluded to this earlier on, that when we have tamoxifen-treated tumors, ER levels go down. In the main, they don't make those tumors ER-negative, but I think that there probably are some low ER-positive tumors that would become ER-negative in those circumstances. So we may be overestimating the ER-negative number in the tamoxifen-treated group in P01. Similarly in the MORE study, raloxifene will have that same effect: in a short term presurgical study with raloxifene, we showed reduced ER expression. We may be getting an anomalous result there owing to the pharmacological effect of the compound in these tumors, which would phenotypically be ER-positive. I don't think that is a major issue. But I wanted to say that these data on ER are only partly useful in helping us select the target population, because we don't know what the receptor status is until the tumor presents. So the question is then: Can we predict the women that are more likely to produce the ER-positive tumors as opposed to the ER-negative tumors? We don't seem to be terribly successful in our current strategies. We should consider the following:

1. Trevor (Powles)'s point about the contralateral breast cancers, if they are from a previously ER-negative patient there may be no prophylactic effect of tamoxifen.
2. The fact that when we treat patients with hormone replacement therapy (HRT) we know when the tumors present that they are more likely to be ER-positive.
3. The fact that in the Raloxifene/MORE study, we find that the prevention of breast cancer is greatest in those women that had the higher estrogen levels initially.

All this suggests that the patients who have the higher estrogen levels, that are at higher risk of breast cancer [as Paul (Goss) has alluded to], are the ones that are most likely to have the higher levels of ER-positivity. This is good news, because this is the group that we want to actually target with our treatment. I am more and more persuaded by the position that Paul (Goss) was taking, that using plasma estradiol levels, and perhaps these surrogate measures of bone and breast density, that we should be using these to enter patients into our prevention studies. I end up with a question for Paul (Goss). Rather than titrating estrogen down, would he consider using an aromatase inhibitor to flatten estrogen levels and then titrate the estrogen back, which might actually be pharmacologically easier to do?

P. Goss: I think we have discussed that and I think that it is a very doable idea. It is probably a little easier practically to just give letrozole in the usual clinical doses, with all the backup data that are needed to do such a thing. Wipe out the estrogen completely, then just give an exact add-back therapy. You can precisely titrate in your patient's level rather than trying to fiddle with the dose on a day-to-day, week-to-week basis. I think this is one possible way to do it.

A. Bhatnagar: It is much more difficult to get flat levels of estradiol using transdermal administration to add it back in again than it is to use a drug like letrozole or anastrozole, which has a fairly long half-life, to give you a steady-state level in about 2–4 weeks, which actually keeps the estrogens fairly flat, and it is much easier to titrate with one drug alone than it is with two for the add-back.

M. Pike: To go back to what Trevor (Powles) was talking about—he was saying how cautious we have to be (I think that is true), but the point is that it is not against nothing. In premenopausal women, what you are trying to do is to find something that is better than the birth control pill, and that is a much easier thing to do, because you have to then demonstrate that your protection against cancer of the ovary is better. It is not so obvious how to do that, by the way, but there are few things you can look at (e.g., What is cell proliferation like in a patient with benign ovarian cystadenomas who is on LH-RH agonists? Is it affected by estrogen? Is it blocked by progesterone? What is the effect of the pill on that?). So you can actually think of ways to take each system and ask, "Is this better than oral contraceptives?" In that way you are just making something better than something that is already on the market. That is much easier than trying to take something from nothing, which is very difficult.

C. Benz: I would like to ask Malcolm (Pike) another question: Do you think that in your strategy for intervention early on that you will actually have an impact on breast cancers arising in women under age 40? And will your chemoprevention strategy affect only a subset of cancers, like those that are ER-positive?

M. Pike: I can't answer that. I guess that in the long term it will have an effect on everything. I believe that to be true because of what happens, for example, when the Japanese move to Hawaii breast cancers increase at all ages, and I still think that it is all steroid control in the end, but it takes a long time to come about. The strategy that we have adopted is that we have hundreds of patients now being treated for fibroids with LH-RH agonists—it's of course totally effective. It completely cures them. Now we're actually looking at what is happening with their bones. What is happening with everything else? The same thing is true if you use a LH-RH agonist against endometriosis. So I believe that we can actually do this without spending hundreds of millions of dollars if we take specific, small problems and try to solve them by saying: Can we make therapy better than what we currently have?

A. Howell: Malcolm (Pike) you say that with LH-RH agonists we can eliminate all breast cancer, but at what age do you think that chemoprevention should start?

M. Pike: I believe that most young women start oral contraceptives in their teens, and they certainly start them by the age of 21. I actually think that there is no reason to suspect that we cannot replace the pill in 21-year-old women. You can take organ systems one at time and show that in fact we can do better than the pill. That is all we have to do.

A. Howell: Mitch (Dowsett) made the point, and there are data in the literature (I don't know if anybody knows it well) for the risk factors for ER-positive and ER-negative tumors. Does anybody know those data? [No response.]

C. Benz: Do you have any data that suggest that ER-negative tumors are affected at all by any endocrine strategy? I am certainly impressed by the unpublished results that Trevor (Powles) mentioned. That is, when your first tumor is ER-negative, tamoxifen will not provide any apparent chemoprevention benefit. This observation raises several important questions. Do women with multiple tumors develop tumors more frequently with a given receptor phenotype? Are these ER-negative tumors induced by a genotoxic mechanism as opposed to an estrogen-promoting mechanism?

J. Forbes: The Swedish randomized trial—2 years of tamoxifen versus 5 years of tamoxifen (which has been published)—had data on ER status, contralateral breast cancer, and primary breast cancer, and there was actually substantial discordance: ER-positive primary tumors had an ER-negative relapse (contralateral new primary and vice versa). So I don't think that it's yet clear-cut that an ER-negative primary breast cancer derives no protective benefit in terms of contralateral cancer from tamoxifen. I think that is still an open question.

A. Howell: They had ER-negative tumors in that trial; and was there any reduction in contralateral breast cancer when they got ER-negative tumors?

J. Forbes: I don't know that.

A. Bhatnagar: I have a question for Joachim Liehr. Do you think that the estrogen initiation process (the genotoxic process) gives rise only to ER-positive tumors? Or would it give rise to both? And if it doesn't give rise to both, then what sorts of other mechanisms would you propose for ER-negative tumors?

J. Liehr: I don't know; I cannot answer that question. The data that I cited from Jose Russo seemed to indicate that at least in human mammary cells, the induction of ER expression is a rather late process in the transformation process. So I don't know.

I wanted to come back to your point, Malcolm (Pike). It is fairly easy to come up with improved, less carcinogenic estrogens that are better than the current birth control pill. The concept that I tried to illustrate is that carcinogenic activity and hormonal potency are not inherently connected but can be separated. It is fairly easy to actually synthesize such compounds. In the late 1980s, I took a patent on 2-fluoroestradiol, because at that time I was convinced that it was a safe, noncarcinogenic estrogen. I worked for a while with Ely Lilly, and they told me that they were not interested in this compound because, first of all, there needs to be proof that estrogens actually induce tumors in humans (in the 1980s, this needed proof). But this isn't the only problem. In addition, there needs to be convincing evidence that this new estrogen actually prevents this carcinogenesis process. The studies are basically impossible to do. If estrogens induce tumors with a low frequency (are weak carcinogens) and have a long latency period, then it is practically impossible to establish the lack of carcinogenic activity of novel estrogens in humans. The only way to do this for a new estrogen, for a novel and poorly carcinogenic estrogen, is to prove lack of carcinogenic activity in preclinical animal studies, where this can easily be shown, and then come out and market this new birth control pill without any additional claims about human carcinogenicity. Then, 50 years later, you'll probably be able to have the data by epidemiological studies and demonstrate that this novel estrogen is also a poor carcinogen in humans.

One more point concerning prevention for a large population, I think, is that it has to be almost diet-based. If we look for a moment at our experience with tobacco smoking and lung cancer incidence, we can reduce incidence, but only very slowly and over a long time. I think that cancer prevention has to be a minimally invasive procedure. I doubt it can be a pill. I don't think you can convince a 15- or 18-year-old to take a pill for more than 40 years until age 60 in order to prevent tumors, because at that age, people are not even thinking about tumors.

R. Tekmal: In response to Ajay (Bhatnagar) and to the question raised by the chair, our preclinical model using aromatase overexpressing transgenic mice has shown that the preneoplastic changes, such as hyperplasia and dysplasia, initiated as a result of increased tissue estrogen are always ER-positive, and ER expression goes up, as does, also, the expression of PR in these mice. Some growth factors that are known to be under estrogen control—such as TGF-α EGF, and their receptor EGFR—go down with continuous estrogenic stimulation.

The last speaker suggested that if we can titrate aromatase inhibitors without affecting physiological responses, we may able to use aromatase inhibitors for chemoprevention. We have presented some of our studies at the aromatase congress held in Port Douglas, Australia (and these are also being published in the *Journal of Steroid Biochemistry and Molecular Biology*), which showed that we could titrate the dose of letrozole in such a way that we can selectively block the conversion of androgens to estrogen in breast tissue without affecting normal physiology. Using 0.25 to 0.5 μg of letrozole per day per mouse, we could abrogate all the preneoplastic changes in breast tissue without affecting the circulating estrogen levels or FSH. Other uterotrophic markers like lactoferrin and progesterone receptor levels were also not affected in these animals, and uterine and ovarian histology appeared to be normal. Not only were normal physiological changes unaffected in these animals after they were treated with letrozole for 6 weeks, but the mammary neoplastic changes had gone down, and these mice could undergo pregnancy and lactation. The litter size and weight of the pups and morphological features were normal. Whether these changes revert or not remains to be seen, since we are still aging these animals after discontinuing letrozole treatment. In summary, the aromatase inhibitor letrozole can be used to selectively block the conversion of androgens to estrogens in breast tissue without affecting normal physiology and the estrogen-mediated changes found in breast tissue can be blocked without affecting normal physiology.

C. Benz: Let me get back to one practical question. Trevor (Powles), if you were to do this all over again, what population would you pick to target for intervention and chemoprevention using an endocrine agent? Could you be more specific, given the facts in hand? How might you do this again?

T. Powles: I would just like to make one point first that relates to that. I am attracted by the idea that you have to reduce the estrogen levels only a bit to reduce the incidence of breast cancer quite markedly, both in premenopausal women probably and in post-menopausal women. If we look at the levels of estrogen where you have, say, the top quartile versus the bottom quartile of estrogen levels in breast cancer risk, that is at a much higher level than at the top quartile versus the bottom quartile for risk of osteoporosis. I am concerned, as you can see, about the use of aromatase in-hibitors—full-blown aromatase inhibitors—that are taking estro-gen levels down maybe 100-fold below the level at which you start to get osteoporosis. I am also a little worried about the add-back—Mitch and I have spoken about this many times—to look at two things that are variable is much more difficult than looking at one. Now we must have some information related to the use of these aromatase inhibitors in premenopausal women. I don't know what we have got, but we must have anastrozole or letrozole given a lit-tle bit? I had asked Malcolm (Pike), (a) Had we used these agents in premenopausal women? (b) What sort of levels of estrogen do we get [following on from what Paul (Goss) said]? and (c) Is that enough for what Malcolm (Pike) wants? Can we take 1000 pmol down to 150 pmol in a premenopausal woman with one-tenth of a dose of anastrozole, and do we need to add anything back then? And in the postmenopausal women, can we reduce the dose? I have never thought of this before, but what is very attractive to my mind is to be using a much smaller dose of these now very potent aro-matase inhibitors to see if we can take the estrogen level to where it is still protecting against bone and other normal tissues but is at the level where you have a half or a quarter of the breast cancer in-cidence. We should almost be able to titrate that. If that is the case, I can start to answer the question about who we should be doing it in. I haven't got a problem with using an aromatase inhibitor if we could halve breast cancer incidence at an estrogen level that still protects normal tissues. I have got a problem if we are going take it down to 50 or 100 times below what we normally need to protect bone or brain or the like.

C. Benz: I think Bill (Miller) mentioned the answer to the first question earlier this morning. There has been some experience looking at estradiol levels in premenopausal women on aromatase inhibitors. Is that not true?

A. Bhatnagar: There aren't any real clinical data using, for example, letrozole in premenopausal women. But there are some data that we published before, which were presented at endocrine meetings (rather than at cancer meetings), that showed that with fadrozole (another aromatase inhibitor) we were able in nonhuman primates (bonnet monkeys) to reduce the overall exposure of estrogen in a menstrual cycle by about 25–30%, without affecting cyclicity or ovulation. As a consequence, we get, in the luteal phase, normal amounts of progesterone, but the area under the curve for estrogen in the follicular phase and in the luteal phase is down by about 25–30%. We were looking for a dose of aromatase inhibitor that would allow normal cyclicity but with a reduced exposure to endogenous estrogens. That has been published and that was possible to do.

C. Benz: How long do you think you would have to administer an agent that produces only a 25% reduction in total estradiol level to achieve a chemoprevention effect? Malcolm (Pike)?

M. Pike: But would someone take it? They can take the pill and not get pregnant at the same time.

T. Powles: I understand your sympathy for using the pill, but what about answering the question: If we reduce the estrogen level by 25%, what impact would that have on breast cancer incidence? How long would you need to give such an agent?

M. Pike: It depends. That would make you like the rural Japanese. We know what happens with them; it would reduce your risk by half, but you have to take such an agent forever. We can tell from tamoxifen what happens in the short term when you are really blocking things hard. It is like being oophorectomized. If you oophorectomize a woman, there is an immediate, huge effect, just like there is with tamoxifen, because you have completely changed the hormonal milieu. We shouldn't expect any estrogen level reductions that didn't last for decades to have any effect that is as big as that with tamoxifen unless you do this really early on. Now the approach that we are taking is not to reduce the estrogen level by 25%; we are reducing the estrogen level by 70%, and we are almost abolishing progesterone. Dr. Liehr talked about estrogen alone, but in fact progesterone, in my opinion, is a major part of the problem. So the reason that we believe that we will get huge effects is because we are tackling both.

I. Smith: Sometimes I wear a lung cancer hat, and in lung cancer, of course, it is easy. We know what causes lung cancer. We can't prevent it. Regrettably, smoking is going up among teenagers and young women, and that is because they feel "immortal." Therefore, any strategy in breast cancer prevention based on very young women doing something won't work, so forget it.

M. Pike: I believe that it also has to be a contraceptive.

P. Goss: Can I just comment on one of the other failed drugs that I have worked with, vorozole? It was given to premenopausal volunteers at full doses in a small study. It caused significant ovarian cyst formation and pelvic ovarian hyperstimulation syndrome with abdominal pain and fluid in the pouch of Douglas. So that is one of the earliest reasons I think why at least that company didn't pursue the compound at full dose in premenopausal patients. I think that Ajay (Bhatnagar)'s point that low doses may be possible is conceivably true.

P. Lønning: A comment on what Trevor (Powles) was saying about suppressing estrogen levels to very low levels: This is a concern about adjuvant therapy with aromatase inhibitors. This question is addressed properly in the study that we are conducting in Norway now. There is randomization between exemestane and placebo for 2 years in low-risk patients and 1 year of follow-up. So we will have that answer in $3\frac{1}{2}$ years.

T. Powles: I think the problem with exemestane is that it's a steroidal aromatase inhibitor. What I'm concerned about are the nonsteroidals. They are more powerful. Am I right on that?

P. Lønning: I agree with you. I asked all the drug companies who might be interested in participating. Only Pharmacia was interested, and now the results that we get cannot be extrapolated to nonsteroidal aromatase inhibitors. So they need to do their own studies.

A. Howell: Obviously there will be bone density data from the ATAC trial and very careful quality-of-life data, so we will have some data by the time we meet in San Antonio.

T. Powles: But it won't be placebo-controlled, Tony (Howell).

A. Howell: It will be tamoxifen-controlled.

T. Powles: Yes, it will be informative, but not completely.

J. Forbes: A question for Malcolm (Pike). The German clinical trials group have done a study in adjuvant therapy using anastrozole. A direct randomization with cytoxan/methotrexate/5-fluorouracil (CMF) chemotherapy and LH-RH agonist given for 2 years to ER-positive premenopausal patients. When it ended, menstruation recommenced in the majority of women; yet in ER-positive patients, the LH-RH therapeutic effect was not different from the CMF effect, which we know is a real effect in that group of patients. There seems to be a living experiment, where short-term reduction in estrogen levels presumably has some effect on whatever cancer was already present, so it does seem plausible, I think, that a shorter-term reduction in estrogen level may be important. Maybe the area under the curve is important and a massive reduction for a short time might be almost as good as a partial reduction for a long time. What do you think about that?

M. Pike: You know that I don't know. It's a possibility, but I don't know how we are going to find out. When we are trying to understand this, we have to follow the literature that most of us don't follow. For example there is a new contraceptive that has just been licensed which is an intravaginal ring, that contains ethinyl-estradiol and norgestrel. This is going to be very important for us all to watch, because it will potentially tell us that if you don't take these compounds by mouth, you can avoid the deep vein thrombosis and a whole set of problems related to cardiovascular disease. It is going to be very important that we learn from these other fields. When you have the next meeting like this we need cardiovascular disease people here.

L. Bradlow: I would just like to point out that there is a very easy way to lower active estrogen levels in people. You have to remember that the major metabolite of estrogen is 2-hydroxy-estrone, and it had been shown that such things as vigorous exercise, low body weight (which decrease breast cancer risk), and omega 3 fatty acids all raise 2-hydroxylation. We have shown in animals that raising 2-hydroxylation will prevent breast cancer just as it does in papillomavirus-induced cancers. This can be readily raised by a number of nutraceuticals: green tea will do it, cruciferous vegetables will do it, omega 3 fatty acids in the diet will do it, as well as vigorous exercise. It is perfectly easy to get a marked decrease in circulating estradiol. For example, women who exercise very vigorously, as in participating in eight-oar crew, will lower their estrogen enough by raising 2-hydroxy estrone that they stop menstruating until they stop rowing in the fall. As soon as they gain a couple of pounds of fat in the fall, their 2-hydroxylation goes down and they start menstruating again. It's a perfectly safe procedure. In addition, we have shown that in women with breast cancer, those with higher $2/16\alpha$ metabolite ratios live longer than those with ratios below the median level.

G. Kelloff: To follow up on Trevor (Powles)'s point and Paul Goss's discussion about a mild titration of estrogen levels—I'd like to comment on what has been said today, in terms of a reduction of breast cancer risk of 2.6-fold with just a 20% drop in estrogen levels, and the fact that estrogen reduction reduces breast cell proliferation, which is as good a short-term marker as we have for cancer risk. About 20–30 years are required in most epithelial populations to go from clonal mutation, to clonal selection, to clonal evolution, and that rate of evolution is driven as much by cell turnover rates as by anything else that you can possibly measure. You certainly have to take into account apoptosis to see which cells you are losing. If one is interested in quality surrogate markers in terms of drug development issues and one looks at the estrogen serum levels—say, compared with cholesterol—one actually has a better fit in the causal pathway of the disease of interest, than exists for cholesterol and heart disease. I have been looking at the cholesterol data because we are interested in how those drug approvals were actually obtained and just how good the data are when one looks at large populations of people and serum cholesterol levels. So I think, in summary, that a lot of the concepts that have been put out this afternoon do make sense for a mild lowering of blood estrogen levels, in that Malcolm (Pike) shows that it reduces breast cancer risk, especially if sustained for 20–30 years. This is very sound in that proliferation rates drive latent periods for invasive cancer, and estrogen lowering drops proliferation rates.

W. Miller: I am now persuaded that aromatase inhibitors in pre menopausal women may be good for chemoprevention, but I want to challenge Malcolm (Pike) about whether all you have to do is reduce estrogens by 20% and you're there. I am just a little bit concerned that you're basing this upon international populations in which differences in risk are associated with differences of 20% in circulating estrogens, but the chemoprotective effects of tamoxifen on contralateral breast cancer are probably mediated in part by preventing the appearance of occult tumors that are there, and the benefits of tamoxifen (or an aromatase inhibitor) will be linked to slowing this growth rate down. I just wonder if this is the case, unless there is some difference in sensitivity, why a 20% reduction in estrogens is enough to slow the rate of occult tumors, yet when tumors become overt, we really want to minimize circulating estrogens to the bottom of range.

M. Pike: I believe for the rural Chinese or Japanese, where their estrogens are reduced by about 20%, that this would relate to about a 20% reduction in cell proliferation, not a 2.5-fold, just a 20%. The fact is that the 20% reduction lasts for a long time, and because of the multistage nature of cancer, you get this huge effect. When we're giving tamoxifen, as in the P01 trial or Trevor (Powles)'s trial or something, we are trying to achieve huge effects rapidly. You can't do that by just reducing things a little; you have to reduce things a lot by that time if you want to get an effect. These are not contradictory.

Part VI

CONCLUSION

Panel Discussion 5

Final Discussion and Wrap-Up

James N. Ingle and Ajay Bhatnagar, *Chairmen*
Tuesday, June 26, 2001

J. Ingle: Welcome to this discussion session. This has been a very exciting, productive, and provocative meeting. We have four major bulleted items to discuss, so we have our work cut out for us. I would like to show several slides to start.

This is a woman I saw about 25 years ago. She was about 60 years old when she presented. Ten years before she had breast cancer and 8 years before she had been put on low-dose Premarin. She came to see me when I had just joined the staff. I said that she should stop the Premarin. She agreed, and 3 months later there was resolution of the malignant pleural effusion and a response in bone metastasis. She had a durable response lasting about 18 months. Obviously we all know that estrogen is the issue here.

We talked about estrogen receptors. Clearly, estrogen is the best predictive marker that we have in breast cancer. We talked about ER-positivity. Here are two images of tumor biopsies (from our laboratory) showing ER-positivity. These stains were done on two different tumors; they were embedded in paraffin and handled the same way, yet there is clearly a difference in their staining.

There is clearly heterogeneity in tumors that is real. The definition of what is hormonally sensitive is perhaps open to discussion.

Dr. Brodie is here. Her model has not been presented, but with her permission I will present several slides. She has an ovariectomized nude mouse, given androstenedione and injected with MCF-7 cells transfected with the aromatase gene. The ordinate shows the tumor volume and the abscissa shows days of treatment. There are data for control, tamoxifen, anastrozole, and letrozole, and you can see clearly the superiority of the aromatase inhibitors. If tamoxifen is added to either of the aromatase inhibitors, the reduction in tumor size is no more than with the aromatase inhibitor alone.

This next slide is a crossover study. Mice were given tamoxifen and then switched to letrozole, then back, and back again. Each time with the aromatase inhibitor, the tumor shrinks, and each time with tamoxifen, the tumor grows. Again, tamoxifen plus letrozole is no better that letrozole alone. It was this slide that prompted me to say to Dr. Baum that I didn't think that the combined arm of ATAC (Arimidex Tamoxifen Alone or in Combination) was going to work. We'll see.

The first topic is breast cancer prevention. You have seen these data. This is P01. Tamoxifen is associated with a lower rate of invasive breast cancer than placebo. This slide shows the hazard rates over time. The rates stay low with tamoxifen therapy at least until 6 years.

The vascular events associated with tamoxifen are among the side effects that lead us to look at alternative therapies. This slide shows the vascular events. As you know, STAR (Study of Tamoxifen And Raloxifene) is currently active. There is one other issue that Dr. Liehr raised—that of estrogen-induced carcinogenesis. In addition to estrogen working through the estrogen receptor, there is also the hypothesis that it could work through its metabolism to 4-hydroxy-quinones, leading to depurinating DNA adducts.

There are a number of questions for discussion. We should break this into post- and premenopausal discussions. We'll start with postmenopausal. Is there a role for aromatase inhibitors? What are some of the issues? What are the approaches to address these issues? What should the trial designs be?

J. Liehr: I would like to tighten this task a little bit. Obviously there is a role for aromatase inhibitors in breast cancer prevention in those cases where you deal with an excess of estrogen and where an excess of estrogen has been measured first. If indeed it is clear that a woman has a marked excess of circulating or of tissue estrogen, then an aromatase inhibitor, as Paul Goss proposed, probably plays a legitimate role. In those cases where estrogen levels are already low or where aromatase inhibitors may markedly interfere with the woman's normal hormonal balance, one may want to go to other approaches.

J. Ingle: So you would say that the population to consider studying would be those women who by some marker had elevated estrogen levels?

A. Bhatnagar: Since you (Dr. Liehr) say there is a role for aromatase inhibitors, what are the sorts of strategies that we need to express and how should those strategies be translated into trial design? Which markers should one use: estrogen levels, breast density, mammograms?

J. Forbes: I don't think it should go outside of postmenopausal women at the present time. Second, the risk based on estrogen levels is one issue, but the risk of breast cancer by other defined factors is also important because you are looking at the ratio. Third, it would be, based on all the data that we have so far, with single agents not combinations, at least until there is more information.

A. Howell: The design of the IBIS-2 trial will be tamoxifen versus anastrozole versus placebo. Women with low bone density can't get in. All of these other comments are interesting. Would others say that women with estradiol levels in the lower tertile shouldn't get into this trial?

J. Ingle: So eligibility criteria will include some measure of estrogen level?

A. Howell: Well, the question is: Should we do that? Should we factor this in? The study is due to start either in September or early next year, and obviously we're worried. We have a cognitive function protocol, we have a bone protocol, but the real question is: Should we be excluding women on the basis of their estradiol levels?

J. Ingle: I think this is a fine point right now. We should say at least that properly selected women at high risk for developing breast cancer could be considered for a study of prevention utilizing a third-generation aromatase inhibitor.

A. Bhatnagar: Yes, there should be some sort of assessment of how you consider them high risk, whether it be estrogen levels or breast density or whatever.

M. Dowsett: I think what we have done today is to discuss something rather novel. The risk factors for entering patients into these studies based on the Gail model are fairly well established. But the new question is (as Tony Howell was saying), should we in fact be using indices of estrogen exposure, be it estrogen itself or bone density or whatever? This is a real possibility that is going to extend the subject as well as improve its targeting. But we haven't really discussed the issue of the accuracy or predictability of these measures. Plasma estradiol is really quite tough to measure accurately and precisely in postmenopausal women. I think perhaps this will happen, but we need to sit down and think about the predictability and the tools that we have to make it happen.

J. Ingle: Can I just ask you Mitch (Dowsett), do you think we are ready to design a phase III trial, or would it be prudent to design pilot studies looking at parameters relating to estrogen, such as breast density or estrogen levels, before considering a phase III study?

M. Dowsett: One thing that we are trying to do is to retrieve blood samples from the IBIS trial and also from Trevor (Powles)'s Marsden trial from the patients that have actually developed breast cancer against those that haven't in the two arms, to see whether or not we can confirm what has been shown in the MORE study, that those patients with the higher estrogen level do get greater protection with tamoxifen. That would encourage us to move into the phase III setting that you are talking about. With the issue of titration: What are the best surrogate markers to allow you to develop that idea? The presurgical model again would be an opportunity to manipulate the estrogen in a controllable fashion. The only caveat I would have, and I would like Ajay (Bhatnagar)'s response to this, is what drugs are we going to use in that? If we use letrozole in its conventional dose, we're going to flatten estradiol levels. If we use it at 4% of its conventional levels, we're probably still going to get undetectable levels (of estradiol).

J. Ingle: So you say that there are issues with respect to dose and monitoring that would indicate the need to do intensive small pilot studies before phase III?

M. Dowsett: Yes.

W. Miller: I would just like to suggest that in terms of a surrogate marker, maybe we should concentrate on the breast. Mitch (Dowsett) has raised the point that in postmenopausal women, circulating estrogens are very hard to measure, also reproducibility is a problem, and what we also know is that levels in the breasts of postmenopausal women do not necessarily reflect those in the circulation. If what you are trying to do is influence a breast event, then I think you should build into these trials something that actually reflects breast levels. In the absence of taking out breast tissue, I think, the mammographic pattern is probably reasonable. Maybe one ought to do a definitive study to determine whether in fact the mammographic pattern relates to circulating estrogen.

J. Liehr: If you want to go into a phase III trial, I think one of the things that has to be done or considered is to try transdermal delivery rather than oral and circulatory, to affect the mammary levels of aromatase. Therefore, I would suggest the transdermal delivery of aromatase inhibitors to affect mammary levels of aromatase and mammary levels of estrogens.

A. Howell: Do we know anything about what transdermals would do?

W. Miller: It's a very interesting hypothesis, but the infusion studies performed by Mike Reid and myself show that in certain tumors it is local uptake that determines endogenous levels, whereas in others it is local synthesis.

J. Ingle: I think that is a fine point that is worthy of consideration, but not now.

J. Forbes: In terms of strategy, if the ATAC trial showed that any of the arms lowered contralateral breast cancer to an order of magnitude similar to tamoxifen or plausibly greater, then I think that would clear the way much more readily for a phase III aromatase trial. One other comment: any effect of aromatase inhibitors in the ATAC trial is transferable across the class of drug from the point of view this horizon here, and if the ATAC trial is a positive trial, it would save a lot of work to prove a principle.

T. Powles: I didn't follow that last bit. Are we saying, then, that a full-blown phase III chemoprevention study of an aromatase inhibitor should go ahead? Is that what we are saying?

J. Ingle: Not yet.

M. Dixon: We need some comparative studies looking at different drugs and we need some comparative studies looking at different doses, because we have got it into our heads that the dose we are going to use for prevention is the same as the dose we are using for treatment. That might not be true, because we know that the three current drugs have different aromatase capabilities and milligram for milligram, 2.5 mg of letrozole is not equivalent to 1 mg of anastrozole. We have to think a bit more laterally. Trevor (Powles)'s point, I think, is tremendously important: we want the maximum effective dose with minimal side effect and we may be overdosing many of our patients.

D. Hayes: With reference to pilot trials, before Matthew Ellis left Georgetown, he and I tried to perform some trials of chemoprevention. We have taken both the preoperative approach that was suggested and we have also taken high-risk women and tried to perform serial biopsies and serial MRIs of otherwise normal breast tissue. At least in the United States, the preoperative approach has just not been feasible. One problem is that we only have 2 weeks between diagnosis and definitive surgery for most patients rather than the 4 weeks they seem to have in Canada. We screened 267 or so patients and enrolled 30 patients over 2 years to study two novel drugs, perricyl alcohol and exemestane. I have really abandoned this approach, and I think looking at high-risk women is a much better way to do these studies if you can get serial biopsies or serial ductal lavage.

J. Ingle: The second part of the prevention discussion involves the premenopausal patient, which is somewhat more problematic. Dr. Pike and others certainly raised some very provocative thoughts. Are we ready to make any recommendations? I think this is an investigator-initiated area where work is going to continue, but where unless someone has a proposal, I think that one should concentrate on the postmenopausal setting first. Are there any contrary opinions?

J. Liehr: Pharmaceutical companies must have tens of thousands or hundreds of thousands of compounds on the shelf, and I would love to see an exploratory study to see if there are any good estrogen 4-hydroxylase inhibitors that can be identified. I think, before such a study, there is not much that we can do in terms prevention.

J. Ingle: Dr. Bhatnagar mentioned the fadrozole, and that may be an interesting possibility.

A. Bhatnagar: I think that becomes one of the strategies. You have the strategy of estrogen lowering or antagonism. You also have now the strategy of 4-hydroxylase inhibition. I think that becomes part of a long-term strategy.

H. Mouridsen: Just one very conservative comment. If it appears that the ATAC trial is completely negative in terms of prevention of secondary breast cancer with anastrozole, would we then proceed with a phase III prevention trial?

J. Ingle: I'm not so sure that would absolutely proscribe proceeding to investigate the aromatase inhibitors in the prevention setting.

A. Howell: Some may disagree with me, but I think if we don't see any superiority of anastrozole over tamoxifen in ATAC, in terms of relapse rate, but also if we don't see any reduction in contralateral cancers . . .

J. Ingle: What if they're the same?

A. Howell: Or if they are the same, then I think we would have to sit down and have a big rethink.

D. Hayes: The BIG (Breast International Group) trial will also have data for this, probably in five or six years. That is such a huge trial that there'll be several endpoints rolling along (with letrozole). So you'll have two big studies.

A. Howell: Just one point about trial designs. I think we can only do pilot studies at the moment. Malcolm Pike has been an inspiration and showed the pilot studies that are going on in Europe and Australia at the moment of LH-RH inhibition plus some sort of add-back: the add-back of raloxifene in the United Kingdom, the add-back of tibolone in Holland, and the add-back of a bisphosphonate in Germany. Those are small exploratory trials, and that is all we should do at the moment.

J. Ingle: Great. We should now move on to neoadjuvant therapy.
 This is Dr. Ellis's study. You'll remember 024's schema. There appeared to be some superiority for letrozole over tamoxifen and interest has been expressed in exploring this in the neoadjuvant setting and developing translational research programs around these

trials. We have heard two potential schemas. Matt (Ellis) presented them. One was a straight comparison of tamoxifen versus letrozole. The second was a protocol involving chemotherapy. Now remember the neoadjuvant, at least the way I think what we are thinking about initially, would be in more locally advanced women. Normally they would get chemotherapy unless there were some extenuating circumstance such as age or frailty.

M. Ellis: The first trial plan is to look at ER-positive and ErbB1- and/or ErbB2-positive breast cancer purely in an adjuvant context, so that the question is: Did our findings in the neoadjuvant setting concerning the large advantage in the neoadjuvant setting pan out in the adjuvant setting? There continues to be a lot of controversy about the role of HER-2 in tamoxifen resistance, particularly in the adjuvant setting, so I believe that this question is important enough to be finally settled in a prospective adjuvant study.

　　The second trial I proposed is the neoadjuvant chemotherapy versus neoadjuvant letrozole study. It may be that this trial does not have the right design as yet, and we can obviously continue to have spirited discussions over that. I certainly like the idea that around this table we have investigators from North America, Europe, and Asia. It's therefore a wonderful forum to consider ways to improve the therapy of postmenopausal women with breast cancer, not only with improved endocrine therapy but also with better targeting, so that we can avoid chemotherapy in those that are really cured by the endocrine therapy.

J. Ingle: Can we take the second situation? I think there was some discussion of an alternative schema where everybody starts off with letrozole and after some short period of time there may be a randomization of those that are responding. I don't think we can possibly get into the specific details of the design, but a study of this type, I think, seems to be an appropriate and very logical next step in this area. Any comments?

J. Forbes: Just to underline the point I made earlier, I think the proof of the principle of getting a better outcome based on neoadjuvant response to therapy can't be tested in this way. Matt (Ellis)'s design will select out a group of responders, and of course they'll do better. The correct design is to compare strategy A with strategy B, where strategy A is neoadjuvant therapy and treatment is not based on response, versus strategy B, which is the same neoadjuvant therapy and an outcome that is based on the outcome thereafter, but they're randomized after they have their surgery.

J. Ingle: But at least a study looking at the concept of integrating neoadjuvant hormonal therapy into the management of patients?

J. Forbes: Absolutely. Particularly neoadjuvant endocrine therapy; but my caution is simply that apart from the short-term activity, the trial designs will be very difficult to interpret.

J. Ingle: So work would have to be done on the trial designs.

H. Mouridsen: To me the key question in this context is to see whether response in the primary tumor predicts late outcome. I think it is very important to design the trial so that we can answer that question. I would be very happy with letrozole followed by postoperative letrozole. The only patients who would be excluded postoperatively would be the 10% who progress during preoperative treatment. You could then still have the distinction between no change and remission patients during the early phase and see whether that relates to outcome. If we can't avoid chemotherapy, you could primarily randomize patients to either letrozole (followed by postoperative letrozole) or to chemotherapy (followed by postoperative letrozole). That trial might answer two questions: (a) whether early response predicts late outcome and (b) whether the addition of chemotherapy to letrozole adds anything.

J. Ingle: Regarding the advanced stage of disease, with the recent presentation of the Intergroup study by Kathy Albain at ASCO, I would like to talk about those very briefly. Even though the absolute survival difference is only 5% at 5 years, it means that chemotherapy, at least in the United States, is a consideration in patients with locally advanced disease. Given that, the design could be such that this could be taken into account.

H. Mouridsen: But I don't think that we can extrapolate those data from this trial here. It should be limited (as far as I have understood from this afternoon's discussion) to patients with receptor-rich tumors. I think that these patients would not benefit at all, or only very little, from the addition of chemotherapy. These are not standard receptor-positive patients; they are patients with receptor rich tumors.

A. Howell: Could I just point out that we have never done the proper preoperative trial in endocrine therapy? This is an opportunity to do it in older women (over 70 or 75 years) with ER-rich tumors. Treatment could be 4 months of preoperative letrozole followed by 5 years of letrozole after surgery compared with 5 years of letrozole without the neoadjuvant component. We need to answer the question of whether neoadjuvant therapy improves survival. That would be an important study as far as I am concerned.

J. Ingle: At what stage would you put those patients in?

A. Howell: Well, whatever you like if you are dealing with older women. Trevor Powles has been leading the field here. He puts in women with tumors over 2 cm or more into neoadjuvant studies. You could do that in the elderly population, I would have thought, quite easily.

J. Ingle: There is clearly room for several potential studies here.

M. Ellis: I think we can basically break them down into young postmenopausal, where there is a question of adding chemotherapy, and old postmenopausal, where you would not give chemotherapy anyway. Then you can perform exactly the study that was described.

W. Eiermann: I would add letrozole to the chemotherapy arm from the very beginning, because this answers the question: Does chemotherapy in receptor-positive patients add anything to endocrine treatment? It would be another very important question answered.

J. Ingle: There are clearly two questions that need to be answered. The first relates to neoadjuvant therapy as a predictor of late outcome and the second—Ajay (Bhatnagar) could you repeat your question?

A. Bhatnagar: My question is whether the neoadjuvant setting is an acceptable setting in which to do experimental work that can then be applied to a wide variety of questions later on in the breast cancer area.

J. Ingle: I think the answer is yes.

A. Bhatnagar: There was controversy this morning when we were discussing putting patients into highly experimental situations without having additional information.

J. Ingle: I think you have to be able to defend that you are giving the patient a reasonable therapy and I think you can do that as long as you select the situation.

M. Ellis: Clearly the toxicity and some of the efficacy issues have to be worked out in the metastatic setting before you would go to the neoadjuvant setting. What we envisage is that you can have a parallel modeling approach in animal studies as well as metastatic disease trials that define safety and dose. Then, before you go to the adjuvant setting, which is what we traditionally do, one would do a neoadjuvant study just to be sure that in the early disease setting we are looking at a potential improvement in treatment.

M. Gnant: I believe that this setting is optimal for testing compounds coming out of the pipeline. Given that safety and toxicity data are available, I think it's perfectly OK to use standard preoperative therapy *not* substituting for any accepted treatment, and doing serial biopsies at 2–3 week intervals, sample testing, and having a look at the molecular changes these compounds produce in the neoadjuvant setting.

A. Howell: These short-term assays could even be put into DCIS (Ductal Carcinoma In Situ). We have a study with Iressa and DCIS. Iressa, as Matt Ellis mentioned, has got to be tested. It has been tested in large numbers of patients for safety, and you can put it further up front like that or you could, if you are thinking about using it for prevention, do ductal lavage before Iressa or whatever you would like to use.

M. Dixon: I think that we need to have two different settings. We need a preoperative setting similar to that for which Dan Hayes has had trouble recruiting, and the neoadjuvant setting. As a clinician, I would not be happy putting any patient into a neoadjuvant study if I had not got clear evidence in a series of patients with breast cancer of proof of principle that the drug works and does something to the cancer which we think is beneficial. The first thing we need to do with a new compound is to evaluate it in a preoperative study where patients get 2–3 weeks of treatment between diagnosis and surgery.

Once it is clear that the drug is doing something to the cancer and that the effect is beneficial, we can at that point think about introducing it to the neonadjuvant setting. These patients trust us to give them compounds that are effective, and we have to be convinced that they work before drugs are given to patients.

J. Ingle: Early-stage breast cancer in postmenopausal patients: you will all remember the data from the 2000 overview. In studies of tamoxifen versus nil, tamoxifen appears to work in both patients who are not receiving chemotherapy and those receiving chemotherapy, both in terms of reduction of recurrence and death. Also, I'd like to share with you this study which is going to affect many of us, at least in the United States. This is the American Intergroup Study, Kathy Albain's study of tamoxifen versus CAF-plus-tamoxifen (either sequential or concurrent tamoxifen). Just to show you the overall results: disease-free survival showed an advantage for the CAF-plus-tamoxifen arm over tamoxifen alone (9% difference at 5 years); overall survival was greater in the CAF-plus-tamoxifen arm (5% difference at 5 years). If you look at relative reductions, they are substantial (27% and 24%, respectively).

As you know, in the adjuvant setting, we have a lot of studies looking at third-generation aromatase inhibitors in sequence with, in combination with, and instead of tamoxifen.

I would like to open up the issues in the postmenopausal setting, understanding that there are a number of ongoing clinical trials. We have already had one proposal from Dr. Ellis in a small subgroup of patients identified as HER-1/2–positive, ER-positive patients. I would like to open this up for consideration.

A. Howell: May I ask a question first? What was the upper limit of age in the Albain study?

J. Ingle: As I remember, patients were postmenopausal with no upper-limit on age.

D. Hayes: I just saw the data on Saturday. As I recall, approximately 15% of the patients were over 65 years of age. There was a fairly substantial proportion in the upper age groups.

M. Dowsett: One of the issues that is bound to arise, and it may be one of the bigger issues, is whether we can combine our aromatase inhibitors with chemotherapy in the same way that we could see added benefit of tamoxifen and chemotherapy given together. These may not equate to the same thing, of course, but it could be a major issue for us to look at over the next few years.

J. Ingle: I thought you were going to raise the issue of whether now is the time to start looking at new small molecules to bring forward. Does anyone think that should be a high-priority area? That is, looking at inhibitors of related pathways. Did I hear an "absolutely"?

J. Forbes: Just to comment, if we had something akin to the CML (Chronic Myelogenous Leukemia) data, we would certainly consider it, but in the absence of any striking data, it is premature at present.

M. Gnant: In view of the data presented from Kathy Albain's trial, I believe that the effect of chemotherapy in addition to tamoxifen is not equally distributed among all postmenopausal women. I believe trials are needed to prove that benefit, especially for the elderly and especially for patients where the absolute benefit is borderline. It may be numerically significant, but it may still be irrelevant—for example, a 1–2% absolute survival difference. There may be a place for trials of, for example, letrozole or optimized endocrine treatment in patients 65–75 years of age plus/minus CAF or something like that.

D. Hayes: As I remember, all of the subset analyses showed the same finding, although the numbers get so small that you lose all of your power.

J. Forbes: There is ER data in the subsets. In the IBCSG (International Breast Cancer Study Group) study 9, CMF plus tamoxifen versus tamoxifen in the ER-positive patients showed absolutely no difference, but there is also an analysis that was done stepwise with ER level, and there is quite a marked change when the ER level gets to a certain point. Then the tamoxifen is very effective, and below that it is not.

J. Ingle: One of the requirements to get on that study, as I remember (it was started in 1988), was an ER of 10 fmol, as they were not doing IHCs (immunohistochemistry) at that time. So they all should be really strongly ER-positive, but we haven't seen those details yet.

D. Hayes: I think we are all saying the same thing. Even we Americans don't believe that every postmenopausal woman who is ER-positive should get chemotherapy. I don't believe that the selection will be on age. I think it will be on some sort of biological factor, whether it is HER-2 or, as we have said earlier, response to chemotherapy in the first place, or level of ER. These are things that we are certainly going to look at within the Intergroup. In this trial that has finished, we already have. I would argue, to keep this discussion on a global basis (rather than specific trial design), that new trial designs with letrozole plus/minus chemotherapy ought to be based on biological factors that you believe will allow you to select the patients most likely to benefit from chemotherapy. The International Breast Cancer Study Group has done tamoxifen plus/minus chemotherapy, and in ER-negative patients, chemotherapy worked in postmenopausal women. That was a relatively unsophisticated look because of the time when it was started, but that is the kind of trial that I think we need to do.

J. Ingle: Are there other thoughts on general trial designs?

M. Dowsett: I made this comment at the BIG meeting in St. Gallen last year. We are all dealing with local challenges at the moment about the ethical issues of doing these tests, and each nation seems to be coming up with its own judgment on this. My own feeling now is that it is actually unethical that we should not do biological studies when we design these new enormous adjuvant trials and waste the opportunity to get data that would allow us to deliver these treatments appropriately. I think it is unacceptable in modern-day clinical trials to omit such studies. One very brief example is—alluding to the ATAC trial and the letrozole-versus-tamoxifen trial—it is quite plausible that letrozole and tamoxifen will have exactly the same outcome in the adjuvant trials (i.e., time-to-relapse curves that overlie each other). But if we measure intratumoral aromatase or ER concentrations or HER-2 levels or whatever, then an uninteresting trial may become a productive trial, as those arms may come apart in the subgroups. It is just not acceptable nowadays not to store tissue in a retrievable fashion.

J. Ingle: I think this is true in all of the studies.

D. Hayes: One quick comment on that. In the United States, our National Cancer Institute has endorsed this concept and now has built it into every prospective adjuvant breast cancer trial at least (prospective collection of blocks and storage of those blocks).

J. Ingle: But I think that it is about developing trials that take into account what we know.

D. Hayes: As we design those trials, we should consider the fact that there may be unexpected subsets that are more likely to benefit or not, and we need to twist our statisticians' arms and our funders' arms to allow us to overpower the trials. One of the big problems with correlative science (in a trial that is powered to look at overall survival for the group you start with) is that your subgroups are, by definition, going to be underpowered, leaving you scratching your head. I have been arguing that we should prospectively overpower the trials to begin with, so that our subgroups (and we don't even know what they are yet) will at least be good hypotheses if not definitive studies.

J. Ingle: I'd like to move on. I think we have some suggestions for postmenopausal breast cancer. I would like to say a few words about premenopausal breast cancer. You will remember from the 1995 overview that tamoxifen has a substantial benefit in reduction of risk and death in younger patients. Chemotherapy versus nil obviously has an effect. Even when tamoxifen is added, chemotherapy still has an effect. I think that chemotherapy is a force to consider. Ovarian ablation: the data from the 2000 overview of ovarian ablation versus no ablation showed a significant difference, but if you add in chemotherapy this difference disappears. You know that there are a number of studies that have been done looking at goserelin either alone or in combination with tamoxifen versus CMF. One of the problems is that CMF is generally not considered to be the best chemotherapy, and none of these patients in any of these studies had tamoxifen added to the chemotherapy and unfortunately the same was true in Intergroup 0101. I just want to present some data to remind you of the results in premenopausal ER-positive/node-positive women, randomized between six cycles of CAF or CAF followed by Zoladex (5 years) or CAF followed by Zoladex and tamoxifen for 5 years. It was designed at a time when it appeared that tamoxifen was considered to be not of much value in premenopausal women, which is a shame and is a limitation of the study. The overall disease-free survival curve shows that there appears to be some advantage for the combined Zoladex-plus-tamoxifen arm, with 15% difference at 7-year disease-free survival. If you look at overall survival, there is about a 3% difference. If you look at CAF plus Zoladex versus CAF adjusted, there is a significant difference in recurrence, and it is borderline for death. If you look at Zoladex plus tamoxifen versus Zoladex, it is significant for recurrence but not for death. The most interesting data, I think, are if you look at it according to age. In the younger women, you can see a substanial separation of the curves. However, in the older premenopausal women, there is not much difference between CAF and CAF plus Zoladex, but Zoladex plus tamoxifen appears to be better. If we look at risk of recurrence according to estrogen levels after CAF, the findings are as you may expect. In the comparison of Zoladex versus no hormonal therapy, the hazard ratio is 0.7 if you are premenopausal (borderline effect), but there appears to be no benefit if you are postmenopausal (no surprise). The addition of tamoxifen appears to have a greater effect (and the only significant effect) if you are postmenopausal.

I want to move onto the amenorrhea question. How important is it? Multiple retrospective analyses have shown a correlation between amenorrhea and outcome. Chemotherapy-induced amenorrhea is a function of the age of the patient and the chemotherapy regimen and, if you look at some of the reports, there can be rates of amenorrhea of less than 10% in younger women. I mention this as an example of at least one initiative that I personally think is very important. In the United States premenopausal women who received chemotherapy in the adjuvant setting and who remained premenopausal would receive tamoxifen as standard therapy. What about ovarian function suppression? I have had patients whose first question has been, "Should we get rid of these periods?"

The question is: In premenopausal women in the adjuvant setting, are there some areas of research that you would like to address? I want to add one other thing. The CALGB (Cancer And Leukemia Group B) is coming forward with a proposal to do a three-arm study in premenopausal ER-positive women with a randomization between tamoxifen, tamoxifen plus goserelin, or goserelin plus letrozole (looking at aromatase inhibitors in that setting). Dan (Hayes), you were at the CALGB meeting last week. Are there any comments you want to add? This is the type of thinking that is going on right now, at least in the U.S. groups, and I think there are discussions with Novartis about getting the letrozole for this. I think that all of the major companies (Novartis, AstraZeneca, and Pharmacia) are planning premenopausal studies looking at an LH-RH analogue plus their aromatase inhibitor. I will open it up for other comments or suggestions.

M. Dowsett: I am just wondering what the accepted duration of LH-RH agonist treatment is now. Has 5 years been accepted?

J. Ingle: That is the way it is written now, and in the IBCSG it is 5 years too.

D. Hayes: I think the IBCSG is 2 years.

J. Forbes: Yes, it is 2 years.

M. Dowsett: We have spent a lot of time yesterday and a little bit today talking about the bone issues with aromatase inhibitors in postmenopausal women. Is this going to be addressed in all of these trials (on LH-RH analogues)?

J. Ingle: Women's bones are monitored whether they are premenopausal and become amenorrheic after chemotherapy or they are premenopausal and they get an LH-RH agonist, or they are postmenopausal. Women's bones now are monitored, and if they need it, they get bisphosphonates. It has become essentially a nonissue as long as people are aware that it is something that has to be monitored.

M. Gnant: We started a trial of goserelin plus anastrozole versus goserelin plus tamoxifen in premenopausal women with hormone-responsive cancers last year. So far we have recruited 400 patients. One of the things we were worried about was bone mineral density in the no-tamoxifen group, but preliminary safety analyses at 12 and 18 months postrandomization haven't given cause to stop the trial. I believe that a very important trial in this context will be combining aromatase inhibitors with oophorectomy with/without chemotherapy to find out whether it is necessary at all to treat at least the highly endocrine-responsive cancers with chemotherapy in premenopausal patients.

J. Ingle: It is obvious that there are two issues: (a) the importance of ovarian function suppression and (b) the role of aromatase inhibitors in premenopausal women.

J. Forbes: A case could be made, given the data in advanced disease and the data you have just presented from the Intergroup on Zoladex plus tamoxifen plus chemotherapy, that the standard endocrine arm actually is LH-RH agonists or ovarian suppression plus tamoxifen.

J. Ingle: There is no study that shows that, unfortunately. It is all extrapolation from another setting. Most people would think that you are probably going to be right, but at least in the United States, the concensus has been that people are unwilling to automatically switch over to ovarian function suppression. We have had discussions with Dr. Gelber, and when the studies were being designed, the sense was that many of the members of IBCSG would be unwilling to randomize to a tamoxifen-only arm. There are global differences in opinion.

Unless there are other issues, we will move ahead to postmenopausal women with metastatic disease. As you know, there have been paradigm-changing data. The first-line hormonal therapy data came in and really changed things. There are the Faslodex data that have been submitted for approval, Per Lønning's data on exemestane, and we will have the adjuvant therapy studies.

I would like to outline what I think is a reasonable paradigm for the hormonal management of postmenopausal women. Today, tamoxifen for 5 years is the standard. If patients recur within a year, they get a nonsteroidal aromatase inhibitor. If they progress, they get Megace or exemestane. I presented this in January, and it is of interest that most of the American groups would use a nonsteroidal aromatase inhibitor based on the data that had been presented to the U.S. Food and Drug Administration. However, at that time this was not the case for many Canadian oncologists. There have been those who suggest that the patient's status—whether symptomatic or not— should determine which strategy should be used. I believe most people think that this hormonal management plan (containing letrozole) is the way to go at this point in time.

J. Forbes: There are two trials that have had data presented at San Antonio and ASCO. I'm not sure whether they have been published, but they are widely known. These are the second-line comparisons of an aromatase inhibitor, which happened to be anastrozole, versus Faslodex. You could include Faslodex in the paradigm.

J. Ingle: But Faslodex hasn't been approved yet. However, if Faslodex is approved, as shown in this slide, then still the control for adjuvant is tamoxifen. If people recur within 12 months, then it will be either Faslodex or an aromatase inhibitor. I suspect that there will be a great interest in Faslodex, primarily from the patients' financial standpoint. I have a number of patients who say "I wish I had an injectable form, because my insurance company doesn't want to pay the $6 per day." Over here (Europe) it would essentially be the same, I think.

The second contingency, as shown on this slide, is if ATAC is positive, meaning some advantage for anastrozole. I doubt the combination will be positive on the basis of Dr. Brodie's data. If ATAC is positive, anastrozole would become first-line adjuvant hormonal therapy, and this might occur in 2002, because there would likely be an expedited approval, at least in the United States. This is unlikely, but it is a contingency we have to deal with. If there is a recurrence within 12 months, well, I'm not sure—possibly a SERM. If there is recurrence after 12 months, I don't know if it would be exemestane or letrozole or whatever. The whole landscape will change.

Comments please on postmenopausal metastatic breast cancer next-generation studies, keeping in mind that it would take at least 6 months to get a study up and running.

A. Howell: I think it is highly likely that Faslodex might be superior to tamoxifen, and we will know those results later this year. So, to give tamoxifen and then first-line treatment after tamoxifen, I think you are in real trouble. The study would be an aromatase inhibitor versus Faslodex, and it is being planned at the moment.

J. Ingle: So if Faslodex is better than tamoxifen . . .

A. Howell: It will be difficult for you to use tamoxifen in that situation.

J. Ingle: You're absolutely right that this would be another contingency one would have to deal with.

A. Howell: I think it is a likely contingency.

J. Ingle: The metastatic setting has been considered last because all of the emphasis is going to be on the development of new strategies in the earlier settings. This may be the area where there is examination of the addition of new agents for the inhibition of multiple signal transduction pathways. You may see a series of phase II studies. The question is: Are there any obvious phase III studies that you can think of that could be done at this point in time?

If Dr. Brodie in her laboratory corroborates the Zaccheo pre-clinical study showing the combination of tamoxifen and exemestane to be superior to either alone, the American Breast Intergroup has discussed studying that combination. As you remember, the nonsteroidals haven't been superior in combination, so why would the steroidals be? That is the only issue that has at least been discussed. The other issue is that Joanne Mortimer of CALGB has a study of anastrozole alone versus anastrozole plus trastuzimab.

D. Hayes: No, it's a study of treatment with tamoxifen where those who progress on tamoxifen receive Herceptin plus/minus tamoxifen. It's a controversial trial design, but that is it.

J. Ingle: It has been discussed for a number of years.

A. Brodie: We are currently doing the study that Jim Ingle mentioned of exemestane plus tamoxifen, but we don't have those data yet. The slide he showed, though, predicted that tamoxifen was worse than Faslodex, as Tony Howell thought, but letrozole is still better than Faslodex.

J. Forbes: If there are data that comes from the laboratory or anywhere else about the combination, you may need to consider a third arm of Faslodex plus an aromatase inhibitor. Can I just remind you of the definitive study in advanced disease of the EORTC (European Organization for Research and Treatment of Cancer) group that Jan Klijn led, where they took the trouble to have three arms and we have learned so much more from that than any two-arm study? It would need quite a substantial international collaboration with groups, I think.

C. Benz: Another factor that might affect the use of tamoxifen in this trial design is whether any of the eligible patients are HER-2–positive. Given awareness of Matt Ellis's results, there may be less inclination to accept treatment with tamoxifen before that with an aromatase inhibitor.

H. Mouridsen: We are discussing advanced breast cancer, right? We have seen in the past so many trials of chemotherapy plus/minus tamoxifen looking at combinations and sequence. These trials have all been negative. I think the situation may be completely different with the aromatase inhibitors. We have to consider doing all of these trials again, looking at the optimal sequence of endocrine and chemotherapy in receptor-positive patients—i.e., first-line therapy in metastatic disease.

J. Ingle: So you would be looking for an advantage of chemo/hormonal therapy over hormonal therapy alone?

H. Mouridsen: I would like to see whether the sequence we use today is correct, because that sequence is based on trials with chemotherapy and tamoxifen.

J. Ingle: I agree with you Henning (Mouridsen). We have so many of those trials going back, and that was with an inferior hormonal agent. So, why would you think that a newer, more potent hormonal agent would be different? Why would you think that chemo/hormonal therapy would be positive over a hormonal agent alone?

H. Mouridsen: That may also be due to interference between chemotherapy and tamoxifen, which might not be the case with chemotherapy plus an aromatase inhibitor.

D. Hayes: Do you know that would not be the case?

H. Mouridsen: No.

J. Ingle: I think for a study like that, especially a phase III study, you would have to have some preclinical data that would give you a testable hypothesis.

M. Ellis: I would strongly underline that. For combination studies— i.e., hormones plus chemotherapy—to be done, we need preclinical modeling that convincingly shows that adding the hormone to the chemotherapy is an appropriate thing to do. I can show you preclinical models. When you use a cycle-dependent chemotherapy like Taxol, you reduce the cytotoxicity of the Taxol by inducing cell-cycle arrest. It is a very obvious thing. I would urge caution to those who think that adding the hormone to the chemotherapy is a good idea. It is not necessarily so.

M. Dowsett: Just one comment on that. There is work by Texiera looking at the interaction between tamoxifen and doxorubicin, and in the circumstance the downregulation of BCL-2 sensitized the cells to doxorubicin. You can actually argue this either way on preclinical models. You can increase the sensitivity perhaps by increasing the S-phase fraction before hitting it, etc.

M. Ellis: Well this wasn't borne out in the case of SWOG 8814, in which CAF alone followed by tamoxifen was compared with concurrent tamoxifen and CAF followed by tamoxifen with no difference in outcome (although we need an update).

C. Rose: Coming back to the main question. What were the preclinical data supporting the trial you just demonstrated for us, the Intergroup study comparing tamoxifen with CAF plus tamoxifen?

J. Ingle: What was the basis?

C. Rose: Yes, you asked Henning for the basis for such a study. To my mind we have no preclinical data telling us that.

J. Ingle: The basis was that when this study was designed in about 1986, the standard of care was tamoxifen in postmenopausal, node-positive, receptor-positive women, and this study was to see if a doxorubicin-based program was better.

C. Rose: I agree with that; but coming back to the principle of combining chemo- and endocrine therapy, we have rather good data telling us that the combination of CMF plus tamoxifen is actually superior to CMF alone in the advanced setting.

J. Ingle: You're talking about using chemotherapy alone versus hormonal therapy plus chemotherapy, which is a different question.

C. Rose: I am talking about CMF in the original fashion compared to CMF plus tamoxifen. Now I think Henning (Mouridsen) is talking about trying a better form of chemotherapy and combining it with endocrine therapy or vice versa. I think still it is worthwhile pursuing that concept in the metastatic situation.

J. Ingle: I think that our colleagues in the laboratory have become so much more sophisticated that the days of empiricism should be over. Unless there is compelling evidence of substantial additivity or synergy, then I think it would be difficult to come up with a lot of support.

M. Dowsett: Before responding to Matt Ellis's point there, I was going to make a slightly different point. You were talking about what trials we should do. One of the things that has been driving us forward over the last few years has been trying to get better and better estrogen deprivation. We're now talking about the possibility of combining a very effective aromatase inhibitor with Faslodex. All of this is rational if we are trying to get complete estrogen deprivation. If we consider the data that Jan Klijn has derived, this is relatively compelling evidence in the premenopausal setting using tamoxifen, which many of us would not view as a particularly good antiestrogenic agent. There are two trials in the metastatic setting that are really quite important. One is led by Charlie Coombes, which should start soon and is looking at stepwise estrogen deprivation and asking the question: Have we been right to deliver these new highly effective estrogen-depriving agents right up front or are we better controlling the disease in a stepwise fashion? My preference would be for the former, but the question remains to be answered. Then there is the other issue that if we go down to these very low levels, either stepwise or with an immediate drop, returning to perhaps just premenopausal estrogen levels may then be an effective therapy for the patients and again controlling the disease for longer using that manipulation. Those are two interesting studies based on the principles we are looking at in the lab.

J. Ingle: What do you think about a study of letrozole versus letrozole plus Faslodex?

M. Dowsett: I have a worry about this. I believe letrozole is a more effective drug pharmacologically than anastrozole. Therefore if you add Faslodex to anastrozole, you might actually overcome that small deficit in the effectiveness of anastrozole. So now we have got anastrozole and Faslodex combined showing better efficacy than anastrozole alone. You might well not find that when you combine Faslodex with letrozole. Nonetheless I would rather see the study done with letrozole.

A. Brodie: We did compare Faslodex with letrozole and actually it wasn't better in combination than letrozole alone.

J. Ingle: But Angela (Brodie), letrozole is so powerful, could we expect the combination to be much better? I suppose it could be at least as good.

A. Brodie: Yes, it was good, but it wasn't any better than letrozole alone. It was about equivalent in combination with Faslodex. However, we have not yet compared time to treatment failure of the two drugs or different doses of Faslodex.

J. Ingle: I would like to ask Tony Howell a question. Do you have any thoughts along the lines of what Mitch Dowsett was saying or things you would like to propose?

A. Howell: Well, despite Angela (Brodie)'s model not showing superiority to letrozole intermittent with tamoxifen, I still feel that there is room somewhere in here to test the hypothesis that we shouldn't wait for resistance for each of these agents to occur before changing over. We ought to do some sort of alternating treatment before resistance occurs. Second, from the principles we have seen from Dick Santen's data (and others have repeated them), it may be appropriate to lower estrogen levels and raise estrogen levels on an alternating basis for advanced disease. I think it is very hard to put those studies in at the moment because the question that needs to be answered is: What is the best first-line agent after tamoxifen? Is it an aromatase inhibitor or is it Faslodex? However, that study will be going on, and then we have got to think of the next studies to improve further because I don't think we are going to get any better agents coming through now and we have got to use the four classes of SERMs, as I said, and the two classes or aromatase inhibitors more effectively to stop this regression/progression/regression/progression cycle that we do with patients at the moment. We have got to think what we do post-Faslodex and postaromatase inhibitors and think more innovatively.

J. Ingle: Several testable hypotheses have been identified and obviously people should pursue them.

H. Mouridsen: Has anyone planned to compare, in the situation where aromatase inhibitors are indicated, a steroidal with a nonsteroidal inhibitor in a crossover study?

M. Dixon: Pharmacia, I think, have a plan to compare exemestane with anastrozole.

A. Howell: All one would ask, if they did that study, is that they powered it to give a proper result. It is very easy to underpower that sort of study. I think the letrozole/anastrozole that you have in the can is probably underpowered also.

H. Mouridsen: I think the Pharmacia study is restricted to patients with liver metastasis.

J. Ingle: Henning (Mouridsen), is that something that you would make a case for doing?

H. Mouridsen: Yes, I think it should be done.

J. Ingle: To do such a study properly and properly power it, it would be gigantic. In terms of premenopausal breast cancer, we have talked about this the other day, but there is a paucity of data in metastatic disease. Going back, we can look at oophorectomy, tamoxifen, LH-RH agonists, and then the combination. Jan Klijn's study (which was wonderful) showed that even with only around 160 patients you could really make a contribution. The overall survival data show an advantage for the combination. I think one can make a case in the metastatic setting based on a randomized clinical trial that an LH-RH agonist plus tamoxifen is reasonable in premenopausal women. The question comes up in the premenopausal setting: Is there value to looking at the third-generation aromatase inhibitors in conjunction with an LH-RH agonist? It would be interesting to get some data (if data exist) on the third-generation inhibitors alone. A comparative study could take LH-RH agonist plus tamoxifen versus LH-RH plus letrozole. Any thoughts?

M. Ellis: Again, the issue is that so many women in the metastatic setting have seen tamoxifen. So finding tamoxifen-naïve premenopausal women who would be eligible for that study would be very tricky. Klijn's study was done at a time when less tamoxifen was used. I certainly think that an LH-RH agonist plus letrozole would be one arm, but what would be the other arm? Would it be Faslodex alone or an LH-RH agonist plus Faslodex? That might be a more contemporary design which might reflect the populations of patients we actually see.

C. Rose: I think first of all we have to define what the control arm should be for future studies. Up to now an LH-RH agonist plus tamoxifen seems to have been superior. But there are two reasons to question this: first, almost all of these patients have seen tamoxifen adjuvantly, and we now have data showing the superiority of the aromatase inhibitors over tamoxifen in the postmenopausal setting.

I think it is a fair conclusion to draw that a combination of an LH-RH agonist making these premenopausal patients postmenopausal and then adding, let's say letrozole, would be at least as efficacious as the combination of the LH-RH agonist and tamoxifen. To my mind the control arm should be Zoladex plus letrozole. Then comes the question: With what should we compare it?

J. Klijn: I think the same (Zoladex plus letrozole) plus Faslodex: triple therapy with an LH-RH agonist and an aromatase inhibitor to have maximal suppression of estrogen levels in combination with blockade of the estradiol receptor. I think that Faslodex is more suitable for blocking the estradiol receptor than tamoxifen.

K. Tonkin: Aren't you going to get into a situation here of rather small numbers? The number of women who are going to remain premenopausal after current chemotherapy for adjuvant disease when they present with metastatic disease will be small. Given that many of them have already seen tamoxifen, you are going to be talking about a small proportion of eligible women. How many of these women are we going to see? The answer is not very many. If you think of your own practice, how many of the women do you see that you are going to be able to give Zoladex to, if you wanted to? Again, the answer is not very many. I would like to go back to what Henning Mouridsen said about the chemotherapy. In this group of patients, surely we could suggest a chemotherapy element, although I don't think that it makes any sense at all, concurrently, but maybe sequentially. Is there not some possibility of that situation with these women? Almost all of them will have had chemotherapy adjuvantly, so they will have had some chemotherapy, and they will likely have had some tamoxifen as well. Therefore it becomes difficult to decide what options are available.

J. Ingle: This seems to be a particularly problematic subset. There are some interesting questions that could be asked, but for multiple reasons, including the small pool size, it would be difficult to do a randomized study. Laboratory analysis may be more reasonable.

A. Howell: Given the Intergroup data, which look very powerful in the under-40's for adding LH-RH agonists, you are going to have everybody who is menstruating being treated in that way. I think this would be right too. So you are not going to have anybody coming through. However, if you look at the ZEBRA study, there are a lot of oncologists in Europe and perhaps more specifically in Austria who are not convinced about the use of chemotherapy in premenopausal ER-positive women. These patients have been put on Zoladex for 2 years and have been taken off. Then, if they have a relapse, they can go back on Zoladex again. Maybe one or two of the European groups (the Germans and the Austrians) could do that sort of study.

J. Ingle: Do we have any other comments about any of the four topics we have discussed?

A. Bhatnagar: I think we have had an extremely valuable two days. A great deal of information has been discussed. In the final discussion, we have been able to distill out some of the issues that we need to look at in the future and identify the directions that we would like to go. I think it could have been expected that we would not come to a complete consensus, as it is very difficult to get consensus in an area like this. However, considering the fact that we have so many different and varied opinions, I think that the participants have done an excellent job of charting the general direction for future research and helping visualize new horizons. That has been the hallmark of this meeting. As you know, the proceedings of this meeting will be published, as this information is not only very valuable and should be shared with the rest of the medical community but also it should be done as expeditiously as possible. Thank you all for your contributions to a highly productive and successful meeting.

Index

Ablation, *vs.* LH-RH agonists, 116
Ablative endocrine therapy, 5–6
Acquired endocrine resistance, ErbB
  receptors, 237
Actonel, 147
Additive endocrine therapy, 5–6
Adenocarcinoma, endometrial, 288
Adjuvant chemotherapy,
  postmenopausal women, 261
  time period, 117
Adjuvant Tamoxifen Treatment Offer
  More (ATTOM), 137
Adjuvant therapy, new drug testing, 251
Adrenalectomy, 6
  medical, 35
Adriamycin, 20
  plus cyclophosphamide, *vs.* tamoxifen,
  24
Advanced breast cancer,
  aromatase inhibitors, 33–42
  chemotherapy, 345–346

[Advanced breast cancer]
  oophorectomy, historical perspective, 4
  panel discussion, 91–122
  SERMs, 47–69
  tamoxifen, 17–28
    vs. aromatase inhibitors, 25–28
    background, 18–19
    vs. chemotherapy, 24–25
    combined endocrine therapy, 21–23
    current clinical use, 18–19
    early trials, 19
    first-line single endocrine agent,
    20–21
    vs. other endocrine therapy, 21
    combinations, 23
    tolerability, 19
    trial endpoints, 20
Age,
  endocrine therapy chemoprevention,
  320, 322
  ER, 321

[Age]
oral contraceptives, 326–327
PgR, 321
primary endocrine therapy, 98
Age-incidence curve,
ER-negative/PgR-negative tumors, 321
non-hormone-dependent cancer,
269–270
Alendronate (Fosamax), 147
Alzheimer's disease, 149–150, 166
Amenorrhea, 352
Aminoglutethimide,
development, 34–35
vs. tamoxifen, 25
with tamoxifen, 23
Amphiregulin, 232
Anastrozole, 36, 39, 355
vs. atemestane, 360–361
vs. faslodex, 121
future role, 68–69
vs. letrozole, 107–108, 109–110
long-term administration, 108–109
percentage response rates, 105–106
vs. tamoxifen, 23, 26–27, 37, 106,
107–108, 142
metastatic disease, 138
thromboembolic events, 113
Androgen-androgen receptor (AR), 4
Androgens, 6
Angiogenesis, 250
endocrine therapy response, 225
Angiostatin, 84–85
Antiestrogens,
breast cancer prevention, 303–307
future trials, 306
pure, 64–68
Antiprogestins, 82–83
ANZ 7801, 24
ANZ GCTG trial, 20
Apoptosis, 160–163, 216, 218, 244–246
AR, 4
Arimidex, 66–67
Arimidex Nolvadex (ARNO) trial, 142
Arimidex Tamoxifen Alone or Combined
(ATAC), 23, 120, 141, 355

ARNO trial, 142
Aromatase antibodies, 256–257
Aromatase enzyme, transcription
regulation, 137
Aromatase gene, MCF-7 cells, 338
Aromatase inhibitors, 6
advanced breast cancer, 33–42
atypical hyperplasia, 315
biochemical efficacy, 39
bone mineral density, 147
bone resorption, 167
cancer prevention, 294, 309–316,
327
trials, 314–315
cost, 174
cross-resistance lack, 40–41
development, 34–35
dosage, 328
early breast cancer, 135–143
rationale, 137–138
efficacy, 40
estrogen, 312
evaluation, 106
future directions, 41–42
vs. gestagens, 111–112
liver, 41
long-term toxicity, 138
metabolic complications, 166–167
metastatic disease, 138
ongoing trials, 139–142
evaluation, 142–143
reporting order, 142
osteoporosis, 328
overall success, 112
palliation, 92
postmenopausal women, 338–340
preclinical models, 143
premenopausal women, 119, 329
response, 205
second generation, 35
vs. SERMs, 146
selection, 321
vs. tamoxifen, 25–28, 94
early trials, 25
third generation, 26–27, 36, 37–39

[Aromatase inhibitors]
transdermal delivery, 341
Aromatic hydrocarbon carcinogens,
288
Arzoxifene, 48, 61–62
Ascorbic acid, 290
Asian women, 269, 275–276
ATAC, 23, 120, 141, 355
Atemestane, 83
vs. anastrozole, 360–361
ATTOM, 137
Atypical ductal hyperplasia, 320
Atypical hyperplasia, aromatase
inhibitors, 315
Australian New Zealand Breast Cancer
Trials Group (ANZ GCTG)
trial, 20

Bcl-2, 218
endocrine therapy response,
225
neoadjuvant tamoxifen response,
226–227
Beatson, George Thomas, 4
Benign ovarian cystadenomas, cell
proliferation,
LH-RH agonists, 324
Betacellulin, 232
BHA, 290
BIG/FEMTA trial, 139–140
Biomarkers,
breast cancer risk, 311–312
drug therapy *vs.* tumor
manipulation,
245–246
estrogen, 311–312
Letrozole 024 Neoadjuvant Study,
188–189
preoperative setting, 176
tests, 83–86
Biopsy, timing, 247–251
Birth control pills (*see* Oral
contraceptives)
Bisphosphonate therapy, 140
Bone demineralization, 138

Bone mineral density, 140,
166
aromatase inhibitors, 147
estrogen exposure, 311
Bone resorption, 167
BRCA1, 311
mutations, 279
BRCA2, 311
Breast,
conservation, 259
density,
estrogen exposure, 312
letrozole, 315
Breast cancer,
chemoprevention, panel discussion,
319–333
ErbB receptors, 235–236
ER primary, tamoxifen, 325
heterogeneity, 228
incidence, modeling, 272–276
intertumor variability, 228
morphological changes, following
neoadjuvant chemotherapy,
215–216
natural history, 175–176
prevention, 338–343
antiestrogens, 303–307
aromatase inhibitors, 309–316
estrogen genotoxicity inhibition,
287–295
hormonal therapy, 267–281
minimally invasive procedure,
326–327
premenopausal women, 342–343
strategies, 293–295
young women, 330
residual,
assessment, 215–216
following neoadjuvant
chemotherapy, 216
risk, 270–271
biomarkers, 311–312
defining, 320
ERT, 310
estrogen levels, 323

Breast-cell labeling index, 273
Breast International Group, 139–140
Buserelin, 80
 vs. tamoxifen, 21–22
Butylated hydroxyanisol (BHA), 290

CAF, with tamoxifen, 131
Cancer cells,
 circulating, detection, 97
 total protein levels, 98
Candidate genes, identification, 250
Castration,
 chemical, 6
 surgical,
  cost, 118
  vs. LH-RH agonists, 116
Catecholestrogen (CE), 289–292
 metabolic redox cycling, 289–292
Catechol-O-methyl transferase (COMT),
  294–295
CCEPRT, 276–277
cDNA arrays, 248
CE, 289–292
 metabolic redox cycling, 289–292
CEA assays, 176
Cell cycle, 253–254
 following neoadjuvant therapy,
  226–227
C-erbB$_2$, endocrine therapy response, 225
Charcoal assay,
 dextran-coated, 95
Chemical castration, 6
Cholesterol, 332–333
 tamoxifen, 19
Chromatin clumping, 216–217
Chronic myeloid leukemia, 84
CKIs, 236–237
Clemarson's Hook, 329–330
Clinical trials,
 design, 252–253, 349–351
 doses, 342
Clomiphene, 278
CMF,
 with epirubicin, *vs.* tamoxifen, 129
 plus tamoxifen, 25, 130–131

Cognitive function, 149–150
Colorectal cancer, age-specific incidence
  rates, 270
COMT, 294–295
Continuous-combined estrogen-
   progestin replacement therapy
   (CCEPRT), 276–277
Copenhagen Breast Cancer Trials, 126
Cost,
 aromatase inhibitors, 174
 goserelin, 118
 surgical castration, 118
 United Kingdom, 173
Crossover study, tamoxifen *vs.* letrozole,
  338
Cyclin kinase inhibitors (CKIs),
  236–237
Cyclophosphamide, 20
 plus doxorubicin, *vs.* tamoxifen, 24
Cyclophosphamide/ methotrexate/5-
   fluorouracil (CMF),
 with epirubicin, *vs.* tamoxifen, 129
 plus tamoxifen, 25, 130–131
Cyclophosphamide/adriamycin/fluoro-
   uracil (CAF), with tamoxifen,
   131
CYP1B1, 294
CYP19 gene polymorphism, 311
Cytokeratine immunostain, 99
Cytoplasm, vacuolization, 217

DCIS, tamoxifen, 18, 320
Deep vein thrombosis (DVT),
 avoidance, 331
 tamoxifen, 173
DES, 48, 50–51, 182
 vs. tamoxifen, 51
Dextran-coated charcoal assay, 95
Didronel, 147
Diet, 326
Diethylstilbestrol (DES), 48, 50–51,
  182
 vs. tamoxifen, 51
DNA damage, estrogen-induced,
  292–293

Docetaxel, *vs.* paclitaxel, 251
Doxorubicin (adriamycin), 20
   plus cyclophosphamide, *vs.* tamoxifen,
      24
Droloxifene, 48, 56–58, 83, 150
   clinical efficacy, 59–60
   ErbB-2, 96–97
Duct carcinoma in situ (DCIS),
      tamoxifen, 18, 320
DVT,
   avoidance, 331
   tamoxifen, 173

E$_2$, 288–289
   serum concentrations, 273
   tumor initiation, 290–292
Early breast cancer,
   aromatase inhibitors, 135–143
   panel discussion, 171–177
   SERMS, 145–153
   surrogate markers, 157–167
   tamoxifen, 125–132
      vs. chemotherapy, 129
      with chemotherapy, 130–131
      duration, 129–130
      ER-negative tumors, 127–129
      ER-positive tumors, 127–129
      node-negative tumors, 127
      node-positive tumors, 127
      postmenopausal women, 126
      premenopausal women, 126
      prognostic factors, 132
Early Breast Cancer Trialists'
      Collaborative Group, 126
Economics (*see* Cost)
Effective mitotic rate, 274
EGF, 232
EGFR, 83
   endocrine therapy response, 225
   overexpression, 104
EM-800, 48, 62–63
EMA, 216
Endocrine axes, 4
Endocrine resistance, ErbB receptors,
      236–237

Endocrine therapy,
   ablative, 5–6
   additive, 5–6
   advanced tumors, selection, 228–229
   chemoprevention,
      approaches, 319
      population, 320
      risk assessment, 320
      strategy, 320
      targeted, 320–321
      timing, 319
   vs. chemotherapy, 94
   decision making, 92–93, 96–97,
      102–103
   ER-directed, clinical toxicity,
      10–11
   historical perspective, 4–5
   metastases, 112
   preoperative,
      trial, 346
      tumor triage, 262–263
   primary, decision making, 98
   prior, 100
   rationale, 3–11
   resistance, 7–9, 231–238
      ERs, 7–8
      HER, 8
      non-ER markers, 8
      non-ER mechanisms, 9
      overcoming, 9–11
      tamoxifen long-term administration,
         8–9
   response, ER, 224
   targeted, chemoprevention, 320–321
Endometriosis, LH-RH agonists,
      324
Endometrium,
   adenocarcinoma, 288
   cancer, 19, 138, 277
Endostatin, 84–85
Epidermal growth factor (EGF), 232
Epidermal growth factor receptor
      (EGFR), 83
   endocrine therapy response, 225
   overexpression, 104

Epiregulin, 232
Epirubicin, with CMF, *vs.* tamoxifen,
    129
Epithelial hyperplasia, aromatase
    inhibitors, 315
Epithelial membrane antigen (EMA),
    216
EPRT, 269, 276–277
    breast cancer risk, 272
Equivalency trial, 253
ER (*see* Estrogen-estrogen receptor)
ERα, 234
ERA-923, 63–64
ErbB, 235
    breast cancer, 235–236
    letrozole, 188–189
    tamoxifen, 188–189
ErbB1, 232
ErbB1⁺, letrozole, neoadjuvant
    endocrine therapy,
    189–190
ErbB2, 232
    breast cancer, 235–236
    cell-cycle effectors, 237
    droloxifene, 96–97
ErbB2⁺, letrozole, neoadjuvant endocrine
    therapy, 189–190
ErbB3, 232
    breast cancer, 235–236
ErbB4, 232
    breast cancer, 235–236
ErbB receptors, 232–233
    acquired endocrine resistance, 237
    breast cancer, 235–236
    mammary gland, 233–235
    polypeptide ligands, 232–233
    pregnancy, 235
ER-directed endocrine therapy, clinical
    toxicity, 10–11
ERE, 7
ER-negative/PgR-negative tumors,
    age-specific incidence curve,
    321
    vs. ER-positive/PgR-positive tumors,
    321

ER-negative tumors, 93
    endocrine therapy chemoprevention,
    325
    tamoxifen, 127–129
ER-positive tumors, 93
    vs. ER negative tumors, prediction,
    323
    HER-2, 97
    nonresponders, 95–96
    premenopausal women, 352–353
    tamoxifen, 127–129
ERT,
    vs. antiestrogen therapy, 51
    breast cancer risk, 310
    early application, 10
    risks, 269
Estradiol (E₂), 288–289
    serum, 273
        Japanese, 275
        measurement, 340
    tumor initiation, 290–292
Estrogen,
    biomarkers, 311–312
    dual action, 289–290
    exposure, indices, 340
    genotoxicity, 287–295
        mechanism, 291
    high-dose, 50–52
    historical perspective, 4–5
    initiation process, 325–326
    levels,
        breast cancer risk, 323
        elevated, 339
    lifetime exposure, endocrine therapy
        chemoprevention, 320
    mammary gland, 233–235
    vs. oral contraceptives, 326
    preventing effects, 312–314
    serum concentrations, estrogen
        exposure, 311–312
    synthesis, 311
    vs. tamoxifen, 21
Estrogen-estrogen receptor (ER), 3, 83
    age, 321
    assays, antihormonal drugs, 98

[Estrogen-estrogen receptor (ER)]
  endocrine therapy,
    decision making, 102–103
    resistance, 7–8
    response, 224
  genetic experiments, 289–290
  Letrozole 024 Neoadjuvant Study,
    185–186
  mutations, 136–137
  prediction, 93, 96–97
Estrogen 4-hydroxylase inhibitors,
    342–343
Estrogen-induced DNA damage,
    292–293
Estrogen-progestin hypothesis, 272,
    276
Estrogen-progestin replacement therapy
    (EPRT), 269, 276–277
  breast cancer risk, 272
Estrogen-related genes, 247
Estrogen replacement therapy (ERT),
  vs. antiestrogen therapy, 51
  breast cancer risk, 310
  early application, 10
  risks, 269
Estrogen response elements (ERE), 7
Estrone, 288–289
Ethinylestradiol, 50–51, 290, 331
Etidronate (Didronel), 147
Exemestane, 36, 39
  after tamoxifen, 141
  vs. anastrozole, 360–361
  evaluation, 106
  in nonsteroidal failures, 40
  percentage response rates, 105–106
  vs. tamoxifen, 141

Fadrozole
  estrogen, menstrual cycle, 329
  vs. tamoxifen, 25
Farnesyl transferase inhibitors, 85, 258
Faslodex, 23, 92, 120–121, 136, 137,
    354–355
  vs. anastrozole, 121
  with letrozole, 359

[Faslodex]
  study, 258
  surrogate markers, 160–161
Ferrous solutions, 97
Fibroblasts, 244
Fibroids, LH-RH agonists, 324
Fine needle aspiration, 99–100
Flaxseed,
  cancer prevention, 312–313
  structure, 313
Fluoroestradiol, 290, 326
Formestane,
  in aminoglutethimide failures, 40
  vs. tamoxifen, 25
Fosamax, 147
Fulvestrant, 53, 64–67
  clinical efficacy, 60
  clinical studies, 64–67

Gail model, 311
  risk factors, 340
Gastrointestinal stromal tumors (GIST-
    tumors), 84
Gene expression, xenografts, surgical
    expression, 245–248
Gene microarrays, 227
Genotoxic process, 325–326
GEP, 279–280
German Adjuvant Breast Cancer Group,
    129
Germline aromatase genes,
    polymorphisms, 257
Gestagens, vs. aromatase inhibitors,
    111–112
GIST-tumors, 84
Gliveec, 84
Glucocorticoid-glucocorticoid receptor
    (GR), 4
Glutathione transferases (GST), 295
Gn-RHA, 278–279
  ovarian cancer, 279
  plus tamoxifen, 281
Gonadotropin-releasing hormone agonist
    +estrogen-progestin (GEP),
    279–280

Gonadotropin-releasing hormone agonist
    (Gn-RHA), 278–279
    ovarian cancer, 279
    plus tamoxifen, 281
Goserelin,
    premenopausal women, 351
    with tamoxifen, 10
Goserelin plus anastrozole, *vs.* goserelin
    plus tamoxifen, 353
Goserelin plus tamoxifen, *vs.* goserelin
    plus anastrozole, 353
GR, 4
GST, 295
GW5638, 48, 59

HB-EGF, 232
Hematoma, mammotome, 249–250
Heparin-binding EGF (HB-EGF),
    232
HER, 4
    endocrine therapy resistance, 8
HER-1, 232
HER-2, 232
HER-3, 232
HER-4, 232
Herceptin, 85–86
High-dose estrogen, 50–52
Hormonal chemoprevention,
    epidemiological basis, 267–281
    future developments, 281
    ovarian cancer, 268
Hormone replacement therapy (HRT),
    267, 276–277 (*see also* Estrogen
    replacement therapy)
    after breast cancer, 148–149
    cognitive function, 149–150
Hprt gene mutation, 293
HRT, 267, 276–277
    after breast cancer, 148–149
    cognitive function, 149–150
Hyalinosis, 218–219
Hydroxyestradiol, 290
Hydroxyestrone, 290, 332
Hydroxyguanine, 292
Hyperchromasia, 216–217

Hypophysectomy, 6
Hypothesis, microarrays, 255

IBCSG Trial VII, 130–131
IBIS, 306
IBIS-2, 315
Idoxifene, 48, 58
    surrogate markers, 160–161
IGF 1, 159
IGFR, 4
Immunicon, 97
Immunostaining, 101
IMPACT trial, 259
Inflammatory cells, 244
Insulin-like growth factor-1 (IGF-1),
    159
Insulin-like growth factor receptors
    (IGFR), 4
International Breast Cancer Intervention
    Study (IBIS), 306
International Breast Cancer Intervention
    Study-2 (IBIS-2), 315
International Breast Cancer Study Group
    (IBCSG) Trial VII, 130–131
International Union Against Cancer,
    response assessment criteria,
    202–203
Intratumoral aromatase model, 113–114
Intrauterine contraceptive device
    (IUCD), 277
Intravaginal ring, 331
Invasive lobular carcinoma, 199–200
Iressa, 86, 347
Ischemic heart disease, 166
Italian National Trial, 306
IUCD, 277

Japanese, breast cancer rates, 274–276

Ki67, 160–163, 246, 289
    antibodies, 234
    labeling index, 218, 220
KiS1, neoadjuvant tamoxifen response,
    226–227
KiS1, protein, 218

Lasofoxifene, 59
Leiden Factor V, 172–173
Letrozole, 36–37, 39
vs. anastrozole, 107–108, 109–110
BIG/FEMTA trial, 139–140
blood levels, 248
bone resorption, 167
breast density, 315
cancer prevention, 294, 327
clinical trials design, 253
ErbB1, 188–189
ErbB2, 188–189
evaluation, 106
favorable outcome, clinical factors,
98
future role, 68–69
vs. letrozole plus faslodex, 359
local progression rate, 260
long-term administration, 108–109
MA17, 140–141
vs. megestrol acetate, 110
neoadjuvant endocrine therapy,
ErbB1⁺, 189–190
percentage response rates, 105–106
premenopausal women, 119
vs. tamoxifen, 26, 37–38, 93–94,
100–101, 106–107, 338, 343–344
metastatic disease, 138
thromboembolic events, 113
Letrozole 024 Neoadjuvant Study,
183–189
biomarkers, 188–189
eligibility, 184–185
ER, 185–186
PR, 186–188
LH, 6 (*see also* Luteinizing hormone-
releasing hormone (LR-RH))
with tamoxifen, 17–18
Liarazole,
estrogen, 314
structure, 314
Liver,
aromatase inhibitors, 41
metastases, 103
pathological enzymes, 103

Lobular carcinoma, invasive, 199–200
LR-RH agonists (*see* Luteinizing
hormone-releasing hormone
agonists)
Luteinizing hormone (LH), 6
with tamoxifen, 17–18
Luteinizing hormone-releasing hormone
(LR-RH) agonists, 80–82
vs. ablation, 116
benign ovarian cystadenomas, 324
endometriosis, 324
fibroids, 324
vs. oophorectomy, 118–119
plus aromatase inhibitors, *vs.* LH-RH
agonists plus tamoxifen, 120
plus tamoxifen, *vs.* LH-RH plus
aromatase inhibitors, 120
premenopausal women, 115
vs. surgical castration, 116
time period, 117
Luteinizing hormone-releasing hormone
(LR-RH) analog, with tamoxifen,
22

MA17, 140–141
Magnetic resonance imaging (MRI),
202
Mammary carcinogenesis, causes,
288–289
Mammary gland,
ErbB receptors, 233–235
estrogens, 233–235
Mammotome, hematoma, 249–250
Markers, endocrine therapy
chemoprevention, 320–321
Mastectomy, neoadjuvant endocrine
therapy, 206
Matrix metalloproteinase inhibitors,
84–85
Matrix metalloproteinase type 2
(MMP-2), 84
MCF-7 breast tumor cell model, 237,
246, 248–249
MCF-7 cells, aromatase gene, 338
Medical adrenalectomy, 35

Medroxyprogesterone acetate (MPA), 6,
     277
Megestrol acetate, 6
  vs. letrozole, 110
  postmenopausal women, 39
Menarche, early
     breast cancer risk, 271
  Japanese, 275
Menopause,
  early, breast cancer risk, 270
  primary endocrine therapy, 98
Metabolic redox cycling, 292
Metastases,
  biopsy, 104
  endocrine therapy, 112
  neoadjuvant endocrine therapy,
     190–193
  postmenopausal women, 354–360
  premenopausal women, 115
Methotrexate/fluorouracil (MF), with
     tamoxifen, 130–131
MIB-1, detection, 99
Mib1, neoadjuvant tamoxifen response,
     227
Microarrays, 244, 247
  alternatives, 250
  hypothesis, 255
Micrometastasis, analysis,
     244
Mifepristone, 83
Minimally invasive procedure, cancer
     prevention, 326–327
MMP-2, 84
Molecular biological techniques, future
     prospects, 86
MPA, 6, 277
MRI, 202
Muc1 assays, 176
Mucinous carcinoma, 202

Naphthoflavone, 290
National Cancer Institute of Canada,
     315
National Institute of Canada-Clinical
     Trials Group, 140

National Surgical Adjuvant and Breast
     Project B20 (NSABP B20), 130
National Surgical Adjuvant and Breast
     Project B33 (NSABP B33), 141
National Surgical Adjuvant and Breast
     Project (NSABP), 10, 127,
     304–305
N-CoR, 236–237
Neoadjuvant, definition, 243
Neoadjuvant anastrozole, tumor
     downstaging
     response, 204–205
Neoadjuvant aromatase inhibitors,
  biological markers, 218
  pathological changes, 218–220
  vs. tamoxifen, pathological changes,
     218–220
Neoadjuvant chemotherapy,
  vs. neoadjuvant letrozole, 344
  PCR, 262
  prognosis, 208
  surgical perspectives, 197–210
  tumor reduction, 210
Neoadjuvant endocrine therapy,
     181–193
  with aromatase inhibitors, 183–189
  breast cancer pathology, 213–220
  excision completeness, 205–206
  historical perspective, 182
  letrozole, ERBB1+, 189–190
  mastectomy, 206
  metastases, 190–193
     vs. preoperative chemotherapy,
     190–192
  oncologist's perspective, 181–193
  prognosis, 208
  randomized trial, *vs.* preoperative
     chemotherapy, 191–193
  response assessment, 201–203
  surgery, cosmetic outcomes, 209
  surgical perspectives, 197–210
  treatment duration, 203
  tumor downstaging, response,
     204–205
  tumor reduction, 210

Neoadjuvant exemestane, tumor
  downstaging response, 204–205
Neoadjuvant letrozole,
  vs. neoadjuvant chemotherapy, 344
  vs. preoperative chemotherapy,
    randomized trial, 191–193
  tumor downstaging response,
    204–205
Neoadjuvant systemic therapy,
  breast-conserving surgery, local
    recurrence, 207–208
Neoadjuvant tamoxifen,
  cell cycle changes, 226–227
  historical perspective, 182
  treatment duration, 203
  tumor downstaging, response,
    204–205
Neoadjuvant therapy, 343–351
  cell cycle changes, 226–227
  late outcome predictor, 346–347
  panel discussion, 243–264
  patient selection, 197–201
  response prediction, 223–229, 264
    ER, 224
    future perspectives, 227–229
  surgical perspectives, 197–210
Neoadjuvant trials, rationale,
    260–261
Neuregulins, 232
Node-negative tumors, tamoxifen,
    127
Node-positive tumors, tamoxifen,
    127
Nolvadex, response rate, 18
Non-hormone-dependent cancer, age-
    incidence curve, 269–270,
    272–274
Norgestrel, 331
NSABP, 10, 127, 304–305
NSABP B20, 130
NSABP B33, 141
Nuclear antigens, detection, 99
Nuclear receptor corepressor (N-CoR),
    236–237
Nutrition, estrogen, 312–313

Oltipraz, 294
Oophorectomy, 6
  advanced breast cancer, historical
    perspective, 4
  vs. goserelin, 115
  vs. LH-RH agonists, 118–119
  vs. tamoxifen, 21, 115
Oral contraceptives, 268, 272, 324
  age, 326–327
  vs. estrogens, 326
ORG 31710, 83
Organochlorines, 288
Osteoporosis, 60–61
  aromatase inhibitors, 328
  SERMs, 146–147
Ovarian ablation, premenopausal
    women, 351
Ovarian cancer,
  Gn-RHA, 279
  hormonal chemoprevention, 268
Ovarian cystadenomas, benign, LH-RH
    agonists, 324
Ovarian cysts, 330

P21, 236–237
P27, 236–237
P53, 83
  detection, 99
  endocrine therapy response, 225
Paclitaxel, vs. docetaxel, 251
PAI-1, 84
PCR, neoadjuvant chemotherapy, 262
PDGF receptors, 84
Pelvic ovarian hyperstimulation
    syndrome, 330
Pesticides, 288
PET, 202, 250
PgR (see Progesterone-progesterone
    receptor)
Phase III trials, 340–342
Plasminogen activator inhibitor type 1
    (PAI-1), 84
Platelet-derived growth factor (PDGF)
    receptors, 84
Pleural cell effusion cytology, 99–100

Polymerase chain reaction (PCR),
  neoadjuvant chemotherapy,
  262
Polymorphisms,
  CYP19 gene, 311
  germline aromatase genes, 257
Polypeptide ligands, ErbB receptors,
  232–233
Positron emission tomography (PET),
  202, 250
Postmenopausal women,
  adjuvant chemotherapy, 261
  aromatase inhibitors, 39, 338–340
  metastases, 354–360
  tamoxifen, 126
  therapeutic choices, 120
Pregnancy, ErbB receptors, 235
Premenopausal women, 114–117
  aromatase inhibitors, 119, 329
  breast cancer prevention,
    342–343
  chemoprevention, 278–281
  chemotherapy, 351
  ER-positive tumors, 352–353
  LH-RH agonists, 115
  metastases, 115
  tamoxifen, 126, 278
  therapeutic choices, 120
  vorozole, 330
Preoperative endocrine therapy, tumor
  triage, 262–263
Preoperative setting,
  biomarkers, 176
  definition, 243
  utilization, 257–258
Preoperative trial, endocrine therapy,
  346
Primary tumor,
  ER status, 228–229
  response, late outcome, 345
Prior therapy, 113–114
PRMs, 82–83
Progestasert, 277
Progesterone antagonists, 82–83
  serum concentrations, 273

Progesterone-progesterone receptor
  (PgR), 4, 83
  age, 321
  assays, 94
  endocrine therapy, decision making,
    102–103
  endocrine therapy response, 225
  prediction, 96–97
Progesterone-progesterone receptor
  (PgR+), letrozole, neoadjuvant
  endocrine therapy, 189–190
Progesterone receptor modulators
  (PRMs), 82–83
Progestin, 277
  breast cancer risk, 271–272
  vs. tamoxifen, 21
  with tamoxifen, 23
Proliferation, 244–246
PS2, 83
  endocrine therapy response, 225
Pulmonary embolism, 19
Pure antiestrogens, 64–68

Quinone reductase, 294

Radiation exposure, 288
Raloxifene, 48, 60–61, 137, 147, 150
  breast cancer prevention, 268,
    306–307
  cancer prevention, 293
  ER expression, 322–323
  surrogate markers, 160–161
Receptor positivity, 98
Receptor tyrosine kinases (RTKs),
  231–232
  inhibitor, 101
RECIST, 105
Residual breast cancer,
  assessment, 215–216
  following neoadjuvant chemotherapy,
    histological grade, 216
Response Evaluation Criteria in Solid
  Tumors (RECIST), 105
Retinoids, estrogen, 314
Risedronate (Actonel), 147

Rituxan, 84
Royal Marsden Prevention Trial,
    305–306
  risk assessment, 320
RTKs, 231–232
  inhibitor, 101

Selective estrogen-receptor modifiers
    (SERMs), 6, 7
  adjuvant therapy, 68–69
  advanced breast cancer, 47–69
  vs. aromatase inhibitors, selection,
    321
  breast cancer prevention, future trials,
    306
  cancer prevention, 293
  cardiovascular effects, 147–148
  cognitive function, 149–150
  early breast cancer, 145–153
    vs. aromatase inhibitors, 146
  estrogen, 312
  fixed-ring, 60–64
    clinical efficacy, 63–64
  future role, 68–69
  nonsteroidal, 53–54
  novel, 52–68, 150–151
    vs. tamoxifen, 150–151
  osteoporosis, 146–147
  triphenylethylene, 55–60, 150
  tumor sampling, 174
SEPRT, 276–277
Sequence, 113–114
Sequential estrogen-progestin
    replacement therapy (SEPRT),
    276–277
SERMs (*see* Selective estrogen-receptor
    modifiers)
Signal transduction pathways,
    254
Steroid hormones, 288
  categories, 5
Steroid receptors, prediction, 100
Surgical castration,
  cost, 118
  vs. LH-RH agonists, 116

Surrogate markers, 174
  breast, 341
  early breast cancer, 157–167
  larger trials, 176
  treatment benefit, 159–165
  treatment complications, 165–167
Swiss Group for Clinical Cancer
    Research, 98

Tamoxifen, 49–50, 83
  with aminoglutethimide, 23
  vs. anastrozole, 23, 26–27, 37, 106,
    107–108, 142
  vs. aromatase inhibitors, 94
    metastatic disease, 138
    third generation, 37–39
  bone density, 166
  breast cancer prevention, 268, 293,
    304–306
  vs. buserelin, 21–22
  with CAF, 131
  vs. CAF plus tamoxifen, 358
  cholesterol, 19
  vs. CMF, with epirubicin, 129
  DCIS, 320
  vs. DES, 51
  DVT, 173
  ErbB1, 188–189
  ErbB2, 188–189
  ER primary breast cancer, 325
  estrogen, 312
  vs. exemestane, 141
  exemestane after, 141
  failure, 137
  with goserelin, 10
  HER-2 positive, 356
  interacting with doxorubicin, 357–358
  ischemic heart disease, 166
  vs. letrozole, 93–94, 100–101,
    106–107, 338
  with LH, 17–18
  with LH-RH analog, 22
  limitations, 136
  long-term administration, 108–109,
    136–137

[Tamoxifen]
endocrine therapy resistance, 8–9
vs. neoadjuvant aromatase inhibitors,
pathological changes, 218–220
vs. novel SERMs, 151
palliation, 91–92
pathological changes, 217–218
plus CMF, 25
plus Gn-RHA, 281
premenopausal women, 278
with progestin, 23
response prediction, 83–86
thromboembolic risk, 172–173
Targeted endocrine therapy,
chemoprevention, 320–321
TAT-59, 59
Taxol, 357
Teardrop appearance, 217
Terminal deoxynucleotidyl transferase-
mediated dUTP-biotin nick endlabeling (TUNEL), 216, 218
Testosterone, 50
TGF, 232
endocrine therapy response, 225
Thromboembolic events, 113
Thromboembolic risk, tamoxifen,
172–173
Thymidine kinase (TK), 83
Time points, tumor sampling, 245–246
Time to progression (TTP), 33, 93
Time to second progression, 109
Tissue storage, retrievable, 350
TK, 83
Toremifene, 48, 55–56, 150
clinical efficacy, 57, 59–60
TP53 mutations, 83
Transforming growth factor (TGF),
232
endocrine therapy response, 225
Trastuzumab (Herceptin), 85–86
Triphenylethylene SERMs, 55–60, 150
TTP, 33, 93

Tumor,
excision, alternatives, 250
sampling, time points, 245–246
triage, preoperative endocrine therapy,
262–263
Tumor-free interval, primary endocrine
therapy, 98
TUNEL, 216, 218

UGT2B7, 295
United Kingdom, cost, 173
UPA, 83–84
UPAR, 84
Urokinase-type plasminogen activator
receptor (uPAR), 84
Urokinase-type plasminogen activator
(uPA), 83–84

Vascular endothelial growth factor
(VEGF), 83–84
Venous thrombosis, 19
Vitamin C, 290
Vorozole,
adverse effects, 330
bone resorption, 167
premenopausal women, 330

World Health Organization (WHO),
response assessment criteria,
203

Xenografts, 86
surgical procedures, gene expression,
245–248

Young women, breast cancer prevention,
330

Zoladex, 279
plus letrozole plus faslodex, 362
premenopausal women, 351–352
time period, 117–118